BMA

Urology
Lecture Notes

D1352923

This title is also available as an e-book.
For more details, please see
www.wiley.com/buy/9781118471050
or scan this QR code:

Urology
Lecture Notes

Amir V. Kaisary

Consultant Urological Surgeon and Honorary Senior Lecturer
The Royal Free Hospital NHS Trust and Medical School
London

Andrew Ballaro

Consultant Urological Surgeon
Barking, Havering and Redbridge University Hospitals NHS Trust
Essex

Katharine Pigott

Consultant Clinical Oncologist and Radiotherapist
The Royal Free Hospital NHS Trust and Medical School
London

Seventh Edition

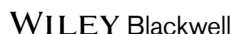
WILEY Blackwell

This edition first published 2016 © 2016 by John Wiley & Sons, Ltd

Previous editions: 1976, 1977, 1982, 1989, 1998, 2009

Registered Office
John Wiley & Sons, Ltd, The Atrium, Southern Gate, Chichester, West Sussex, PO19 8SQ, UK

Editorial Offices
9600 Garsington Road, Oxford, OX4 2DQ, UK
The Atrium, Southern Gate, Chichester, West Sussex, PO19 8SQ, UK
111 River Street, Hoboken, NJ 07030-5774, USA

For details of our global editorial offices, for customer services and for information about how to apply for permission to reuse the copyright material in this book please see our website at www.wiley.com/wiley-blackwell

Library of Congress Cataloging-in-Publication Data

Kaisary, Amir V., author.
　Lecture notes. Urology / Amir Kaisary, Andrew Ballaro, Katharine Pigott. – Seventh edition.
　　　p. ; cm.
　　Urology
　　Preceded by Lecture notes. Urology / John Blandy, Amir Kaisary. 6th ed. 2009.
　　Includes bibliographical references and index.
　　ISBN 978-1-118-47105-0 (paper)
　I. Ballaro, Andrew, author.　II. Pigott, Katharine, author.　III. Blandy, John P. (John Peter), 1927–
Lecture notes. Urology. Preceded by (work):　IV. Title.　V. Title: Urology.
　　[DNLM: 1. Urologic Diseases. WJ 140]
　　RC900.5
　　616.6–dc23
　　　　　　　　　　　　　　　　　　　　　2015034623
A catalogue record for this book is available from the British Library.

Wiley also publishes its books in a variety of electronic formats. Some content that appears in print may not be available in electronic books.

Cover image: iStock/janulla

Set in 9/11.5pt Utopia by SPi Global, Pondicherry, India
Printed in Singapore by C.O.S. Printers Pte Ltd

1　2016

Contents

Preface

It is nearly more than 40 years ago that John Blandy published *Lecture notes in Urology*. He hoped that medical students might find it helpful and simplicity in presentation can aid easy understanding and appreciation. Urology has changed immensely over the years and continues to do so with new technologies and improved understanding of all urology disease stages including aetiology, sophisticated basics in science, cellular biology, immunology and genetics. For a book to be published, time is needed and the chance of being "old news" is always threatening. Electronic communications offer rapid delivery of knowledge. This new edition aims to deliver current various topics as a springboard to sources of continuous medical education. Readers are encouraged to get into the habit of making use of up-to-date urology guidelines available from the European Urology Association (EAU), American Urology association (AUA) and British Urological Association (BAUS). A plethora of resources offered by various publishers and other bodies allow access to up-to-date publications, debates and presentations in various forms including teaching videos. As an example, Wiley Online Library is one resource, out of many, which can offer information that is immediate.

I would like to express my thanks to many friends and colleagues, particularly my co-editors, KP and Andrew. I hope that this book will enable doctors and medical students to embrace urology.

Amir V. Kaisary

Acknowledgements

During preparation of this new edition we were both helped by advice and contributions from many colleagues for which we register our thanks.

Mr David Ralph, MS, FRCS
Consultant Urological Surgeon
St Peter's Andrology Centre
The Institute of Urology &
University College Hospital
London, UK

Professor Pierre Bouloux, BSc, MD, FRCP
Director, Department of Neuroendocrinology
University College London Hospitals
London, UK

Mr Rizwan Hamid, FRCS (Urol), MD (Res)
Consultant Urological Surgeon
University College London Hospitals and
London Spinal Injuries Unit
Stanmore, London, UK
(Chapter 12)

Dr Ranju T. Dhawan, DRM, MSc, FRCR
Consultant Radiologist, Imperial College NHS
Healthcare Trust and Clinical Lead
Hybrid Functional Imaging
Wellington Hospital
London, UK

Dr Tara Barwick, MRCP, MSc, FRCR
Consultant Radiologist and Nuclear Medicine
Physician and Honorary Clinical Senior Lecturer
Imperial College Healthcare NHS Trust
Imperial College
London, UK

Mr Marc Laniado, MD, FEBU, FRCS (Urol)
Consultant Urological Surgeon
Frimley Health NHS Foundation Trust
Frimley, UK

Professor Chris Foster
Consultant Pathologist
Bostwick Laboratory
London, UK

Part 1

Meet the patient

1

Assessment of the urological patient: History and examination

Assessment of the urological patient involves taking a complete and detailed history, a thorough physical examination and analysis of a urine sample. As with all history taking the enquiry should include details of the presenting complaint and its history, the relevant past medical history and a family and drug history. The examination should include the abdomen, external genitals and a digital rectal examination in men and a vaginal examination in women, if clinically indicated. The urinalysis is most readily performed by dipstick testing; a formal microscopic analysis may be required to investigate any abnormality.

History

Communication skills

It is perhaps even more important with urology than with other specialities, because of the personal nature of some of the symptom complexes, for the clinician to create a personal rapport and a warm environment to facilitate enquiry into sometimes intimate problems. Stand up to greet the patient and welcome him/her warmly. Introduce yourself and make an initial assessment of the patient's age, built, demeanour, intelligence and socio-economic group and adapt your consultation style accordingly, based on your experience, in an attempt to make the patient feel comfortable. An ice-breaker such as 'I hope you haven't been waiting too long' or 'Did you manage to park easily?' can help the patient to relax. Aim to project a caring, experienced and open but professional image that will put the patient at ease and facilitate communication.

Then begin with, 'How old is your patient and what is his/her occupation? How can I help', or 'Your GP has written to us saying you have a problem with...please tell me about it', which are good open questions to start the consultation. Look out for signs that the patient may not be able to describe the problem due to anxiety or embarrassment or a language barrier. Then listen. Listen until you are clear on the nature of the problem, or the patient has gone off on a tangent and you feel you have to gently redirect him/her. Once you are clear on the presenting complaint, obtain a history of it and ask more specific questions aimed at eliciting the important diagnostic points. The following are common complaints initiating a consultation.

Urology Lecture Notes, Seventh Edition. Amir V. Kaisary, Andrew Ballaro and Katharine Pigott.
© 2016 John Wiley & Sons, Ltd. Published 2016 by John Wiley & Sons, Ltd.

Basic symptoms

Haematuria

The presence of blood in the urine is termed hae-maturia. Haematuria has many causes ranging from the insignificant to life-threatening cancers and is often a result of urinary tract infection (UTI). The patient should therefore be asked whether the blood was accompanied by symptoms of urinary tract inflammation such as dysuria, pain, urinary frequency or whether the urine smelled offensive. In all patients with a history of haematuria, the urine should be examined by dipstick and cultured if this suggests infection (see later). The extent of investigation required for a confirmed infection is guided by patient characteristics; however, all patients with symptomatic infections should be treated with appropriate antibiotics and the urine retested for blood once the infection has resolved. It is important to remember that UTI itself can be the first sign of serious urinary tract pathology. Uncommonly, urine discolouration that is reported as haematuria may be caused by myoglobinuria, beetroot intake and drugs such as rifampicin. It is generally advisable to investigate for haematuria anyway. Haematuria may be visible or non-visible and associated with other LUTS or asymptomatic, and this is the starting point for subsequent enquiry.

Visible haematuria

Visible haematuria is arguably the most important symptom in urology as it implies urological cancer until proven otherwise, and all patients including those with demonstrated infection should undergo investigation. The patient may notice the blood at the beginning, throughout or at the end of the urinary stream, and this sign may give an indication of its origin and cause. Initial haematuria often originates from the prostate or urethra and as such is less likely to reflect bladder or upper urinary tract pathology, whereas haematuria throughout the stream implies the blood emanates from the bladder or above. Terminal haematuria may indicate upper tract bleeding. This differentiation is unreliable, however, and all patients require the same investigation with upper urinary tract cross-sectional imaging by computerised tomography including a urographic phase and cystoscopy as a minimum.

Non-visible haematuria

Non-visible or microscopic haematuria is defined by the presence of more than three erythrocytes per high-power field on microscopy or at least 1+ on dipstick of a fresh midstream urine sample. It is usually detected in the community on routine urine testing or during the investigation of symptoms. A few erythrocytes in the urine are common and often found after heavy exercise. After exclusion of infection as a cause, a single episode of non-visible haematuria accompanied by LUTS or persistent asymptomatic haematuria is clinically significant and should be investigated.

Asymptomatic non-visible haematuria commonly represents early chronic kidney disease, and patients under the age of 40 with no other risk factors for urothelial malignancy should be investigated with urine protein/creatinine ratio and first referred for nephrological rather than urological opinion if evidence of deteriorating glomerular filtration rate, significant proteinuria or hypertension is present. The patient should be asked if there has been a recent upper respiratory tract infection as this may be associated with glomerulonephritis.

Urological investigation with urinary tract ultrasound and cystoscopy of all other patients is recommended, and in some centres computerised tomography is also performed. The incidence of finding a significant urological abnormality in patients with asymptomatic non-visible haematuria is less than 10%.

 KEYPOINTS

- Haematuria has many causes ranging from the insignificant to a range of malignancies. Infection should always be excluded; however, it may also be the first sign of serious pathology.
- Asymptomatic non-visible haematuria is commonly nephrological, not urological.
- Visible haematuria is caused by malignancy until proven otherwise.

Lower urinary tract symptoms

LUTS are a common reason for someone to seek a urological opinion with over a half of the population likely to experience them at some point in their lifetime; the incidence, as might be expected, increases with age. LUTS occur in both sexes, reminding us that these symptoms are not specific to the enlarged prostate and are currently classified as either *voiding* or *storage* symptoms.

Voiding symptoms

Hesitancy – This is a delay in the start of micturition. Normally it takes a second or so to start passing urine.

Intermittency – This is a stop/start pattern that happens involuntarily during micturition and is generally due to prostatic obstruction.

Poor flow – This is a decreased flow of urine and can be due to prostatic obstruction or urethral stricture. This happens over a long period of time.

Straining – This is due to the use of abdominal muscles to empty the bladder.

Terminal dribble – This is passing drops of urine at the end of micturition and is generally an early sign of obstruction secondary to prostatic enlargement.

Feelings of incomplete bladder emptying – This is the feeling of needing to void again soon after voiding.

Storage symptoms

Frequency – A normal adult will pass urine 3–7 times during the day with volumes of around 200–400 mL per void. Urinary frequency is either due to increased urinary output (polyuria) or decreased bladder capacity.

Nocturia – This is getting up at night more than once. It can be due to either increased urine production or decreased bladder capacity. Frequency without nocturia is usually psychological. On the other hand, nocturia without frequency can be related to heart failure or diabetes insipidus.

Urgency – The International Continence Society defines urgency as 'a complaint of a sudden compelling desire to pass urine, which is difficult to defer'.

Dysuria – This is a painful micturition and is generally felt both suprapubically and over the urethral meatus. It is usually a sign of inflammation in the urinary tract.

While often attributed to bladder outflow obstruction and functional bladder problems, LUTS are not disease or organ specific. Storage symptoms in particular may reflect a wide range of pathologies from impaired fluid and solute handling problems to non-specific inflammation of the urinary tract and can also be a sign of underlying malignant processes. Identical storage and voiding symptoms may be caused by either bladder muscle dysfunction or outflow tract obstruction due to benign or malignant prostatic enlargement. It is therefore important to determine the presence of individual voiding and storage symptoms, to quantify their severity and to elucidate other symptoms and signs that may indicate their origin.

Polyuria

Polyuria is the excessive production of urine, usually defined as over 2.5 L/24 h in an adult. It should not be forgotten that someone who drinks large volumes of anything, particularly diuretics such as caffeine-containing drinks and alcohol, is likely to need to void more often due to increased urine production. In addition to the fluid load, caffeine increases bladder smooth muscle excitability directly and can precipitate urinary storage symptoms. A history of fluid intake is therefore valuable. It is also important to remember the impact of non-urological diseases on urinary symptoms, specifically those influencing renal fluid and solute handling such as diabetes mellitus, which causes glycosuria and an osmotic diuresis, and less commonly diabetes insipidus. Random serum glucose and electrolytes should therefore be analysed.

Nocturia

Nocturia is the need to wake from sleep to pass urine at night. In normal health, nocturnal urine output is reduced to less than the bladder capacity so that we don't need to get up to void. Nocturia may be caused by either the functional bladder reservoir volume being reduced, such as occurring in patients with large post-micturition residual urine volumes, or by producing too much urine at night so that the bladder is unable to store it. This may reflect general polyuria, or nocturnal polyuria, a specific entity in which more than a third of 24 h urine production occurs at night. Congestive cardiac failure may cause nocturia through several mechanisms, as can obstructive sleep apnoea. A history of the symptoms and signs of heart failure and the presence of snoring should therefore be sought. As with polyuria, evening intake of pharmacological and non-medicinal diuretics such as caffeine and alcohol is an obvious but often overlooked cause of nocturia.

Nocturia is more common in the elderly, and a loss of the circadian secretion of antidiuretic hormone, which normally reduces nocturnal urine production, may be present. It is therefore important to assess the patient's fluid intake, urine output and voided urine volume to allow identification of polyuria, reduced functional bladder capacity and nocturnal polyuria, and this is performed using a frequency–volume chart.

Overactive bladder syndrome

Overactive bladder syndrome is a condition with characteristic symptoms of 'urinary urgency', usually accompanied by frequency and nocturia, with or without urgency incontinence (i.e. storage LUTS), in the absence of urinary tract infection or other obvious pathology'. The condition may be associated with involuntary contractions of the bladder, and this is termed detrusor over-activity (see Chapter 12); however, these contractions are not always associated and are present in many asymptomatic patients.

Evaluation of LUTS

A detailed history of the speed of onset of LUTS is important: uncomplicated bladder outflow obstruction tends to be insidious, whereas the rapid onset of severe symptoms suggests an alternative diagnosis. A history of previous urological

intervention, including catheterisation, or surgery should be obtained as often a resected prostate may regrow and iatrogenic urethral and bladder neck strictures are common. The presence of specific additional symptoms suggestive of pathology in addition to bladder outflow obstruction should also be determined. These include haematuria, nocturnal enuresis (the involuntary loss of urine at night), which is strongly suggestive of high-pressure chronic urinary retention when occurring in adults, or associated sensory disturbances or back pain, which should initiate investigations to exclude disruption of the bladder's neurological control such as spinal cord compression. Furthermore, symptoms and signs of inflammation of the urinary tract may indicate an inflammatory cause for urinary storage symptoms or bladder outflow obstruction complicated by infection.

In the absence of polyuria and symptoms suggestive of alternative diagnosis, the most likely causes of LUTS are bladder outflow obstruction and bladder dysfunction, that is, either overactive or underactive detrusor contraction. The subsequent management of LUTS is strongly influenced by their severity and the impact on the patient – this is quantified using the International Prostate Symptom Score (IPSS) patient questionnaire. Functional bladder problems and bladder outflow obstruction can sometimes only truly be differentiated from each other by pressure-flow urodynamic studies.

Incontinence

Incontinence is the involuntary loss of urine. It is highly prevalent in the community and occurs more commonly in females in an

---

 KEYPOINTS

Investigation of the patient with LUTS is focused on excluding disorders of fluid handling; detecting a specific infective, inflammatory or malignant urological cause; and quantifying the severity and impact on quality of life of the symptoms. This is achieved using the urine dipstick, the frequency–volume chart and the IPSS questionnaire.

age-dependent manner. Incontinence causes considerable morbidity and expense, and when taking the history the urologist should first determine whether the incontinence is continuous or intermittent – the latter category may be subclassified into stress, urge, mixed stress and urge or overflow incontinence. Symptom questionnaires are useful in documenting symptoms, and a voiding diary of fluid intake and urine output compiled over at least 3 days should be recorded. Further insight into the aetiology of incontinence can be gained by careful history taking.

International Continence Society definitions

- **Stress urinary incontinence:** Involuntary urine leakage on effort or exertion or on sneezing or coughing.
- **Urgency urinary incontinence:** Involuntary urine leakage accompanied by or immediately preceded by urgency.
- **Mixed urinary incontinence:** Involuntary urine leakage associated with both urgency and exertion, effort, sneezing or coughing.
- **Overactive bladder:** Urgency that occurs with or without urgency urinary incontinence and usually with frequency and nocturia. Whether occurring with incontinence (wet) or without incontinence (dry).

Continuous incontinence

Continuous incontinence implies complete failure of the sphincter mechanism, as occasionally occurring after bladder outflow tract surgery and more commonly after radical prostatectomy, or the presence of an abnormal urinary tract allowing bladder or ureteric urine to bypass the sphincter mechanism. This may be a fistula occurring after gynaecological surgery or as is common in third world countries as a result of tissue necrosis after poorly managed childbirth. Rarely congenital abnormalities such as an ectopic ureter may open distal to the urinary sphincter causing continuous incontinence from birth.

Intermittent incontinence

- **Urge urinary incontinence** is the complaint of involuntary leakage accompanied by or immediately preceded by urinary urgency – the feeling of the need to pass urine that is difficult to defer. Urge incontinence may be caused by an overactive bladder, a complex and incompletely defined abnormality of bladder smooth muscle contractility or by bladder inflammation. It is important to determine the cause by assessing the presence of accompanying symptoms and abnormalities on urine analysis. The presence of suprapubic pain, haematuria, dysuria and voiding urinary symptoms all suggest a cause other than idiopathic overactive bladder.
- **Stress urinary incontinence** is the complaint of involuntary leakage on effort or exertion, or on sneezing or coughing. In women this occurs due to weakening of the pelvic floor neuromuscular mechanisms that support the urethra and bladder and can occur after childbirth or in association with aging. It is also a sign of urinary sphincter weakness and may occur after prostatectomy in men. A detailed obstetric history of respiratory disease and smoking, pelvic irradiation and pelvic surgery and bowel habit is therefore required to evaluate stress incontinence.
- Both stress and urge incontinence may occur together for a number of reasons, and management is initially directed according to which type of incontinence predominates. Sometimes determining this requires a pressure-flow urodynamic studies.
- **Overflow incontinence** is characterised by intermittent dribbling of small amounts of urine and nocturnal enuresis – the involuntary loss of urine occurring during sleep. This occurs as the normal inhibitory mechanisms and voluntary sphincter contraction that occurs during the day in an effort to minimise leakage is suppressed in sleep. Overflow incontinence occurs in association with a chronically distended bladder that never empties and is caused by bladder outflow obstruction or neurological disease and may be insidious. When occurring in association with bladder

KEYPOINTS

When evaluating incontinence, the history should focus on determining whether it is continuous or intermittent. Intermittent incontinence is characterised by stress, urge, mixed stress and urge or overflow incontinence. The pathophysiology of the incontinence can subsequently be ascertained with minimal additional investigation.

outflow obstruction, nocturnal enuresis may be a sign of upper urinary tract obstruction and renal impairment termed high-pressure chronic urinary retention.

Urological pain

General

Pain originating from the urological tract is generally caused by either distension of a viscus due to obstruction of the flow of urine, for example, a ureteric stone, or inflammation. The pain caused by inflammation is more severe when the parenchyma of an organ is involved, for example, testis or kidney, as this causes the capsule to be stretched. As with all types of pain, a careful history of its site, duration, type (dull, sharp or burning), radiation, exacerbating and relieving factors and other associated symptoms should be obtained.

Loin pain

The term loin refers to the area between the lower ribs and the pelvis and is used to describe both human and animal anatomy. There are many causes of pain in this area and many of these are non-urological. Loin pain truly originating from the kidney is more accurately referred to as renal angle pain; this is the area between the lateral borders of the erector spinae muscles, the 12th rib and the iliac crest. Renal angle pain results either from distension of the renal pelvis, which occurs with ureteric obstruction, or from distension of the renal capsule, which occurs with acute inflammation of the renal parenchyma in association with pyelonephritis.

The pain associated with renal inflammation is generally constant and severe and may be associated with systemic signs of sepsis. It may also be associated with gastrointestinal symptoms due to the close proximity of the peritoneum and intra-abdominal organs, and a careful history and examination may be required to determine the true origin. Occasionally, loin pain may be caused by small calculi in the renal collecting system, particularly if they are still adherent and blocking a papilla.

Ureteric colic

Ureteric or renal colic refers to the pain that results from acute obstruction of the ureter associated with the passage of a urinary stone. It is historically compared in severity to the pain of childbirth, and in the age of modern obstetric analgesia, renal colic can reasonably be considered the most severe pain one might be likely to suffer other than through trauma. Renal pain is intermittent and intensifies with ureteric peristalsis, which, in the presence of obstruction, causes the intrarenal pressure to rise and characteristically causes the patient to writhe and unable to get into a comfortable position. This feature differentiates it from other, generally more morbid, causes of acute abdominal pain that are generally minimised by lying still.

It is sometimes possible to clinically determine the site of ureteric obstruction from the location of the pain. Pain originating from the upper two-thirds of the ureter (that above the pelvic brim) may be referred to the iliac fossa on either side and must be differentiated from surgical causes. A stone in the lower third of the ureter near the bladder may cause LUTS and strangury: this is an unpleasant sensation of a constant need to void that is not relieved by voiding and suprapubic and urethral pain at the end of voiding. Pain may also be referred to the tip of the penis or labia.

Pain caused by chronic insidious obstruction of the ureter, for instance, by a slow-growing ureteric tumour or gradual extrinsic compression, is considerably less severe than acute ureteric colic and may be a chronic dull ache or not clinically significant. Non-urological causes of loin pain are common and can be difficult to diagnose. Musculoskeletal back pain is common and is typically associated with movement or particular positions; however, it can be difficult to identify. Other less common causes include pain originating from the pleura, gastrointestinal tract, spleen and liver.

Suprapubic pain

Acute distension of the bladder associated with acute urinary retention causes intense pain that is relieved by catheterisation. Chronic bladder distension, however, is painless, and the bladder may contain litres of urine with no discomfort. Constant suprapubic pain unrelated to voiding is unlikely to be urological and may originate from other pelvic organs or distal bowel; intermittent pain associated with bladder filling relates to inflammation most commonly caused by bacterial cystitis. Severe inflammation of the bladder may cause peritoneal involvement and signs of localised peritonitis.

Scrotal pain

Scrotal pain may be acute or chronic. Acute scrotal pain in a child is caused by torsion of the testis or testicular appendage (hydatid of Morgagni) and the resulting ischaemia unless proven otherwise, and urgent surgical exploration of the scrotum generally indicated. Pain due to torsion is generally of sudden onset and may awake the patient. There may be associated vomiting and previous episodes of intermittent pain. The clinical presentation of testicular torsion is varied, however, and pain may be transient and have resolved at the time of examination.

Testicular torsion may present with non-specific discomfort in the lower abdomen or have clinical features of appendicitis; it is therefore imperative to examine the scrotum in any patient presenting with abdominal pain. Urinary symptoms are sometimes present with testicular torsion and cannot, therefore, be taken as indicating urinary infection, which is far less common than torsion in children. No surgeon ever regretted operating on an acutely painful scrotum, and surgical exploration should be regarded as an investigation rather than a treatment.

Acute scrotal pain in adults may also be due to torsion but is more common in this age group caused by infections and trauma. A history of LUTS and those suggestive of infection, as well as a recent change in sexual partners, is therefore important to elicit. Trauma is usually evident; however, a history of trauma does not exclude other causes of the pain such as torsion and tumour. It is not unheard of for an adult to present with testicular pain not resolving after seemingly minor trauma and found to have a torted ischaemia testis requiring removal.

Scrotal pain may also originate from inflammatory conditions affecting the scrotal wall; these include cutaneous abscess, cellulitis and Fournier's scrotal gangrene. Chronic scrotal pain may be caused by chronic epididymitis or non-inflammatory conditions such as hydrocele or epididymal cyst. Varicocele is an abnormally dilated collection of veins draining the testis and characteristically causes a chronic dull ache worse during standing for long periods and relieved by lying. Chronic scrotal pain may also be referred from the retroperitoneum, reflecting the embryological origin of the testis, or an inguinal hernia.

Urethral pain

Pain felt in the urethra is usually caused by inflammation. Dysuria refers to urethral pain that occurs during voiding and is felt at the external urethral meatus. It is commonly caused by lower UTI or inflammation. Urethritis is accompanied by urinary frequency and urgency.

Prostatic pain

Pain originating from prostatic pathology may be difficult to describe and be poorly localised. Pain is often localised to the perineum, between the anus and the scrotum, and may be referred to the testis, suprapubic area or back. Pain on ejaculation is strongly suggestive of prostatic pathology, and there are often associated both storage (due to inflammation) and voiding (due to obstruction) LUTS. Prostatic pain is generally caused by inflammation; locally advanced prostate cancer can cause a similar pain when it invades periprostatic tissues.

KEYPOINTS

By taking a careful history and examination, most causes of urological pain can be elucidated without further investigation.

Distension of a urological viscus and stretching of the capsule of an organ due to inflammation are the main mechanisms of urological pain.

Loin pain has many non-urological causes.

Scrotal pain in children is an emergency and usually necessitates surgical exploration to exclude testicular torsion.

Erectile dysfunction

Erectile dysfunction is the inability or reduced ability to attain a satisfactory penile erection. There are a number of causes, and the history should be aimed at differentiating between them. It is firstly necessary to confirm the problem as truly erectile dysfunction and not another sexual dysfunction such as failure of or pain on ejaculation, anoragsmia or psychological causes in nature; the most important point to elicit here is whether morning erections occur and whether the dysfunction occurs all the time or just in a particular situation. A reduced libido is a sign of both psychological causes and testosterone deficiency.

Erectile dysfunction may be caused by trauma both to the penis itself and the pelvis, and this history is important to elicit as traumatic vascular damage is the only cause that is, sometimes, correctable by surgery. The next step is to identify any reversible causes other than trauma, which although rarely resulting in complete return of erections can often improve the situation and are important to identify for other reasons. The most prevalent of these are smoking and alcohol. It should not be forgotten that erectile dysfunction may be the first symptom of atherosclerotic vascular disease and may predate ischaemic heart disease, and a general assessment of the patients' cardiovascular risk status and lipid profile is indicated. The history should also determine whether the patient is fit cardiovascularly enough to resume sexual activity should his erections be artificially improved.

Urinary tract infections

UTI is the symptomatic inflammatory response of the urothelium to the presence of microorganisms and is usually associated with bacteriuria (the presence of bacteria in the urine). UTIs are a common reason for referral. The presentation may be varied, depending on the organism and site of resulting inflammation, and it is important to elicit the precise symptoms resulting from the purported infection. Bacteriuria itself may be asymptomatic; the urine of most patients with long-term catheters contains bacteria and this only requires treatment when associated with symptoms of inflammation.

Lower UTIs are those in which the inflammation is confined to the urethra and bladder and typically present with dysuria which is the sensation of urethral pain on voiding and commonly referred to as burning urine or passing broken glass. Dysuria is usually accompanied by urinary frequency, urgency and suprapubic pain relieved by voiding when the bladder is inflamed, and the urine may be cloudy or smell bad. This symptom complex is commonly termed cystitis. A substantial proportion of lower UTIs present with visible haematuria and termed haemorrhagic cystitis.

Infections involving the upper urinary tracts (ureters and kidneys) present differently, although lower tract symptoms may also be present if secondary to an ascending infection. Infection of the renal parenchyma promotes a systemic inflammatory response, and the patient is febrile and unwell. The combination of loin pain, tenderness and fever with evidence of bacteriuria or pyuria is termed acute pyelonephritis.

Pneumaturia

Pneumaturia is the presence of air in the urine. It is an uncommon symptom and is almost pathognomonic for the presence of an abnormal communication between the bladder and bowel – a vesico-colic fistula. This occurs in the presence of bowel inflammatory disease such as diverticulitis, or malignancy, and is also predisposed to by pelvic radiotherapy.

Examination

Examination of the urological patient should include a general examination, examination of the abdomen, the external genitalia and when indicated a digital rectal examination and vaginal examination. The urologist should be gentle and sensitive to the patient, and the intimate nature of the examination and verbal permission for each aspect of the examination should be sought. It is wise and mandatory when a male urologist is examining a female patient to have a nurse chaperone present who will record their details in the medical record to document their presence.

General

Non-specific signs of anaemia, cachexia, lymphadenopathy, hepatomegaly and uraemia may all be urologically related, and the abdomen and external genitalia should first be properly inspected. With the increasing advancement of minimally invasive surgical techniques, it is becoming less common to see the large deforming thoraco-abdominal, 'roof top' or extended paramedian scars of the open nephrectomy, and it may be difficult to see the small punctures through which laparoscopic ports are inserted. The combination of two small punctures with a 4–5 cm iliac fossa scar suggests a nephrectomy, whereas three small punctures are created during laparoscopic pyeloplasty or partial nephrectomy. Similarly a series of lower abdominal punctures may conceal a major operation such as radical prostatectomy or cystectomy; a cystectomy may not necessarily involve creation of a stoma if an orthotopic bladder reconstruction has been performed. A lower midline or Pfannenstiel scar may indicate any open pelvic operation and is used during both urological and gynaecological procedures, again less commonly.

Abdomen

Urological examination of the abdomen is focused on detecting an enlarged kidney, suggesting tumour, or bladder, suggesting urinary retention. Traditional signs of an enlarged kidney are a bimanually palpable mass in the loin which moves up and down with respiration, and which you can get above. A normal kidney is palpable in thin individuals (Figures 1.1 and 1.2).

An enlarged bladder may not be palpable if the patient is large, and it is often not possible to reliably differentiate by palpation between an enlarged full bladder and a pelvic mass

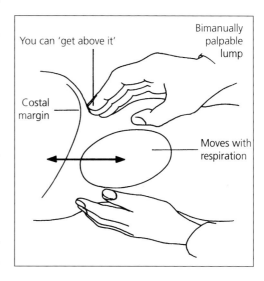

Figure 1.1 Physical signs of an enlarged kidney.

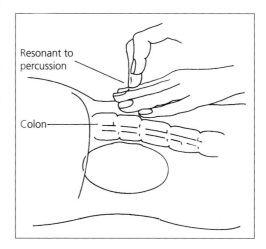

Figure 1.2 There is often a band of resonance in front of the kidney from gas in the colon.

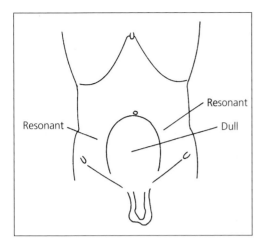

Figure 1.3 The bladder is dull to percussion.

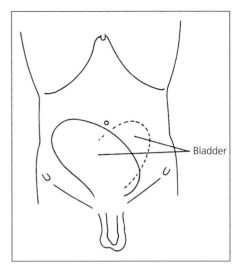

Figure 1.4 An enlarged bladder may go to one or other side.

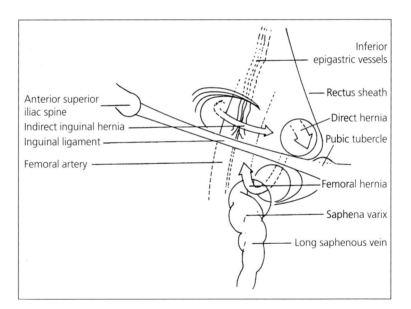

Figure 1.5 Landmarks for groin hernias.

(Figures 1.3 and 1.4). It is therefore important to re-examine the patient after catheterisation, if clinically indicated, as a pelvic mass will still be present. An ultrasound will also reliably distinguish between solid and cystic swellings.

Examination of the groins is an important part of the urological investigation. Although inguinal and femoral herniae are dealt with by general surgeons, they often account for symptoms that initiate urological referral (Figures 1.5 and 1.6).

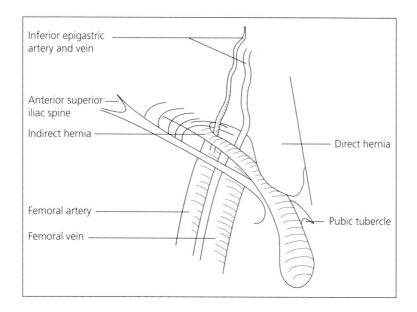

Figure 1.6 Pantaloon hernia.

Inguinal lymph nodes drain the external genitalia and lower limb and may be enlarged in infections or tumours of these regions. Examination of the groin for enlarged lymph nodes is particularly important when there is a penile cancer. Small, so-called 'shotty' nodes, a reference to shotgun pellets, are normally palpable in thin individuals; tenderness or persistent enlargement over 1 cm in size is a sign of concern. Groin nodes may also be involved in metastatic spread from pelvic disease but not testis cancer unless this has advanced to involve the scrotal wall.

External genitalia

Penis

The penis should also be routinely examined. The foreskin may give rise to a number of symptoms, and when inflamed or phimotic (tight and scarred), it can be implicated in the aetiology of UTIs, LUTS, pain and haematuria. The foreskin should be gently retracted after asking the patients permission or alternatively asking the patients to do this themselves to allow inspection of the external urethral meatus. The meatus may

be strictured and involved with a transitional cell carcinoma or ectopic. The glans penis should also be examined, specifically as it may harbour a premalignant skin lesion or overt squamous cell carcinoma. Palpation of the penile shaft will identify the hard localised plaques that cause erectile deformity and dysfunction in Peyronie's disease, and severe strictures of the penile urethra may also be palpated ventrally.

Scrotum

Examination of the scrotum should take place with the patient both lying and standing. The scrotum should at first be inspected with the patient standing, looking for skin lesions and the characteristic bag of worms' appearance of the varicocele (Figure 1.7).

With the patient lying, the scrotum should be gently palpated looking for abnormal lumps. If one is found, the following questions should be answered.

- Can you 'get above' the lump? If you can it must be scrotal, and if not it is probably an inguinal hernia (Figure 1.8).
- Is the swelling solid or cystic? This is tested by determining the presence of fluctuance in

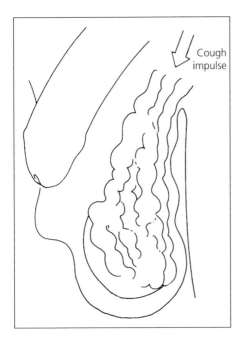

Cough impulse

Figure 1.7 Varicocele: enlarged testicular veins. There is a cough impulse and the swelling disappears when the patient lies down.

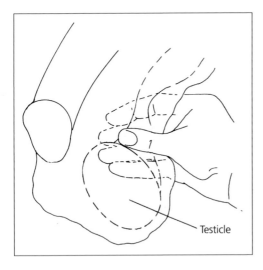

Testicle

Figure 1.8 Lump in the scrotum: can you get above it?

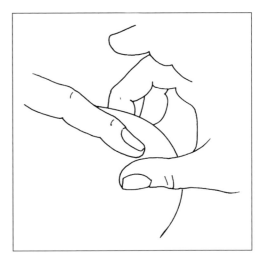

Figure 1.9 Lump in the scrotum: check whether it is solid or fluctuant. Determine fluctuation in two planes.

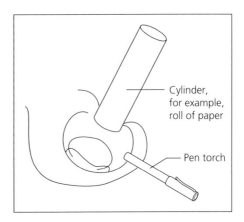

Cylinder, for example, roll of paper

Pen torch

Figure 1.10 To see if light shines through a swelling, it helps to use a cylinder, for example, one made from rolled-up paper.

- Is the lump separate from the testis or not? A cystic swelling inseparable from the testis is probably a hydrocele (Figure 1.11).
- A cystic lump separate from the testis is probably an epididymal cyst (Figure 1.12). In practice it is often difficult to differentiate these two entities; this is not clinically important.
- If the lump is solid, it is crucially important to determine whether it is separate from the testis or not. If it is separate, it is most likely to be an

two planes (Figure 1.9). A cystic lesion also usually transilluminates, that is, lights up if a torch is pressed against it in a darkened room (Figure 1.10).

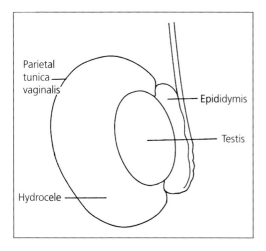

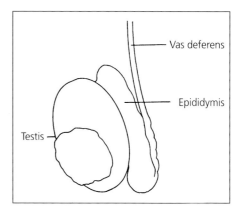

Figure 1.14 A solid swelling in the testis is a cancer until proven otherwise.

Figure 1.11 Hydroceles lie in front of the testis and tend to surround it.

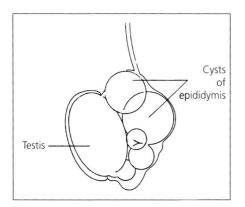

Figure 1.12 Cystic swellings behind the testis are cysts of the epididymis.

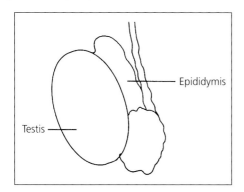

Figure 1.13 Solid swellings in the epididymis are usually inflammatory.

area of inflamed epididymis or sperm granuloma after vasectomy (Figure 1.13). If it is not separate from the testis, it should be considered a testicular tumour until proven otherwise (Figure 1.14), and an urgent ultrasound will confirm.

- The vas deferens lies posterior to the spermatic cord. If it is inflamed, it can feel thickened and firm. If it has been operated upon, for example, vasectomy, it might show a nodule along its course. If multiple knotty swellings are felt, this would strongly suggest tuberculosis (Figure 1.15).

Vaginal examination

Vaginal examination should be performed in women with LUTS or incontinence, haematuria or pelvic pain. The external urethral meatus should be inspected for signs of surgery or stenosis and the patient asked to cough both in the lying and standing positions to assess urethral hypermobility, the presence of pelvic organ prolapse and stress incontinence. Although rare, urethral carcinoma may cause urethral stenosis and first present as LUTS.

Uncommonly, a urethral diverticulum may be palpable. This presents as a cystic mass in the anterior vaginal wall and is associated with persistent dysuria, dyspareunia (painful sexual intercourse) and UTI.

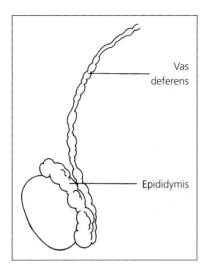

Figure 1.15 Multiple knotty swellings in the epididymis and a 'beaded' are highly suggestive of tuberculosis.

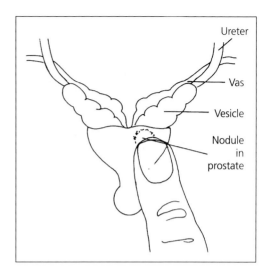

Figure 1.16 Anatomical landmarks that may be felt per rectum.

Digital rectal examination

Rectal examination although included in the general abdominal examination is arguably not mandatory for all urological complaints, although generally advisable when dealing with pelvic or LUTS and haematuria. One may perform a rectal examination in both sexes in the left lateral position. Inspection of the anal margin is mandatory, for anal carcinoma or external thrombosed piles, and always ask the specific permission of the patient and exclude the presence of an anal fissure or painful haemorrhoids first.

Introduce the gloved index finger carefully and slowly with plenty of lubrication. Once inside the rectum, carefully palpate circumferentially to exclude a low rectal tumour. Then palpate the prostate gland, which is found anteriorly. Palpate for nodules, a discrepancy between the two lateral lobes, and firmness (Figure 1.16). The examination will often be uncomfortable but should not be painful; a tender prostate is a sign of inflammation.

A more thorough examination of the pelvis in both sexes may be performed using bimanual

> **🔑 KEYPOINTS**
>
> - As with all surgical examinations, a general and organ-specific examination is required.
> - Great sensitivity should be applied when examining intimate organ systems and specific permission always sought.
> - A chaperone is required during the urological examination.
> - Inspection should precede palpation, including during the rectal and vaginal examination.
> - Vaginal examination is important in women with recurrent infections and unexplained urinary symptoms.

examination under a light general anaesthetic with the patient in the lithotomy position. In the male one finger is placed in the rectum, and in the female two fingers are placed in the vagina, and the organs are examined by compressing them against the other hand placed on the anterior abdominal wall suprapubically.

2

Assessment of the urological patient: Urinalysis and imaging

Urinalysis

Analysis of the urine should be performed in all patients. On inspection the colour of the urine varies from clear to orange depending on the hydration status of the patient. Cloudy urine is commonly caused by the presence of pus cells and infection.

A simple dipstick (Multistix) performed in the clinic can provide a great deal of diagnostic information; however, it is vital that it is collected correctly to reduce contamination. Generally, a midstream specimen is required. The male patient should retract the foreskin, and the female retract the labia and wash the urethra with antiseptic solution. In infants a sterile plastic bag with adhesive collar can be applied to collect urine. The sample should be sampled immediately, and microscopic examination and culture plating should take place ideally within an hour.

Urine dipstick

- Blood

Haemoglobin catalyses a reaction between hydrogen peroxide and chromogen tetramethylbenzidine, which produces a dark blue oxidation product on the dipstick. A positive dipstick for blood may indicate haematuria, haemoglobinuria or myoglobinuria. True haematuria may be distinguished from haemoglobinuria and myoglobinuria by visualisation of intact erythrocytes on microscopy. Haemoglobinuria occurs in extensive burns, haemolytic anaemia and blood transfusions, whereas myoglobinuria occurs during extensive muscle breakdown, for instance, in association with crush injuries and compartment syndromes. The sensitivity of the dipstick to detect haematuria, defined as over three erythrocytes per high-powered microscopy field, is over 90%. False positives are caused by menstrual blood and dehydration.

- Protein

Proteinuria is detected by dipstick impregnated with tetrabromophenol blue, which turns blue on exposure to protein. False negatives occur with alkaline or very dilute urine or when the protein is not albumin. Significant dipstick proteinuria (2+ or 3+ on dipstick) should be followed by analysis of a 24 h urine collection for protein. Up to 150 mg of protein is excreted into the urine in healthy adults; levels significantly above this indicate either renovascular or interstitial renal disease or excessive production of protein due to conditions such as myeloma.

Glomerular proteinuria is common in renal manifestations of systemic disease such as diabetes

Urology Lecture Notes, Seventh Edition. Amir V. Kaisary, Andrew Ballaro and Katharine Pigott.
© 2016 John Wiley & Sons, Ltd. Published 2016 by John Wiley & Sons, Ltd.

mellitus and results from increased permeability of the glomerulus to albumin. Tubular proteinuria results from failure of reabsorption of filtered low-molecular-weight immunoglobulins. The total protein loss in tubular proteinuria rarely exceeds 3 g/24 h in contrast to glomerular disease in which the protein loss may be considerably greater. Determination of the type of protein lost is achieved by protein electrophoresis.

● Glucose and ketones

When the renal threshold for glucose, that is, the capacity of the kidney to reabsorb filtered glucose, is exceeded, glucose appears in the urine. This occurs physiologically after a heavy meal and pathologically in diabetes mellitus. Ketones are detected in the urine during periods of body fat breakdown. This occurs when carbohydrate stores are depleted during diabetic ketoacidosis, starvation and sometimes pregnancy.

● Leucocyte esterase and nitrites

Leucocyte esterase is produced by neutrophils and if present in urine catalyses the hydrolysis of indoxyl carbonic acid, which then oxidises a diazonium salt on the dipstick to produce colour change. It is a sensitive test for leucocytes in the urine. Nitrites are formed from nitrates by the action of many gram-negative organisms and form a red azo dye on the dipstick. When combined with positive nitrite testing, a positive nitrate result on dipstick is highly sensitive for bacteriuria. A major reason for false negative results for both leucocytes and nitrites is contamination.

● Urine pH

The urine pH is determined on the dipstick by two indicators – methyl red and bromothymol blue – which change colour over the pH range 5–9. A urine pH under 5.5 is termed acidic and over 6.5 alkaline. Urine pH generally reflects the

plasma pH, except in renal tubular acidosis when inappropriately alkaline urine is produced by an acidotic patient due to impairment of renal acid–base regulation. Urine pH may also give a clue to the causes of renal stones and infection; with uric acid stones, the urinary pH is normally acidic and alkaline urine in a patient with stones and UTI indicates urease-producing bacteria such as proteus.

Urine microscopy

Microscopic examination of the urine can determine the cause of non-visible dipstick-detected haematuria. Haematuria originating from inflammatory, autoimmune and vasculitis abnormalities of the kidney is almost always accompanied by significant proteinuria. Haematuria from a nephrological cause is also commonly associated with the presence of casts on urine microscopy (Figure 2.1).

Casts consist of physiological mucoproteins that coagulate within the renal tubule. The mucoproteins trap erythrocytes in the presence of tubular bleeding or leucocytes in the presence of tubular inflammation, and these can be differentiated from each other on microscopy. Hyaline casts contain only mucoproteins and are usually of no clinical significance.

The morphology of erythrocytes in the urine under the microscope can give further information regarding their origin. Glomerular bleeding, generally caused by glomerulonephritis, is associated with dysmorphic erythrocytes in the urine. Non-glomerular bleeding is characterised by undamaged circular erythrocytes in the urine in the absence of erythrocyte casts.

In addition to the detection of casts and morphological examination of red blood cells in the

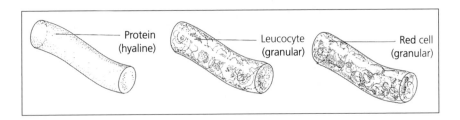

Protein (hyaline) Leucocyte (granular) Red cell (granular)

Figure 2.1 Casts in the urine.

urine, microscopy is employed for the detection of organisms, for which it is more sensitive than dipstick, and crystals, which is particularly useful in managing some patients with stone disease.

Imaging the urinary tract

Plain abdominal X-ray of the kidney, ureter and bladder (KUB)

This is a plain frontal supine radiograph of the abdomen. Check adequacy of the film. It must include the bladder base and the prostate urethral region in order not to miss a urethral stone. Look at each film with four Ss in mind (Figure 2.2):

- Side:
Radiographers, being only human, sometimes put the wrong letter on the film. Always check that the soft tissue shadow of the liver is on the right side and the gastric air bubble on the left.
- Skeleton:
Check the spine, ribs, hips and sacroiliac joints for sclerotic bony metastases. In children with enuresis, careful examination of the lumbosacral spine is essential to exclude spina bifida defects. The film should include the symphysis pubis and the twelfth rib.

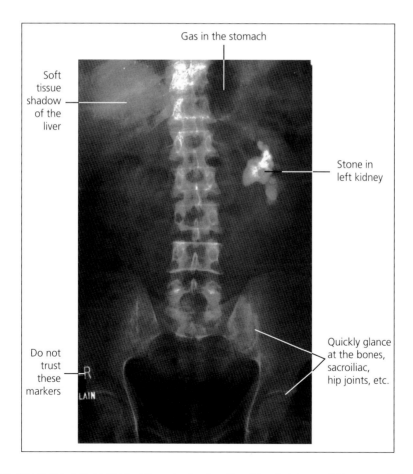

Figure 2.2 Check the plain abdominal X-ray for the four Ss: side, skeleton, soft tissues and stones.

- Soft tissues:

In obese people the kidneys are surrounded by radiolucent fat, which defines their outlines. A distended bladder or an enlarged uterus will fill the pelvis and displace the usual bowel gas shadows.

- Stones:

Any radio-opaque shadow in the line of the urinary tract might be a stone. The ureters start at the lower border of L1, the left slightly above and the right slightly below due to the liver. They descend over the tips of the transverse processes of the vertebrae and enter the pelvis at the sacroiliac joint. Thereafter they deviate laterally towards the ischial spines and then course medially to the bladder entering at a position that projects to just above the pubic rami on the plain film. 'Stones' in the pelvis often turn out to be calcified fibroids or phlebolith. Only 60–70% of stones are dense enough to be visible on radiographs.

Ultrasound

Ultrasonography is easy to perform, non-invasive, inexpensive and therefore widely available. It produces no ionising radiation. An AC is applied to a piezoelectric crystal, which then pulsates and produces a sound wave. The resulting wave penetrates soft tissues and is reflected by interfaces between tissues of different density, for example, renal calices and parenchyma, or a renal cyst and parenchyma (Figure 2.3). The returning echoes are received by the crystal, which reverses the process. The sound is converted into an electrical impulse, which is processed by a computer to give an image. Ultrasound images are more meaningful if you see them moving on a screen yourself. As images are obtained in a real-time mode, it is an excellent guide to interventional procedures, for example, nephrostomy. It is the method of choice in paediatrics. Ultrasound refers to sound waves with a frequency too high for humans to hear. Typically frequencies of between 3.5 and 10 MHz are used. Disadvantages of ultrasound include poor tissue specificity, lack of contrast media, a small field of view and recorded images that are difficult to interpret by others at a later date.

Ultrasound is probably the most commonly performed urological imaging modality in urological patients. It is commonly used for imaging the kidney, where it enables accurate measurement of the size, echogenicity, cortical thickness, identification of scarring, stones, cysts and tumours. It allows excellent imaging of the pelvicalyceal system and is the investigation of choice for the detection of hydronephrosis, which is dilatation of

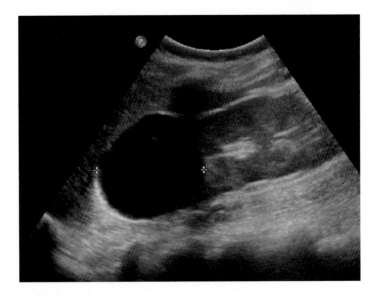

Figure 2.3 Ultrasound image of a kidney containing a cyst in the lower pole.

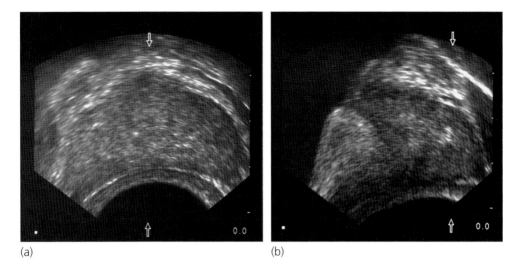

(a)   (b)

Figure 2.4 Transrectal ultrasound (TRUS) examination of the prostate: (a) transverse and (b) longitudinal.

the pelvicalyceal system usually due to urine flow obstruction.

In the bladder ultrasound is commonly used to measure post-micturition urine volumes, evaluate bladder wall thickness and detect tumours and stones. It is used for the evaluation of non-visible haematuria; however, it is not as sensitive for bladder lesions as contrast CT.

Ultrasound of the testis and scrotum has become a routine extension of the clinical examination of these organs; the superficial location of the testis allows the use of a high-frequency probe (5–10 MHz), which allows very good soft tissue resolution and is the imaging of choice for scrotal lumps and suspected testicular tumours.

By inserting a special probe into the rectum (transrectal ultrasound (TRUS)), high-resolution images can be obtained of the prostate (Figure 2.4). This allows geographically mapped guided prostate biopsies. Transvaginal ultrasound has been particularly valuable in the detection of urethral diverticula.

Intravenous urogram or pyelogram

This investigation involved administration of contrast with serial X-rays taken for 4 h afterwards. It allowed good visualisation of the collecting systems and ureters and was historically used to investigate haematuria and ureteric stones and also to determine the ureteric anatomy. Its use has been entirely replaced by computerised axial tomography, which is performed either with or without intravenous contrast depending on requirements.

Contrast media

Its high atomic number makes iodine relatively opaque to X-rays. Free ionic iodine is toxic, but when joined to benzoic acid, it forms organic salts, which can be given in large quantities, usually with safety. In urological investigation contrast is administered either intravenously or intraluminally. It has several drawbacks:

- Chemical irritation:
Occasionally irritation of the vein results in flushing, nausea and vomiting, when the bolus of hypertonic contrast medium reaches the systemic circulation. These effects are not common and seldom serious. Chemical inflammation and necrosis of the skin could result if the hypertonic solution is accidentally injected outside the vein. This is less of a concern now as the contrast media used are nonionic and of low osmolality.

- Allergy:

True allergy to contrast medium is much more serious. It can range from a trivial urticarial rash, which will resolve with an antihistamine, to life-threatening oedema of the glottis, trachea and bronchi, with widespread vasodilatation, hypotension and cardiac arrest. The allergen is the complete iodobenzoate molecule, not free iodine, so it is futile to perform skin tests with iodine. The reaction is not avoided by giving the first few millilitres of contrast slowly.

Millions of intravenous contrast studies are done every year, and fatal reactions occur only in $1:200\,000$. Patient anxiety increases the likelihood of a reaction; thus, quick reassurance to patients by the staff is helpful. Essential precautions are as follows:

Contrast-related precautions

Always enquire about even the most trivial previous reaction to contrast media, food particularly shellfish, drugs or animals. History of asthma and hay fever, recent illness and heart failure is relevant. Never start to give intravenous contrast medium without first making sure for yourself that all the essentials for treating an allergic reaction are to hand and within reach of the X-ray table. There should be the following:

- Adrenaline
- Hydrocortisone
- Oxygen, with face mask and airway
- A 'panic button' that will summon the cardiac arrest team

Particular precautions should be applied when administering intravenous contrast to patients at increased risk of developing contrast-induced nephropathy (CIN). These include those with impaired kidney function (chronic kidney disease), diabetes, heart failure and the elderly. Alternative non-contrast imaging modalities should be used when possible. The patient should be well hydrated and observed for signs and symptoms of CIN, which include feeling tired, loss of appetite and swelling of the feet and face. If contrast is administered, the patient should be well hydrated and observed afterwards.

Intravenous administration of iodinated contrast to patients taking metformin can result in lactic acidosis. This rare complication occurs if the contrast causes renal failure and the patient continues to take metformin. The drug is not excreted by the kidneys and toxic metabolites accumulate. Metformin should therefore be withheld for 48 h after contrast administration and can be restarted if there is no deterioration in renal function.

Computerised tomography

The CAT image is obtained by the computerised calculation of X-ray absorption after thousands of pencil-thin beams of X-rays are transmitted through a patient as a rotating source while the patient moves through the source on a table (hence producing a 'spiral' data set). This technique provides exquisitely good spatial resolution but does involve a high radiation dose. It is the test of choice in urolithiasis, staging of renal cell carcinoma and the evaluation of renal tract trauma (dynamic CT scanning). It can be supplemented with contrast, for example, intravenous dye injections (CAT/IVU combination) (Figure 2.5). Comprehensive urinary tract imaging is provided by the triple-phase CT.

The triple-phase CT

Non-contrast study

A plain CT is needed to image renal calcification and stones in the urological tract as they are obscured by contrast in the collecting system. When imaging of the parenchyma of an organ is required, contrast is given to demonstrate enhancement of tissue. This is particularly important when imaging renal masses; a tumour will enhance with contrast, whereas a cyst will not.

Nephrogram

It takes 15–20 s for the contrast medium to reach the kidney. Contrast medium should be injected rapidly in order to ensure the bolus reaches the kidneys quickly. A scan taken in the first 60 s will catch the contrast as it lies in the glomeruli and proximal tubules where

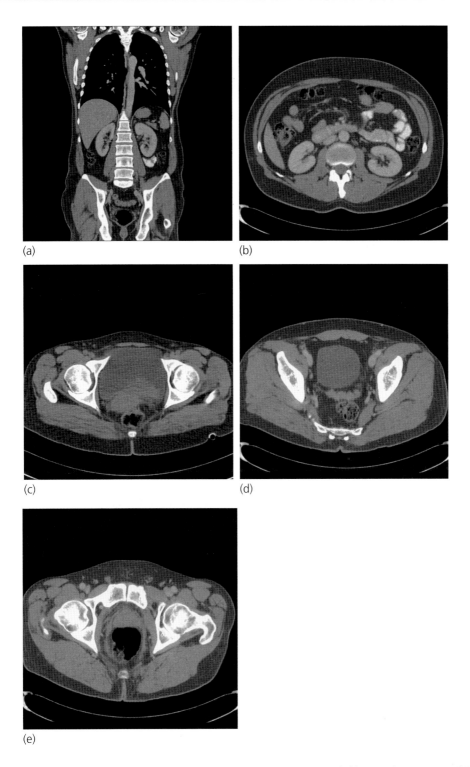

Figure 2.5 Computerised tomography: (a) normal male longitudinal coronal, (b) normal transverse axial at kidney level, (c) normal female transverse axial at bladder and uterus level, (d) normal male transverse axial at bladder level and (e) normal male transverse axial at prostate level.

water is being reabsorbed, so this, the 'imme-diate' or 'nephrogram' film, gives an image of the renal parenchyma. In obstruction the filtrate cannot escape down the tubule, and so the nephrogram is denser and lasts longer. (With a stone blocking the ureter, it is quite common to see the nephrogram persist for 24 h or more.)

Pyelogram

In a normal patient the glomerular filtrate containing the contrast medium quickly reaches the calices and pelvis to give the pyelogram. A scan taken at 5 min will therefore show the relationships of the calices to the renal contour and contrast in an unobstructed ureter and bladder.

Intraluminal contrast studies

Retrograde urogram

This study is used to visualise the internal aspect of the ureter in detail during endoscopic procedures. A fine ureteric catheter is passed up the ureteric orifice through a cystoscope, and contrast medium is injected to outline the ureter, pelvis and calices (Figure 2.6). A bulb-ended catheter jammed in the ureteric orifice allows dye injection up the whole length of the ureter (the ureterogram; Figure 2.7) without possible leak back into the bladder. These retrograde studies are performed under X-ray control.

Antegrade or descending urogram

A fine needle is passed into the renal pelvis under X-ray or ultrasound control. A flexible guide wire is passed through the needle into the pelvis, the needle is withdrawn, and a cannula is slipped over the guide wire into the pelvis to perform a percutaneous nephrostomy (Figure 2.8). This is the first step in a whole range of percutaneous operations on the kidney. Contrast medium injected through the cannula will delineate the renal pelvis and ureter. The pressure inside the cannula can be measured at the same time in the course of investigating obstruction.

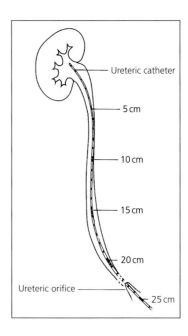

Figure 2.6 Retrograde pyelogram with a ureteric catheter.

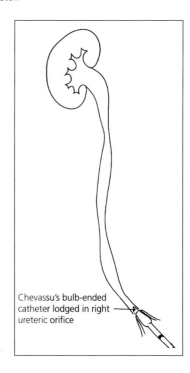

Figure 2.7 Retrograde ureteropyelogram using a bulb-ended catheter.

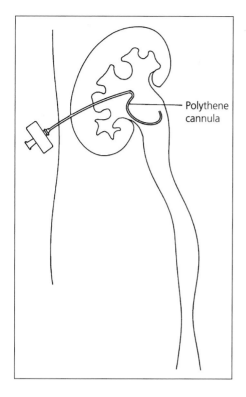

Figure 2.8 Percutaneous nephrostomy to obtain descending or antegrade pyelogram.

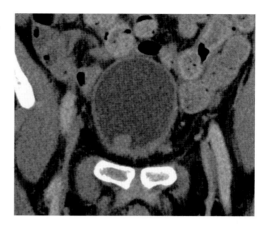

Figure 2.9 The image of the bladder showing a tumour in a standard CT.

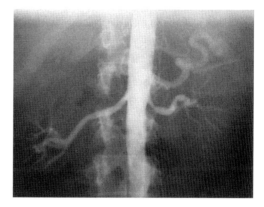

Figure 2.10 Arteriogram showing stenosis of left renal artery.

Cystogram

The image of the bladder in the standard CT will usually show diverticula or large tumours of the bladder (Figure 2.9). If the picture is not clear, or when it is necessary to rule out reflux from the bladder up the ureters, or in order to investigate incontinence, then the bladder is filled with contrast and screened while the patient passes urine. This is often combined with measurements of the pressure inside the bladder and the urine flow rate in a micturating cystometrogram. The cystogram is also used to detect bladder perforation and to test vesicourethral anastomosis after radical prostatectomy.

Urethrography

In investigating strictures and other disorders of the urethra, an ascending urethrogram is made by injecting contrast medium into the urethra with a small catheter. As opacification of the female urethra is technically difficult, this study is predominantly performed in men.

Angiography

A flexible guide wire is passed through a needle in the femoral artery over which a flexible cannula with a curved tip is slipped and guided under X-ray control into the opening of the renal artery. Contrast is then injected into the renal artery or its branches to give an arteriogram (Figure 2.10). This investigation can be of value in the diagnosis of trauma, stenosis of the renal artery and where

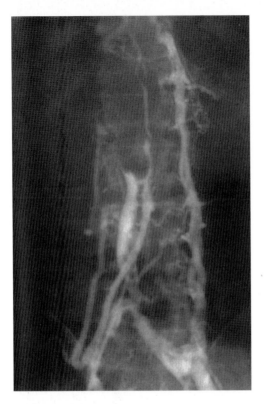

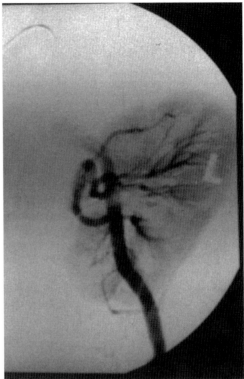

Figure 2.11 Inferior vena cavogram showing tumour in the vena cava.

Figure 2.12 Subtraction angiogram of a renal transplant in the left iliac fossa.

the cause of haematuria proves to be particularly hard to discover. Similar studies are made when it is suspected that there may be extension of tumour into the vena cava (Figure 2.11). The image of smaller vessels in the angiogram can be improved if overlying shadows of bone and bowel gas are removed: this can be done with a computer (Figure 2.12) to give a digital subtraction angiogram. Renal venography has been largely replaced by ultrasonography or contrast-enhanced CAT or MRI. One remaining indication is the cannulation of the gonadal veins with a view to embolisation in cases of scrotal varicocele.

Magnetic resonance imaging

Human cells contain protons and when placed in a strong magnetic field the protons align. Radiofrequency pulses producing an electromagnetic field are transmitted perpendicular to the magnet causing the protons to move out of position. When the protons return to their baseline state, called relaxing, energy is produced, which is translated into images (Figure 2.13). MRI can discriminate between body tissues based on their relative proportions of water and fat and can produce highly detailed images of soft tissues. Relaxation times for protons can vary and two times are commonly measured: T1 and T2. In a T2-weighted scan water, fat and fluid are bright, and these scans are used more often in urology for looking at soft tissue definition and are particularly useful for imaging the prostate.

Current indications for urological MRI include the local staging of pelvic urological cancers, assessing the degree of venous involvement of a renal cell cancer and the detection of renal artery

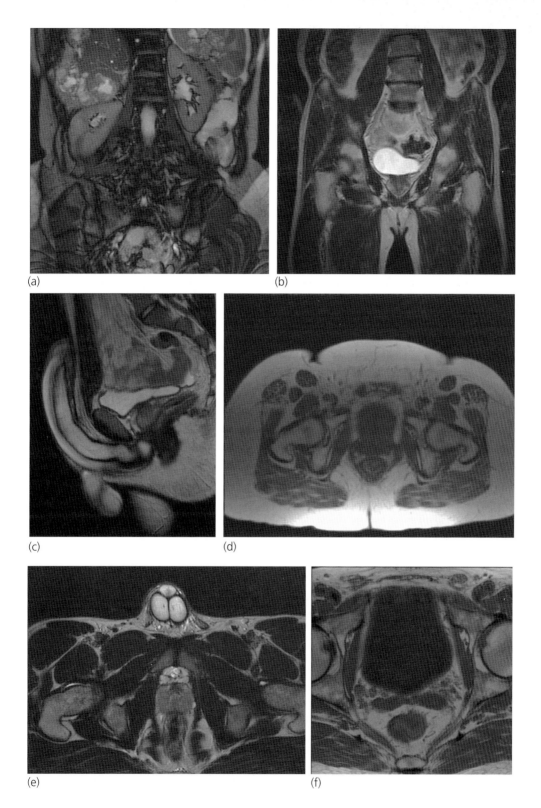

Figure 2.13 MRI scan: (a) normal upper abdomen, (b) normal pelvis, (c) lateral normal male pelvis, (d) transverse normal female pelvis, (e) transverse normal male pelvis at prostate level and (f) transverse normal male pelvis at seminal vesicles level.

stenosis. Some centres use MRI routinely in patients with impaired renal function in whom the use of nephrotoxic contrast medium is inadvisable. Patients who have pacemakers and metal surgical devices are not suitable for this type of investigation.

Radioisotope studies

Radionuclides are tagged on to various pharmaceuticals (often with very long names) to create radiopharmaceuticals. These are administered to the patient to provide functional imaging, and in some cases quantification, of various bodily processes. The radionuclide decays and, as it does so, emits small packets of energy (usually gamma photons), which interact with the detector crystal on a gamma camera, to cause a small flash of light to be emitted. This flash of light is then converted into an electrical current and amplified by an array of photomultiplier tubes on the back of the crystal. The resulting current is then put through a range of electronic wizardry, and a digital image is produced. The more radiopharmaceutical materials are taken up, the brighter the image.

Four radiopharmaceuticals are most commonly used in renal imaging:

1. ^{99m}Tc benzoylmercaptoacetyltriglycerine (more conveniently known as MAG3) is secreted by the proximal tubules into the tubular lumen.
2. ^{99m}Tc diethylenetriaminepentaacetic acid (DTPA) is excreted predominantly by glomerular filtration. Both of these agents are used for dynamic renography, which allows time activity curves to be produced (Figure 2.14) that show how the kidneys handle the tracer and give a good idea of how well each kidney is functioning. The images also give valuable information about the anatomical appearance of the kidneys although in less detail than ultrasound or CAT. Better results in patients with poorer renal function are obtained from MAG3 than DTPA.
3. ^{99m}Tc 2,3-dimercaptosuccinic acid (DMSA) is taken up and 'fixed' by the tissues of the proximal convoluted tubules. This radiopharmaceutical is not used for renography but does provide important information about the

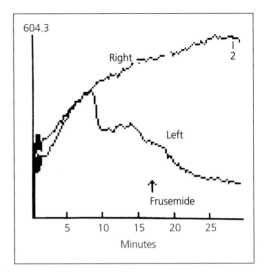

Figure 2.14 DTPA renogram in a case of hydronephrosis showing hold up of contrast on the right side, in spite of frusemide.

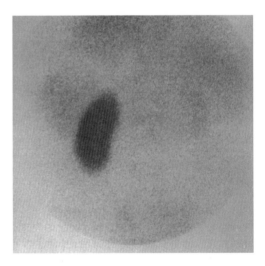

Figure 2.15 DMSA scan showing a normal right kidney but almost no uptake on the left, due to severe scarring.

renal cortex (e.g. detecting renal scars) (Figure 2.15), locating ectopic kidneys and in the evaluation of relative renal function (L:R ratios).

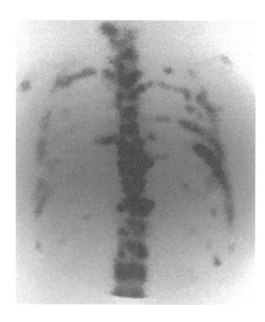

Figure 2.16 Bone scan in a man with carcinoma of the prostate with widespread metastases.

4. ^{51}Chromium EDTA is used to determine the glomerular filtration rate. This test involves only measurements of radioactivity in blood samples after intravenous injection of the radiopharmaceutical. No images are acquired.

Other nuclear medicine tests that are useful in urology include the bone scan. This is usually performed with ^{99m}Tc methylene diphosphonate (MDP), which is taken up wherever there is active bone turnover and gives rise to a 'hot spot'. It is not a very specific test but is extremely sensitive. The pattern of hot spots throughout the skeleton is important. Bony metastases often give rise to a random scatter throughout the axial skeleton and proximal long bones. This appearance is typical of prostate cancer (Figure 2.16).

Positron emission tomography

Positron emission tomography (PET) is a special type of isotope scanning technique in which two high-energy gamma photons (180° apart) are emitted from each atomic disintegration. The isotopes used in the radiopharmaceuticals have short half-lives (typically 10–60 min). The most commonly used radiopharmaceutical for PET imaging is ^{18}F-fluoro-2-deoxyglucose (FDG). This is taken up by any cell, which actively metabolises glucose. Cells that have more active metabolism, for example, many cancers, will take up more than surrounding cells. A PET scan detects the radiopharmaceuticals. Recent advances have made it possible to combine a PET scan with a conventional CAT scan. The patient undergoes a CAT scan immediately followed by a PET scan. The images from both scans can then be fused. This method of scanning beautifully combines functional imaging with high-resolution anatomical imaging so that pathology on a CAT scan effectively 'lights up'. This method is very useful in oncological imaging (see Figure 15.10).

 KEYPOINTS

- Valuable diagnostic information can be obtained from simple urine analysis.
- Ultrasound is the most commonly used urological imaging modality and is safe, non-invasive and easy to use.
- Triple-phase CT scanning gives more detailed images; cautions should be taken to avoid contrast-related complications.
- Functional information is obtained by radioisotope scanning.

Part 2

The kidneys and adrenal gland

3

The kidney: Embryology, developmental errors and cystic disease

Embryology

Primitive vertebrates develop with each somite having a pair of tubules, which allowed fluid from the coelom to drain out into the surrounding fluid. Mammals develop three kidneys during intrauterine growth, the pronephros, the mesonephros and the metanephros, which develop from the most cranial to caudal somites, respectively. In humans the first two serve as temporary excretory organs for the embryo and then regress; in primitive vertebrates they may persist as the end product of development:

1. Pronephros: The pronephros is the earliest stage in humans and corresponds to the mature structure of the most primitive vertebrates. It involves the most cranial somites and is a vestigial structure that disappears by the 4th week of development.
2. Mesonephros: The second kidney develops at the 9th to 10th somite level and serves as a transient excretory organ, while the final kidney develops from the metanephros. The mesonephros corresponds to the kidney of present-day fish and frogs whose mesonephric (Wolffian) duct empties urine into the cloaca. It differs from the pronephros in that a basic glomerulus and Bowman's capsule exist. In humans the mesonephros largely degenerates by the 8th week leaving the mesonephric duct.
3. Metanephros: The definitive human kidneys form most caudally in the sacral region (Figure 3.1). It originates with a ureteric bud growing out from the mesonephric duct. This grows cephalad and interacts with metanephric mesenchyme at 4 weeks of gestation to form the metanephros. The ureteric bud expands within the metanephros to form the renal pelvis, and multiple outgrowths branch into it forming hollow collecting ducts. Mesodermal cells become arranged as vesicles at the end of these ducts and develop into uriniferous tubules. The glomeruli are developed by the 36th week. The nephron therefore develops from the metanephric mesenchyme; the collecting system from the collecting ducts to the ureter is formed from the ureteric bud derived from the mesonephric duct.

Renal ascent and development of the ureter

The metanephros ascends from the level of the 28th somite to the first lumbar vertebrae by term due to active cephalic migration and differential

Urology Lecture Notes, Seventh Edition. Amir V. Kaisary, Andrew Ballaro and Katharine Pigott.
© 2016 John Wiley & Sons, Ltd. Published 2016 by John Wiley & Sons, Ltd.

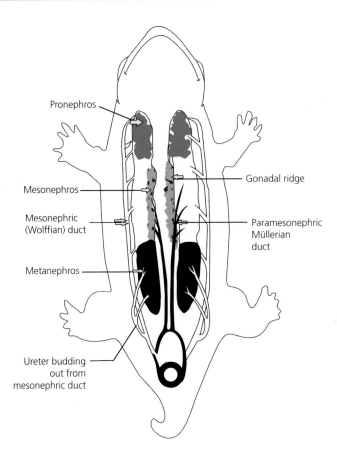

Pronephros

Gonadal ridge

Mesonephros

Mesonephric
(Wolffian) duct

Paramesonephric
Müllerian
duct

Metanephros

Ureter budding
out from
mesonephric duct

Figure 3.1 Embryology of the kidney.

caudal growth of the body. As it ascends, it is vascularised by a succession of temporary vessels sprouting from the aorta. These degenerate as their function is replaced by more cranial vessels, and the final pair persist as the renal arteries. Sometimes a more inferior pair of vessels persist and supply the lower pole of the kidney. The developing ureter, or nephric duct, reaches and enters the primitive urogenital sinus by independent caudal growth and separates it into a cephalad vesicourethral canal, which develops into the bladder and pelvic urethra, and a caudal urogenital sinus, which forms the external genitalia:

Mesonephric (Wolffian) ducts

In humans the mesonephric duct persists as the vas deferens in males and the caudal part of the ureter (Figure 3.2). If the mesonephric duct fails to develop,

then there will be neither ureter, kidney nor a vas deferens on that side – renal agenesis (Figure 3.3).

Paramesonephric (Müllerian) ducts

These are a second pair of ducts parallel with the mesonephric ducts:

- In females, they form the fallopian tubes, which fuse in the midline to form the uterus (Figure 3.4).
- In males, they largely regress but persist as a pit on the verumontanum in the prostatic urethra – the utriculus masculinus – as well as the cyst of Morgagni, which is attached to the upper pole of the testis and sometimes twists on its stalk mimicking torsion of the testicle (Figure 3.5).

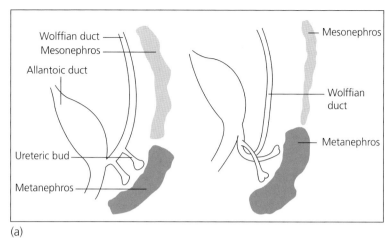

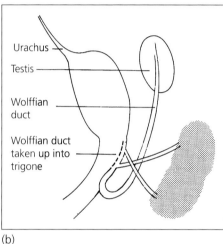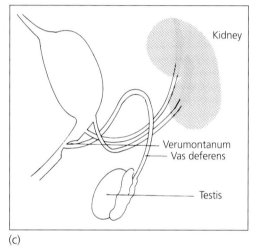

Figure 3.2 (a) Two ureteric buds from the Wolffian duct reach the metanephros, and then the Wolffian duct is bent round. (b) The lower end of the Wolffian duct is incorporated into the bladder. (c) The Wolffian duct becomes the vas deferens.

Congenital errors

Errors of development

Agenesis

If the mesonephric duct fails to develop, there is an absence of ureter, trigone, kidney and (in boys) vas deferens.

Aplasia

The metanephros may not differentiate at all (Figure 3.6).

Dysplasia

The metanephros may develop poorly, with odd-looking tissue including little cysts and lumps of cartilage (Figure 3.7).

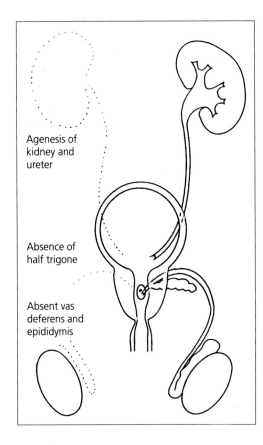

Agenesis of
kidney and
ureter

Absence of
half trigone

Absent vas
deferens and
epididymis

Figure 3.3 Renal agenesis.

Hypoplasia

This is a term to avoid: it implies that the kidney is small but otherwise normal. This is never the case: it is either dysplastic or scarred, or both.

Errors of position

Rotated kidney

A kidney often faces forwards rather than medially. Its outline is then an ellipse and some of its calices point medially (Figure 3.8). This condition is harmless.

Horseshoe kidney

If both the metanephroi get fused together in the foetal pelvis, not only are both kidneys rotated, but also their lower poles are joined in the shape of a horseshoe (Figure 3.9). The cause for this is unknown. As the foetus grows, the joined kidneys are held up by the inferior or superior mesenteric arteries. In operations for aortic aneurysm, the isthmus joining the two kidneys may have to be divided, but otherwise it should be left alone. This condition is often associated with reflux, ureterocele and hydronephrosis.

Each of these conditions should be dealt with in the usual way, without meddling with the isthmus.

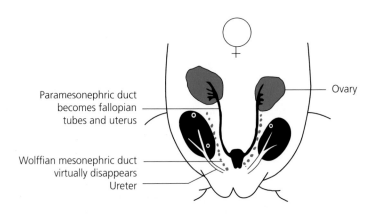

Paramesonephric duct
becomes fallopian
tubes and uterus

Ovary

Wolffian mesonephric duct
virtually disappears
Ureter

Figure 3.4 Female genitalia.

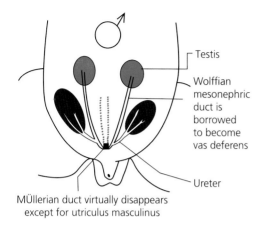

Figure 3.5 Male genitalia.

Testis

Wolffian mesonephric duct is borrowed to become vas deferens

Ureter

Müllerian duct virtually disappears except for utriculus masculinus

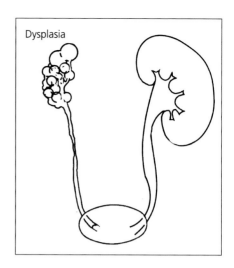

Figure 3.7 Dysplasia.

Dysplasia

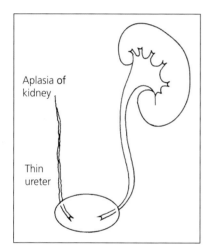

Figure 3.6 Aplasia.

Aplasia of kidney

Thin ureter

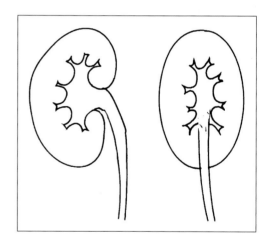

Figure 3.8 Rotated kidney.

Crossed renal ectopia

Instead of being united in the midline like a horseshoe, the two kidneys may fuse together on one side. Their ureters always run along their proper side. As with horseshoe kidney, there is often some other congenital anomaly such as reflux or obstruction (Figure 3.10).

Pelvic kidney

Here the metanephros remains in the pelvis. One might expect it would get in the way of the baby during childbirth, but it hardly ever does. A pelvic kidney is usually detected by chance and seldom needs any treatment unless associated with some other condition such as hydronephrosis. But there is one unexpected and important hazard: at laparotomy for abdominal pain, an unwary surgeon may come across an unusual 'tumour' and go ahead to remove it. In pelvic kidneys the segmental arteries arise directly from the aorta, common and internal iliac arteries. If the condition is not recognised, there can by confusion and bleeding (Figure 3.11).

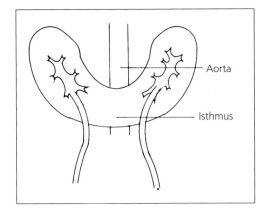

Figure 3.9 Horseshoe kidney.

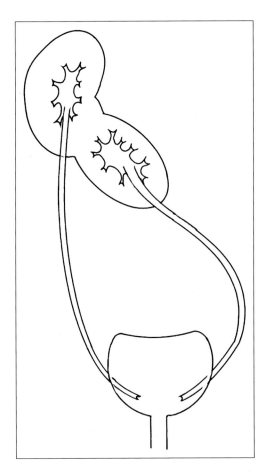

Figure 3.10 Crossed renal ectopia.

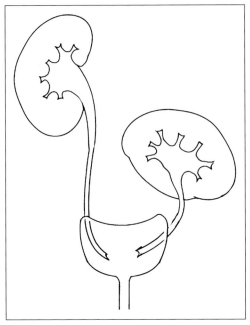

Figure 3.11 Pelvic kidney.

Thoracic kidney

This is not so much an error of development of the kidney as of the diaphragm, where one kidney is carried up into the chest along with other viscera. Such a 'thoracic' kidney is found by chance in a chest radiograph or an intravenous urography (IVU). The kidney is not really in the thorax: a thin layer of diaphragm and pleura always separates the two compartments. The kidney itself needs no treatment (Figure 3.12).

Duplex kidney and ureter

After budding out from the lower end of the mesonephric duct, the ureter usually begins to branch when it gets near the metanephros, but sometimes it divides earlier and may produce a complete double system of renal pelvis and calyces. The overlying renal parenchyma is never completely separated, but a distinct 'waist' marks the distinction between the two halves, as does a prominent bulge in the parenchyma, which may be mistaken for a carcinoma in X-rays (Figure 3.13). The upper half of the kidney has

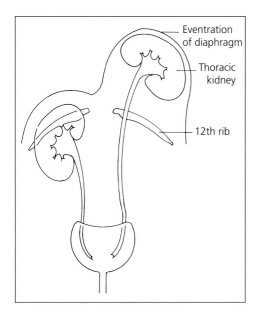

Figure 3.12 Thoracic kidney.

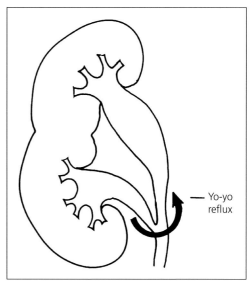

Figure 3.14 Yo-yo reflux.

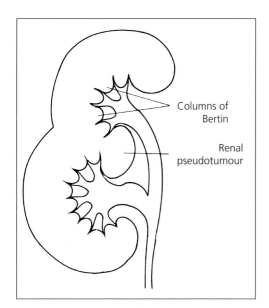

Figure 3.13 In duplex kidney there is often a very prominent column of Bertin.

reflux (Figure 3.14). A duplex kidney is nearly always innocent and symptomless, but it can be associated with three conditions that cause trouble.

1. Ectopic ureter: The ureter draining the upper half of the kidney may open into the vagina, caudal to the sphincter, and gives rise to continual incontinence (Figure 3.15).
2. Reflux: The ureter from the lower half of the kidney has a short course through the wall of the bladder and thus is less efficient as a valve, and urine may reflux from the bladder up to the kidney (Figure 3.16).
3. Ureterocele: If the lower end of the mesonephric duct is incompletely absorbed into the trigone, it may form a balloon just where the ureter enters the trigone – ureterocele. This is most often seen at the lower of two ureteric orifices in duplex. Very occasionally an ureterocele may prolapse out of the urethra as a translucent 'cyst' causing painful acute retention of urine (Figure 3.17).

Cystic disorders of the kidney

The kidney is one of the most common sites for cysts. The cysts may differ in size and location and may be ectatic renal tubules or saccular

two main calyces; the lower half has three and makes more urine.

Urine may be squirted from the lower half up into the upper half, causing distension and pain – yo-yo

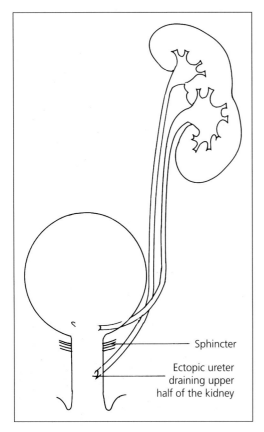

Sphincter

Ectopic ureter
draining upper
half of the kidney

Figure 3.15 If the ureter from the upper half of the
kidney opens below the sphincter in a girl, there is
continual incontinence.

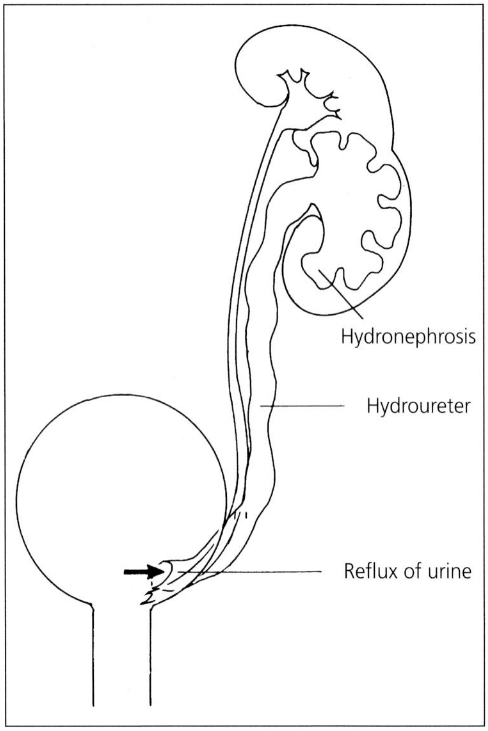

Hydronephrosis

Hydroureter

Reflux of urine

Figure 3.16 Reflux up the upper ureteric orifice
into the lower half of the kidney.

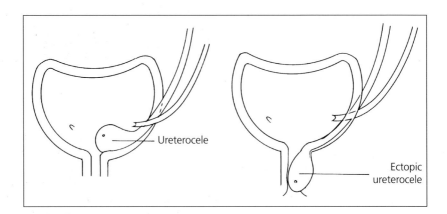

Ureterocele

Ectopic
ureterocele

Figure 3.17 A ureterocele may prolapse into the urethra.

structures that resemble diverticula located off the nephron. They can be classified as genetic and non-genetic.

Non-genetic

Medullary sponge kidney

This is a disorder characterised by cystic dilatation of medullary collecting pre-calyceal ducts in one or more renal papillae (Figure 3.18). It may result from disruption of the interface between the ureteric bud and the mesonephric blastema during embryonic development. Part or all of one or both kidneys may be affected, and the medulla becomes honeycombed with cysts giving the appearance of a sponge. It was previously believed that most cases of medullary sponge kidney were sporadic; however, recent studies show that familial clustering is common and has an autosomal dominant inheritance, a reduced penetrance and variable expressivity.

Medullary sponge kidney is usually asymptomatic but can cause non-glomerular renal bleeding. Repeated attacks of infection in the dilated tubules are soon followed by the development of numerous small stones, which give repeated attacks of ureteric colic and predispose to urinary tract infection. Histologically there are dilated collecting ducts, inflammation of interstitial region and atrophy near the papillary tips. Renal scarring can occur. Progression rarely leads to renal failure. The radiographic appearance is characteristic (Figure 3.19): medullary calcification, radiating linear striations and dilated collecting ducts in renal papillae. This is best shown by contrast pooling studies (IVU) rather than CT or MRI. Associated metabolic abnormalities include absorptive hypercalciuria and distal renal tubular acidosis.

Multicystic dysplastic kidney

Most renal cystic conditions arise from the nephrons or collecting ducts after they have formed. Multicystic dysplasia however arises from abnormal development of the metanephros or obstruction occurring early in development. The kidney comprises multiple cysts with little stroma between them and has the appearance of a bunch of grapes (Figure 3.20). It is associated with

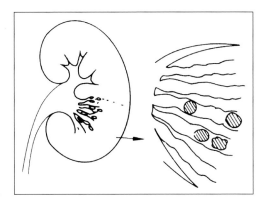

Figure 3.18 Medullary sponge kidney: dilated collecting tubules and stones.

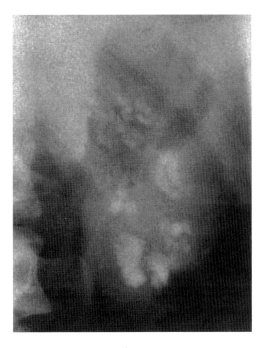

Figure 3.19 X-ray of medullary sponge kidney showing multiple calculi in dilated collecting ducts.

increased expression of genes and growth factors associated with aspects of renal development, and it is thought obstruction during development is the primary insult as there is often ureteric atresia. Multicystic dysplastic kidney is a common cause of an abdominal mass in infants, and the contralateral kidney may also be abnormal with

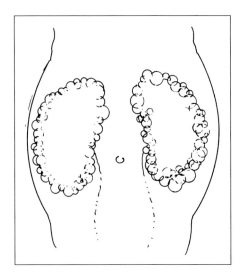

Figure 3.20 Congenital multicystic kidney.

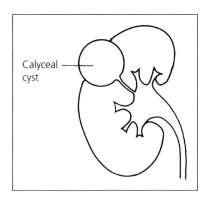

Figure 3.21 Calyceal cyst.

vesicoureteric reflux and pelviureteric obstruction common. The kidney is non-functioning and may involute; it may rarely increase in size after birth and is very rarely associated with Wilms' tumour, so monitoring is required.

Calyceal diverticulum

A single calyx may become obstructed, and the pyramid draining into it becomes converted into a hollow bag, which communicates with the collecting system via a narrow neck. They are associated with infection or stones, which may develop in the cyst (Figure 3.21).

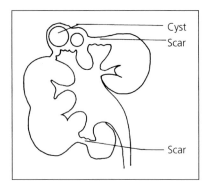

Figure 3.22 Obstructed cysts in pyelonephritic scarring.

Parapelvic cyst

This is a renal cyst that arises from the renal parenchyma adjacent to the renal pelvis. The cyst can abut the collecting system and be misinterpreted as hydronephrosis on ultrasound.

Acquired renal cystic disease

Acquired renal cystic disease is a condition that occurs in patients with end-stage chronic renal failure, whether or not they are receiving dialysis. The obstructed nephrons occasionally become grossly distended with protein (Figure 3.22). The condition results in pain and haematuria and is associated with the development of renal cell carcinoma. Renal tumours develop in a 10th of patients receiving chronic haemodialysis, and this incidence increases to a quarter if acquired cystic disease is present. The cysts in the native kidneys may regress after receipt of a transplanted kidney suggesting a toxin is responsible.

Simple renal cysts

Simple cysts may be single or multiple and are very common incidental findings on ultrasound. The most common type of simple renal cyst arises as a diverticulum from the collecting tubules of the kidney. Simple cysts occur in middle age in almost every normal kidney and are detected by accident in an ultrasound scan (Figure 3.23). Simple renal cysts are seldom seen in children and their incidence increases with age; they are therefore characterised as acquired. They may grow to over 10 cm in size although the

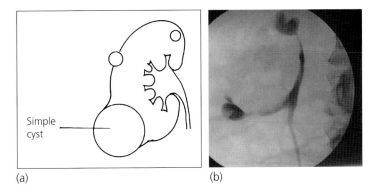

Figure 3.23 (a) Simple cysts of the kidney. (b) Ultrasound showing a simple cyst.

majority are less than 2 cm and when large may cause pain. In this situation they can be surgically marsupialised or de-roofed.

Simple benign renal cysts should be differentiated from complex renal cysts, which have malignant potential, by imaging. Ultrasound criteria include a sharp, thin distinct wall, spherical shape with no internal septa or structure and homogenous content. If these criteria are not met, the cyst is termed complex, and cross-sectional contrast imaging with CT or MRI is required (see Bosniak classification in Chapter 7).

Genetic

Polycystic disease

A bizarre exaggeration of this process is seen in polycystic disease. There are two main forms of this condition: childhood and adult.

Childhood polycystic disease (autosomal recessive polycystic disease)
This type of polycystic disease is inherited as an autosomal recessive characteristic and is secondary to a mutation of the PKHD1 gene on chromosome 6. It may present at four stages:

1. Foetal: Ultrasound in pregnancy reveals that both kidneys have been converted into giant sponges. It is not compatible with survival.
2. Neonatal: A similar condition is discovered in the neonate, who may survive for up to a year, unless a transplant can be found.
3. Infantile: Between 3 and 6 months, these children are found to have uraemia and enlarged

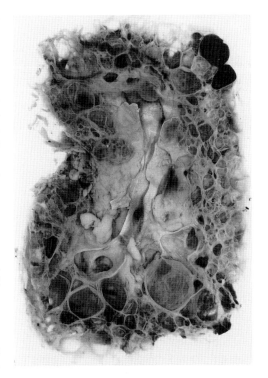

Figure 3.24 Adult polycystic disease.

kidneys, and all children have a degree of congenital hepatic fibrosis.

4. Juvenile: This is discovered in later childhood and is also associated with hepatic fibrosis.

There is no cure and supportive treatment of portal hypertension and heart failure is required to extend life. Haemodialysis and transplantation are generally required.

Adult polycystic disease

This is inherited in an autosomal dominant fashion and occurs due to a mutation on the PKD1 gene on chromosome 16, which codes for proteins important in the structure of renal tubular epithelial cells (Figure 3.24). It may appear in children but is usually diagnosed in adult life and is an important cause of both hypertension and end-stage renal failure. Adult polycystic disease is associated with renal adenomas but not renal cell carcinoma and commonly coexists with cysts in the liver and pancreas and berry aneurysms of the circle of Willis, which cause subarachnoid haemorrhage. Many patients have no symptoms at all. Often the diagnosis is made by accident when an abdominal lump is found on routine palpation or ultrasound scanning.

Multiple malformation syndromes with renal cysts

These include tuberous sclerosis and von Hippel–Lindau disease. Tuberous sclerosis is an autosomal dominant disease characterised by hamartoma formation in the cerebrum, kidneys and eyes and causes mental retardation, epilepsy and adenoma sebaceum. In the kidneys, renal cysts and angiomyolipomas form, and there is a higher incidence of renal cell carcinoma than normal.

Von Hippel–Lindau disease is an autosomal recessive condition associated with cerebellar and retinal hemangioblastomas, renal and pancreatic cysts and a 50% incidence of clear cell renal carcinoma.

4

Kidney trauma

Most of accident and injury patients are now managed by multidisciplinary trauma teams. The urologist will be involved if there is clinical or radiological evidence of renal injury. The most reliable clinical sign is haematuria. It is important to obtain a complete history of the injury, which enables an opinion to be formed of the degree of force and severity of injury likely to have been sustained. Injury to the kidney may be by either penetrating forces or blunt ones.

Penetrating injuries

All penetrating abdominal and retroperitoneal injuries should generally be surgically explored. The kidney may be injured by a knife or bullet wound; in knife injuries the kidney can usually be repaired. In high-velocity injuries the energy of the bullet devitalises a large area of tissue adjacent to the track, and if the kidney is involved, it usually requires nephrectomy.

Closed injuries

Minor closed injuries of the kidney are often seen in sport; more severe direct blunt and avulsion injuries are seen in road traffic accidents. To damage the kidney, the blow has to be quite severe, and so it often fractures the lower ribs and tips of the transverse processes of the lumbar vertebrae (Figure 4.1).

There are five grades of closed renal injury (Figure 4.2):

1. The renal parenchyma is contused but not lacerated, and there may be a contained sub-capsular haematoma.
2. There is a small cortical laceration of less than 1 cm with no urinary extravasation. There is a non-expanding perirenal haematoma.
3. There is a cortical laceration greater than 1 cm with no urinary extravasation or involvement of the collecting system.
4. There is a cortical laceration extending into the medulla and collecting system, or the renal artery or vein is damaged with a contained haemorrhage.
5. The kidney is shattered into several pieces or avulsion of the renal hilum.

Management

The patient should be managed as a trauma patient and carefully examined to rule out other injuries particularly pneumothorax and internal bleeding into the chest or peritoneal cavity from associated injury to the liver or spleen.

After appropriate resuscitation, renal imaging with CT is required for all patients with penetrating injuries when there is suspicion of renal or visceral involvement or any degree of haematuria.

Urology Lecture Notes, Seventh Edition. Amir V. Kaisary, Andrew Ballaro and Katharine Pigott.
© 2016 John Wiley & Sons, Ltd. Published 2016 by John Wiley & Sons, Ltd.

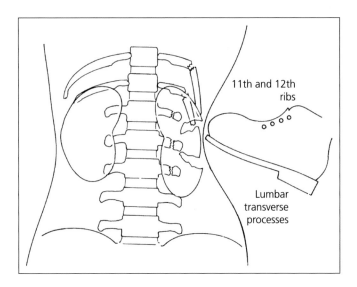

Figure 4.1 The mechanism of closed injury of the kidney.

Grade	Description
I	Contusion: Macroscopic/microscopic haematuria. Urological studies normal Haematoma: Sub-capsular non-expanding. No parenchymal laceration
II	Haematoma: Perirenal non-expanding haematoma Laceration: <1 cm parenchymal depth. No urinary extravasation
III	Laceration: >1 cm parenchymal depth. No collecting system rupture. No urine extravasation
IV	Laceration: Parenchymal laceration through renal corticomedullary junction into collecting system. Or Vascular: Segmental renal artery/vein injury-contained haemorrhage, partial vessel laceration or thrombosis
V	Laceration: Completely shattered kidney Vascular: Avulsion of renal hilum

Figure 4.2 Five grades of renal injury.

With closed injuries CT imaging is indicated when there is visible haematuria, when there is evidence of cardiovascular compromise or when the mechanism of injury suggests significant renal trauma may have occurred.

Patients with low-grade (I–II) blunt injuries who are cardiovascularly stable may be observed with regular observations.

When there is evidence of urinary extravasation (grade III), ureteric stenting and percutaneous

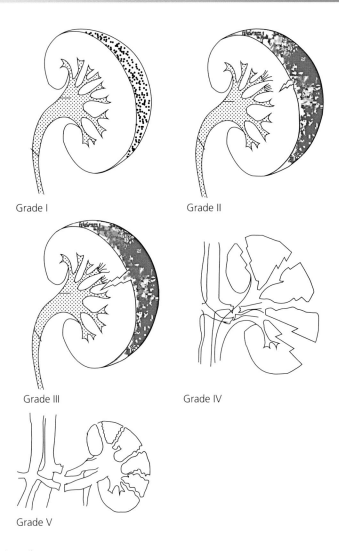

Grade I

Grade II

Grade III

Grade IV

Grade V

Figure 4.2 (*Continued*)

drainage of the urinoma may be indicated and a high index of suspicion for sepsis should be maintained.

Patients with high-grade (IV) injuries should be observed hourly and undergo serial blood tests and CT scans to monitor bleeding.

Radiological selective embolisation of a torn vessel is the preferred treatment option in a cardiovascularly stable patient; with evidence of continued bleeding, occasionally surgical exploration is required (Figure 4.3).

Patients with grade V injuries usually show signs of cardiovascular compromise and require emergency open surgery and usually

nephrectomy. It is sometimes possible to repair and reconstruct a damaged kidney; this is more likely in dedicated trauma centres of excellence.

Complications

1. ***Secondary haemorrhage***: When there has been a severe laceration, the clot that is holding the pieces of kidney together may undergo lysis. Delayed haemorrhage may occur at any time within the first 2 weeks but is exceedingly rare when the initial tear in the kidney was only a small one (Figure 4.4).

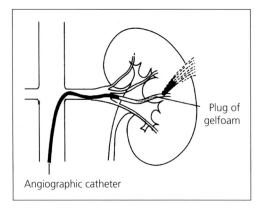

Figure 4.3 Bleeding from a segmental artery can be blocked by injection of gelfoam through an angiography catheter.

Plug of gelfoam

Angiographic catheter

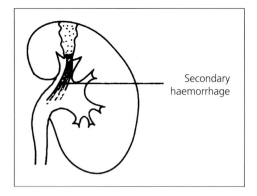

Secondary haemorrhage

Figure 4.4 Secondary haemorrhage.

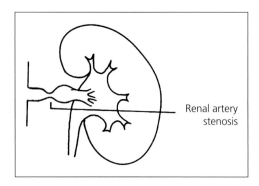

Renal artery stenosis

Figure 4.5 Renal artery stenosis.

2. ***Renal artery stenosis***: A small laceration of the renal artery may heal with stenosis and cause hypertension (Figure 4.5).
3. ***Page kidney***: An organising haematoma may form a thick tough shell around the kidney, which then shrinks, compressing the kidney leading to ischaemia and hypertension (Figure 4.6).
4. ***Pseudocyst or urinoma***: This is a rare complication in the event a tear in the collecting system is not detected during the acute phase imaging. A perirenal urine collection may become surrounded by scar tissue and require delayed drainage (Figure 4.7).

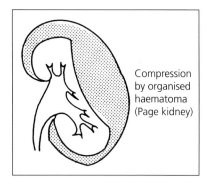

Compression by organised haematoma (Page kidney)

Figure 4.6 Page kidney.

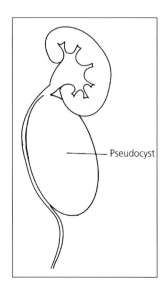

Pseudocyst

Figure 4.7 Pseudocyst or urinoma.

KEYPOINTS

- Multidisciplinary trauma teams now manage most of accident and injury patients.
- The urologist will be involved if there is clinical or radiological evidence of renal injury.
- The most reliable clinical sign is haematuria.

5

Kidney infections and inflammation

There exists a balance between host defence mechanisms and the virulence of pathogenic bacteria, and any factor that upsets this balance may contribute to the development of urinary tract infection. Bacteria may access the kidney by either ascending from the infected bladder or the blood-borne route. Upper tract infections may be categorised into uncomplicated and complicated.

Uncomplicated infections

Uncomplicated infections are those that occur in a structurally and immunologically normal host. The pathogens responsible are a subgroup of *Escherichia coli* spp. with unique adaptations termed virulence factors. These factors enable the bacteria to ascend to the upper urinary tract and evade host defence mechanisms and also contribute to pathogenicity.

Complicated infections

Complicated infections are those that occur in an immunocompromised host or patients with structural abnormalities, urinary tract stones, indwelling catheters or ureteric stents (Figure 5.1). These host factors provide an advantage to

pathogenic bacteria enabling them to proliferate and survive in the urinary tract.

Some bacteria are able to attach to such foreign bodies and form protective biofilms around themselves enabling them to proliferate and survive host defence mechanisms. Additional bacteria to those responsible for uncomplicated infections should be suspected.

Impaired host resistance factors provide an advantage to pathogenic bacteria enabling them to ascend, proliferate and survive in the urinary tract. When complicating factors are present, additional bacteria to *E. coli* species should be suspected.

Ascending infection

Bacteria ascending the ureter from the bladder cause most upper urinary tract infections. Factors that precipitate lower urinary tract infection may therefore predispose also to upper urinary tract infection. The pathogens responsible are a subgroup of *E. coli* spp. with unique adaptations termed virulence factors. These factors differentiate these bacteria from those responsible for cystitis alone by enabling them to ascend to the upper urinary tract, evade host defence mechanisms and also contribute to pathogenicity. The most important factor is the expression of P-fimbriae, which enable the bacterium to adhere to the upper tract urothelium.

Urology Lecture Notes, Seventh Edition. Amir V. Kaisary, Andrew Ballaro and Katharine Pigott.
© 2016 John Wiley & Sons, Ltd. Published 2016 by John Wiley & Sons, Ltd.

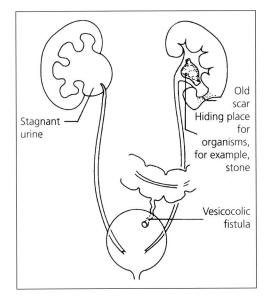

Figure 5.1 Factors contributing to complicated infections.

Blood-borne infection

Less commonly, blood-borne infection may carry microorganisms to the kidney where they may form single or multiple abscesses in the renal parenchyma or diffuse infection, depending on the causative organism. Blood-borne infections are more often than not complicated, specifically involving a generally immuno-compromised host, and may be caused by a wider range of pathogens than uncomplicated ascending infections including viruses, yeasts and multiple bacterial strains.

Acute pyelonephritis

Clinical features

Acute pyelonephritis is an acute generalised bacterial infection of the renal parenchyma. It classically present with signs of renal inflammation and sepsis characterised by pain and loin tenderness and acute onset of high fever with rigours reflecting an early systemic response. These signs are often accompanied or preceded

 KEYPOINTS

Impaired host resistance is encountered in:

1 Diabetes mellitus

2 Acquired immune deficiency syndrome (AIDS)

3 Immunosuppression: for transplantation or during cancer chemotherapy

by those of lower urinary tract infection, when infection occurs by the ascending route.

Severe renal inflammation may involve the adjacent peritoneum and bowel causing abdominal pain, localised peritonism, nausea, vomiting and diarrhoea. The patient may be ambulatory or very unwell with severe pain and sepsis. There is usually a high white cell count in blood and urine samples. Bacteria may be grown from blood cultures and, provided there is no ureteric obstruction, from the urine.

Management

Some patients with uncomplicated pyelonephritis are suitable for ambulatory care; others require hospital admission for parenteral antibiotic treatment depending on fitness and clinical presentation. Ambulatory patients in whom no complicating factors are suspected do not require immediate imaging; however, the facility for this must be available should there not be an early response to treatment.

In unwell patients and those in whom a complicated infection is suspected, early urinary tract ultrasound is required, and contrast-enhanced computerised tomography (CT) should be performed to further characterise any ultrasonography abnormality. Ambulatory patients may be managed with NSAIDS and an initial dose of parenteral antibiotics followed by oral treatment; hospitalised patients should have parenteral fluids in addition.

The antibiotic of choice is determined by urine and blood cultures, and until the results of these are available, the broad-spectrum combination of a quinolone or aminoglycoside and penicillin is most commonly prescribed. A urine Gram stain may guide early treatment.

Acute pyelonephritis is usually uncomplicated and resolves with no sequelae if treated

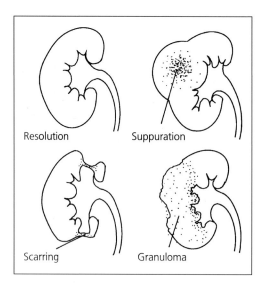

Resolution

Suppuration

Scarring

Granuloma

Figure 5.2 Four possible outcomes from renal infection.

appropriately. In patients who show no clinical response to treatment, re-imaging to exclude a complicating factor and a change of antibiotics should be considered.

End result of urinary infection

Infection in the kidney, like infection anywhere else, can be followed by one of four processes (Figure 5.2):

1. Resolution
2. Suppuration
3. Scarring
4. Granuloma

Complicated renal infections

Focal nephritis

Bacterial infection of the kidney may also be localised to a single or several areas or the renal parenchyma. This may be uncomplicated but

occurs more commonly in diabetic than non-diabetic patients and has a similar clinical presentation to pyelonephritis.

The causative bacteria are usually similar to those responsible for pyelonephritis. Ultrasonography findings are non-specific, and CT imaging typically shows wedge-shaped areas of decreased enhancement. Treatment is with parenteral antibiotics and fluid resuscitation; if there is no clinical improvement, development of a renal abscess should be suspected.

Renal abscess

Renal abscess occurs due to failure of resolution of localised or generalised bacterial renal parenchymal infection and should be suspected if the patient remains febrile for more than 4 days after treatment with appropriate antibiotics. Renal abscess is predisposed to by host anatomical abnormalities such as renal damage caused by stones, previous inflammation and vesicoureteric reflux.

Blood-borne infections of a structurally normal kidney in an immunocompromised host may also result in multiple small abscesses, which grow and coalesce to produce if not treated (Figure 5.3).

The abscess is best imaged using contrast CT, and treatment is, as with all abscesses, drainage. This can be performed by needle aspiration, by placing a temporary percutaneous drain or in severe cases by open incision and drainage. Small abscesses may resolve with parenteral antibiotics without surgical drainage.

Before drainage it is important to differentiate a parenchymal abscess from infection in an obstructed calyceal diverticulum. In this situation removal of the drain risks recurrence, and either percutaneous or retrograde surgical dilatation of the diverticulum neck with or without ablation of the diverticulum urothelium and stent placement is required.

Perinephric abscess

Perinephric abscess is the presence of pus between the renal capsule and Gerota's fascia. This occurs due to either rupture of a renal

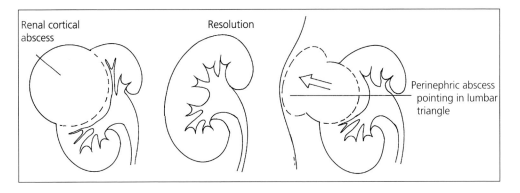

Figure 5.3 Blood-borne infections may give rise to cortical infection, which may resolve or proceed to an abscess.

abscess through the capsule or infection by blood-borne organisms of a perinephric haematoma caused by trauma or surgery.

Perinephric abscess is predisposed to by focal obstruction within the renal collecting system. Untreated infections distal to stones obstructing renal calyces result in pus tracking under pressure through the often atrophic renal parenchyma and capsule to the perinephric space.

The clinical findings are similar to that of a renal abscess, contrast-enhanced CT is the imaging method of choice with all suspected renal abscess, and treatment is with appropriate antibiotics, drainage of the pus and correction of the underlying cause.

Emphysematous pyelonephritis

Emphysematous pyelonephritis is an uncommon complicated form of acute pyelonephritis characterised by severe necrotising infection of the renal parenchyma caused by gas-forming organisms in diabetic patients.

The condition is predisposed to by several factors: infection with organisms that form gas by fermentation of glucose through the glycolytic pathway such as some strains of *E. coli*, *Klebsiella pneumoniae* and *Proteus* and rarely *Clostridium* species, high tissue glucose levels, impaired immune response and impaired tissue perfusion. Gas formation in the tissues is detectable

on CT, and there is rapid destruction of the renal parenchyma so that the kidney is often rendered non-functioning.

The patient with emphysematous pyelonephritis is extremely unwell with systemic sepsis and requires urgent resuscitation and broad-spectrum antibiotics. Nephrectomy is usually required after the patient is stabilised.

Pyonephrosis

Pyonephrosis is the presence of infected urine in an obstructed pelvicalyceal system. The most common cause is a ureteric calculus with proximal urine infection; the accumulation of infected pus under pressure causes destruction of renal parenchyma and endotoxin-medicated septicaemia from pyelolymphatic and pyelovenous passage of infected urine into the bloodstream.

An infected and obstructed pelvicalyceal system is a surgical emergency, and the patient is extremely unwell with high fever rigours and loin pain and tenderness. Renal ultrasound or CT may show hydronephrosis. Resuscitation, broad-spectrum antibiotic treatment and surgical decompression and drainage of the renal pelvis by percutaneous nephrostomy or, if the patient is fit enough for anaesthetic, retrograde insertion of a ureteric stent should be performed as soon as the diagnosis is made as tissue destruction is rapid.

Clinical sequelae of renal infections

Urinary sepsis and septic shock

Sepsis is the clinical syndrome characterised by the presence of a systemic inflammatory response (SIRS) in response to infection. Sepsis occurs when the host inflammatory response to a localised infection becomes generalised and blood-borne resulting in involvement and damage to distant organs.

Septic shock occurs when untreated sepsis is complicated by organ failure and circulatory collapse. Sepsis and septic shock may be caused by many infections and are a common sequelae of Gram-negative urinary infections.

Septic shock is primarily mediated by a lipopolysaccharide virulence factor. This is a component of the Gram-negative bacterial cell wall, which activates host immunological defence mechanisms involving the complement system, cytokines and clotting pathways.

The widespread activation of these pathways results in a complex interaction between inflammatory mediators causing vasodilatation and increased endothelial permeability. The function of the myocardium is also depressed, and the result is hypoperfusion and subsequent failure of vital organ systems.

Anticipation and early recognition is vital, and ITU admission for aggressive resuscitation, fluid balance monitoring, antibiotic treatment and organ support with inotropes is required.

Acute kidney injury

The function of an infected, inflamed renal parenchyma may be temporarily impaired; this may manifest as acute kidney injury (AKI) if there is pre-existing contralateral renal impairment. Furthermore the treatment of renal infections typically involves administration of potentially nephrotoxic agents such as NSAID and aminoglycoside medication and intravenous contrast during CT, and a high index of suspicion for AKI should be maintained in all hospitalised patients. Tissue destruction during emphysematous pyelonephritis or pyonephrosis results in permanent renal damage. Urinary sepsis also causes AKI by pre-renal mechanisms as discussed earlier.

Chronic upper urinary tract infections and inflammation

Chronic pyelonephritis

Chronic pyelonephritis refers to the clinical picture of a shrunken, scarred end-stage kidney with histological features of chronic inflammation. The condition is often asymptomatic, although there may be chronic loin pain and history of recurrent bacterial pyelonephritis, and presents with renal failure and characteristic radiological findings.

The cause of the chronic inflammation is repeated urinary infections in a functionally or structurally abnormal urinary tract. The most important changes seem to result from infections of the developing kidney during infancy, with subsequent insults causing cumulative damage.

Although recurrent pyelonephritis may cause permanent renal impairment, infection of structurally normal adult kidneys does not result in the scarring that is characteristic of chronic pyelonephritis.

The most common structural abnormality associated with chronic pyelonephritis is vesicoureteric reflux.

Granulomatous disease

Xanthogranulomatous pyelonephritis

This is an unusual but severe chronic infection of the renal parenchyma associated with renal calculi causing focal obstruction and chronic infection within the kidney.

It results from a granulomatous host response to recurrent unresolved infections and is characterised morphologically by an accumulation of lipid-filled macrophages in a grossly enlarged fibrotic pus-filled non-functioning kidney.

Macroscopically, the renal mass consists of a firm, yellow and lobulated tissue, which resembles renal cell carcinoma. The clinical presentation is of a long history of intermittent fever, malaise, weight loss, loin pain and persistent bacteriuria with the radiological findings of an enlarged kidney usually with large calculi.

Treatment is with stabilisation of current infection and nephrectomy. Nephrectomy may involve extensive excision of perinephric granulation tissue and has a high morbidity due to loss of the normal tissue planes and involvement of adjacent retroperitoneal structures in the inflammatory process (Figure 5.4).

Tuberculosis

Pathophysiology

There are many non-bacterial infections of the urinary tract; most are seldom seen in developed countries. Tuberculosis (TB), however, is widespread worldwide and is clinically important in the United Kingdom. The emergence of multi-drug-resistant TB is proving to be a new challenge to physicians worldwide.

Mycobacterium tuberculosis bacilli are inhaled through the lungs, where they are phagocytosed by polymorphonuclear leucocytes and macrophages. Some bacilli are carried to the region's lymph nodes and enter the

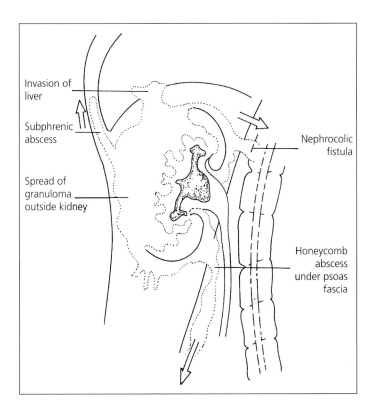

Figure 5.4 Xanthogranuloma burrows into the surrounding tissues.

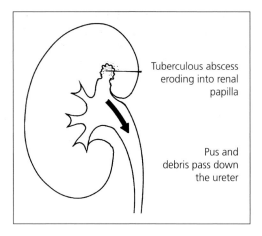

Figure 5.5 Tuberculous abscess in a renal papilla.

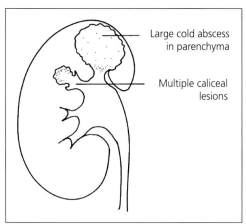

Figure 5.6 Extension of the tuberculous abscess to the calyx.

venous blood during the initial infection seeding of different organs.

Effects on the urinary tract

In the kidneys, granulomas form at the site of metastatic foci and may remain inactive for decades, becoming active due to failed host immune response (Figure 5.5).

Although both kidneys are seeded, clinically significant disease, which is caused by capillary rupture and delivery of proliferating bacilli into the proximal tubules, usually develops in only one kidney. Granulomas grow and eventually erode into the calyceal system (Figure 5.6).

The inflammation may narrow the neck of one or more calyces, which then fill with calcified debris (Figure 5.7), and eventually the entire kidney can be converted into a bag of calcified caseation tissue, which has a striking appearance in the plain X-ray (Figure 5.8). Erosion into the collecting system allows the bacilli to spread to the renal pelvis, ureters, bladder and other genitourinary organs.

Depending on the status of the patient's defence mechanisms, ureteric fibrosis and strictures may develop with chronic abscess formation. Extensive lesions can result in non-functioning kidneys. Hypertension is common. The disease may extend to the ureters and bladder, causing strictures, obstructive uropathy and nephropathy and bladder fibrosis and contraction. Shortening of the

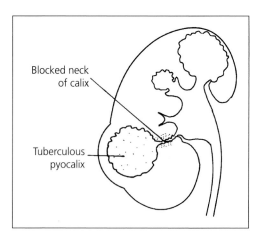

Figure 5.7 Multiple tuberculous pyocalyces.

healed tuberculous ureter can produce a 'golf-hole' ureteric orifice appearance (Figure 5.9).

In males urinary TB may be accompanied by TB of the prostate, seminal vesicles, epididymis and vasa deferentia. In females there may be involvement of the fallopian tubes and uterus.

Diagnosis

It needs suspicion to diagnose genitourinary TB. Patients with urinary tract TB classically have sterile pyuria, high urine leucocyte counts and usually microhaematuria. One good rule is to insist that every patient with pus in the urine,

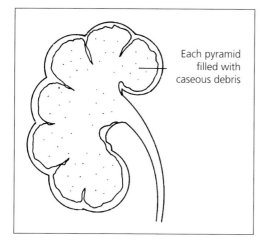

Figure 5.8 The end-stage kidney.

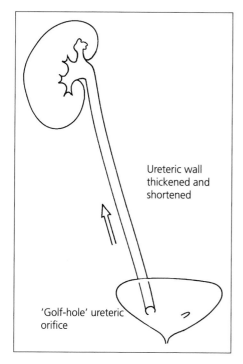

Figure 5.9 Shortening of the tuberculous ureter.

Urine may be cultured; however, mycobacterium bacilli are intermittently excreted and very slow growing, so three samples of early morning urine are required, and the culture, which should be on Löwenstein–Jensen medium, takes 6 weeks.

Molecular methods for involving polymerase chain reaction may speed the diagnosis. Treatment of genitourinary TB is systemic, with localised management of the urological complications.

Treatment

TB is a systemic disease. The patient often has active disease in the chest. The disease must be notified so that contacts can be traced. In practice this means you should summon the help of a colleague, usually a chest physician, who can treat the whole patient and will be expert in the dosage and details of combination chemotherapy.

With small lesions in one or two renal papillae, one expects a complete resolution with, at worst, a fleck of calcification to mark the site of the tuberculous granuloma. Healing may lead to stenosis of the ureter, and to detect this, imaging must be repeated within 2 weeks of starting treatment.

Early stenosis of the ureter may be prevented by means of a double-J splint for a few weeks, and so long as the sensitivity of the mycobacteria is certain and antibiotics are being given, steroids may assist in the prevention of scarring.

When the narrowing is near the bladder, the ureter may need to be re-implanted. If the entire length of the ureter is stenosed, it can be replaced with ileum. A contracted bladder can be enlarged by one or other types of cystoplasty.

 KEYPOINTS

- Urinary tract infections are among the most prevailing infectious diseases encountered in humans.
- Bacteria reach the urinary system tract via the bloodstream, lymphatic channels or transluminal.
- There exists a balance between host defence mechanisms and the virulence of pathogenic bacteria.

not explained by bacterial infection, must have TB excluded.

A history of TB infection can be confirmed by the tuberculin test within 2–3 days; however, this does not always mean that TB is currently active.

6

Urinary tract calculi

Epidemiology

Operations for urinary stones were well known in the time of Hippocrates, whose Oath enjoined young doctors to not 'cut for stone' but to 'leave the operation for specialists in this art'. The lifetime risk of renal calculi is approximately 12%, with men being twice as likely as women to experience a stone episode due to hormonal influences on renal oxalate excretion.

The peak age of a stone-related clinical episode in men is in the third decade, and in women stones are more common in the early post-menopausal years. The incidence of stone also varies in different populations, a reflection of the fact that both environmental and patient factors contribute to stone-forming activity.

Patient factors

The prevalence of urinary stones is directly correlated with body mass index, and the incidence has doubled since the 1970s as obesity in developed countries has increased. There are both direct and indirect relationships between urinary stones and obesity; poor eating habits and a diet rich in salt and animal fats and low in fruit predispose to both independently, and the metabolic factors related to obesity (dyslipidaemias, insulin resistance and hypertension) may be associated with free radical-mediated renal tubule damage, a likely important first step in stone formation.

Environmental factors

A seasonal variation in the incidence of stone-forming activity exists with a higher prevalence in the hotter summer months, and there is marked geographic variation in the prevalence of stone disease with higher numbers in countries with hotter, drier climates. Stones are more common in those whose work causes them to become dehydrated and therefore form more concentrated urine. It is probable that the incidence of bladder stones in children in underdeveloped countries is a manifestation of infantile diarrhoea and dehydration.

Pathophysiology

Supersaturation of urine

There are many factors contributing to the formation of renal calculi. Central to these is the presence of a concentration of stone-forming salts high enough to supersaturate the urine.

Salts added to urine continue to dissolve until no more will do so. At this point the concentration of the ions making up the salt is termed the solubility product. Below the solubility product, crystals and stones cannot form.

Urology Lecture Notes, Seventh Edition. Amir V. Kaisary, Andrew Ballaro and Katharine Pigott.
© 2016 John Wiley & Sons, Ltd. Published 2016 by John Wiley & Sons, Ltd.

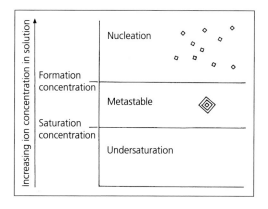

Figure 6.1 Increasing ion concentrations and urine saturation.

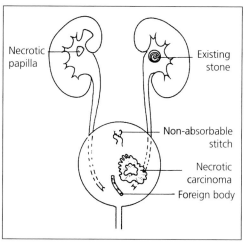

Figure 6.2 Many things can act as a nucleus for stone formation.

In urine a metastable solution of ions may form at concentrations above the solubility product. Whether or not crystals precipitate depends upon the presence of various inhibitory and promotional factors.

If the concentration exceeds that of the metastable region, crystals precipitate to make their own nuclei irrespective of the presence of any inhibitors. At this point the concentration of ions is termed the formation product (Figure 6.1).

Inhibitors of stone formation

The most important inhibitors of stone formation are citrate, Tamm–Horsfall protein and osteopontin. The latter two are both inhibitors of calcium oxalate crystal aggregation. Citrate in the urine binds with calcium, reducing its ability to combine with urinary oxalate, and also inhibits the aggregation of calcium oxalate crystals.

Promoters of stone formation

In addition to the presence of inhibitors, the metastable state is influenced by temperature, the presence of colloids, the rate of flow of the urine and the presence of anything that can act as a nucleus, for example, dead papillae, necrotic carcinoma, a non-absorbable suture, a fragment of catheter or a previously existing fragment of stone (Figure 6.2).

The pH of the urine may also be an important influence on the formation of calculi; magnesium ammonium phosphate is insoluble in alkaline urine and is precipitated by infection with *Proteus mirabilis* and other urea-splitting organisms. Uric acid is insoluble in acid urine but may dissolve if the urine is made alkaline.

Anatomical factors

Crystals grow better in the presence of a stagnant substrate; any factor causing obstruction to the urine flow may therefore be regarded as calculogenic. Congenital anatomical abnormalities are associated with stone formation for the same reason. These include pelviureteric junction obstruction, horseshoe kidney, calyceal diverticula and medullary sponge kidney. It is often not clear, however, whether the urinary flow obstruction alone or the metabolic abnormality that usually coexists with these malformations when they are associated with stone forming is the cause of the stone formation.

Crystal aggregation and stone growth

It is not clear whether the initial crystallisation that leads to stone formation can occur in pure solution, the *free particle theory*; crystals large

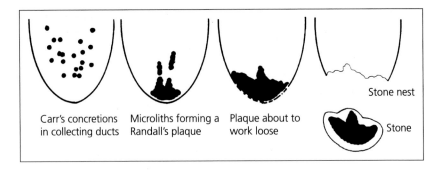

Carr's concretions in collecting ducts | Microliths forming a Randall's plaque | Plaque about to work loose | Stone nest | Stone

Figure 6.3 Formation of calculus in a renal papilla.

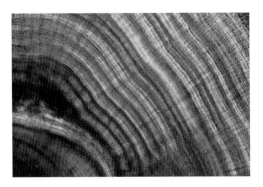

Figure 6.4 Cross section of a stone showing its laminations.

Table 6.1 **Stone composition and approximate occurrence rates**	
Calcium containing	
Calcium oxalate (monohydrate/dehydrate)	60–80%
Mixed calcium oxalate–calcium phosphate	20%
Pure calcium phosphate	Rare
Non-calcium containing	
Magnesium ammonium phosphate (struvite)	20%
Uric acid	5–10%
Cysteine	1–3%
Indinavir/xanthene	Rare

enough to be retained in a renal tubule have been shown to form experimentally. Alternatively, crystallisation may only occur in association with an anchoring site on the tubule wall, the *fixed particle theory*. More evidence exists to support the latter.

It is likely that the first step in stone formation is the precipitation of a plaque of calcium apatite (calcium complexed to a group of phosphate minerals) on the basement membrane of a renal tubule that has been previously damaged by lipid peroxidation. The plaque grows within the renal parenchyma and erodes through the urothelium of the renal papilla to act as a stable surface for the nucleation of supersaturated compounds in the urine. These 'Randall's plaques' may be easily seen on the papilla (Figure 6.3). The stone continues to grow as layer after layer of calcium salts, together with protein matrix, is laid down (Figure 6.4).

Stone-specific factors

Stone composition

Each stone is composed of the named crystalline components and a small amount of non-crystalline matrix, which is made up of mucoproteins including Tamm–Horsfall protein, nephrocalcin and glycosaminoglycans of renal origin (Table 6.1):

Calcium-containing stones

Hypercalciuria is an excess of calcium in the urine (over 4 mg/kg/day) and is the most common abnormality detected in calcium stone formers. Although not all patients with hypercalciuria form stones, high urinary calcium levels lead to saturation of urine with calcium salts and calcium stone formation. Hypercalciuria appears to be a genetic disease and affects 50% of first-degree relatives although the causative genes remain to be identified.

Hypercalciuria has been historically classified into three types, with the term idiopathic hypercalciuria applied when the cause was difficult to determine. It is now apparent that urinary calcium levels are influenced by a complex interaction between the gastrointestinal tract, the kidney, the bone, multiple hormones and tissue vitamin D response and distinct types of hypercalciuria cannot be defined as separate entities. The three types may be still used for descriptive purposes however:

1. **Absorptive hypercalciuria** refers to increased intestinal absorption of calcium and is the most common type. It is caused by an increase in the rate of dietary calcium absorption due to either excessive dietary intake of calcium, vitamin D supplementation or possibly abnormalities of the gut vitamin D receptor causing an exaggerated response to vitamin D. Increased absorption of calcium leads to transient periods of increased renal calcium excretion mediated by PTH suppression and peaks of hypercalciuria. Overall serum calcium levels remain within normal range.

2. **Renal hypercalciuria** is the impaired renal reabsorption of calcium, resulting in increased urinary levels. The loss of calcium causes secondary hyperparathyroidism; the mechanism of the calcium leak is unknown.

3. **Resorptive hypercalciuria** is due to the loss of calcium from the body's normal stores in the bony skeleton and is typically found in primary hyperparathyroidism (Figure 6.5). In this condition, calcium is released from the bone in response to excessive serum PTH levels causing significant hypercalcaemia, and the kidneys are forced to excrete the extra calcium into the urine.

Other causes of hypercalcaemia such as malignancy, vitamin D intoxication, sarcoidosis

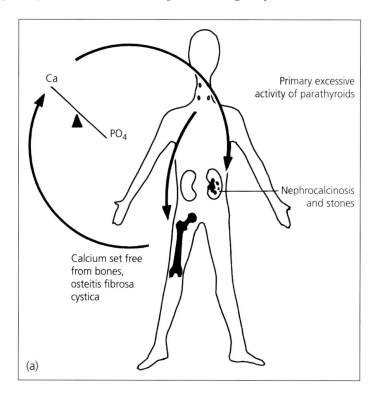

Ca

PO$_4$

Primary excessive
activity of parathyroids

Nephrocalcinosis
and stones

Calcium set free
from bones,
osteitis fibrosa
cystica

(a)

Figure 6.5 Primary hyperparathyroidism: (a) pathway

and tuberculosis also result in this type of hypercalciuria.

Oxalate-containing stones

1. *Primary (hepatic) oxaluria* is due to a rare autosomal recessive disorder of metabolism where an inherited liver enzyme deficiency leads to an excess of oxalates in the urine.

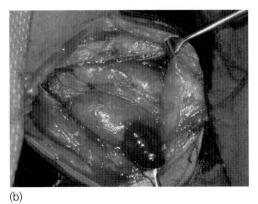

(b)

Figure 6.5 (*Continued*) (b) parathyroid adenoma.

Oxalates precipitate in the collecting tubules and eventually lead to renal failure due to nephrocalcinosis (Figure 6.6).

2. *Secondary (enteric) oxaluria* is the most common cause of hyperoxaluria and is due to increased absorption from the bowel. This condition is associated with diseases causing chronic diarrhoea in which malabsorption of fatty acids occurs. These include small bowel resection, bacterial overgrowth syndromes, fat malabsorption, chronic biliary or pancreatic disease, intestinal bypass surgical procedures and inflammatory bowel disease.

   The excess fatty acids in the bowel lumen bind by a process called saponification with calcium, thereby reducing the amount of calcium available to complex with dietary oxalate (calcium oxalate is not reabsorbed by the gut) and increasing the oxalate available for reabsorption (Figure 6.7).

3. *Dietary hyperoxaluria* may occur with excessive intake of oxalate-rich foods. These include nuts, chocolate, black tea, spinach,

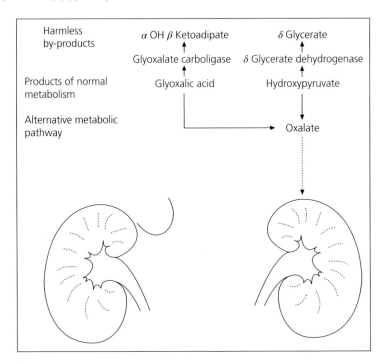

Figure 6.6 Primary hepatic oxaluria.

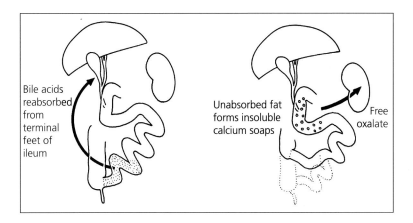

Figure 6.7 Secondary enteric (ileal) oxaluria.

broccoli, strawberries and rhubarb. Other factors may predispose to dietary hyperoxaluria; reduced dietary calcium may increase the free oxalate available for absorption, and increased animal protein can also increase the amounts of both calcium and oxalate in the urine predisposing to stone formation. A genetically inherited abnormality in oxalate metabolism may also contribute to dietary hyperoxaluria.

Uric acid stones

In humans and higher primates, uric acid is the final breakdown product of purine metabolism and is excreted in urine. The Dalmatian dog has a genetic defect in uric acid uptake by the liver and kidneys and, uniquely among other mammals, also forms uric acid stones.

The solubility of uric acid in the urine is closely related to urine pH. At higher pH uric acid is present as the more soluble sodium urate; solutions with pH under 6, physiological levels of uric acid production result in urine supersaturation and uric acid precipitation.

The primary causes of uric acid stone formation are low urine pH, low urine volume and increased uric acid production (hyperuricaemia), with the first two of these being more prevalent. Low urine pH is linked to the metabolic syndrome and insulin resistance and

also diet rich in animal protein. The causes of hyperuricosuria include inherited metabolic disorders, increased tissue breakdown and protein catabolism in association with chemotherapy for certain malignancies, drugs and diet.

Pure uric acid stones are radiolucent; commonly they act as a nidus for calcium oxalate and calcium phosphate precipitation in which case they become variably radio-opaque.

Treatment of hyperuricosuria consists of encouraging a high water intake, together with bicarbonate to keep the urine alkaline and, as second line, allopurinol to inhibit xanthine oxidase and inhibit the formation of uric acid.

Cystine stones

Cystinuria is an autosomal recessive disease caused by mutations in two genes that encode a transporter protein for the freely filtered positively charged amino acids cystine, ornithine, arginine and lysine in the proximal convoluted renal tubule. This results in increased concentrations in the urine and precipitation of cystine, which is the most insoluble.

Cystine stones are harder than most other stones and produce a characteristic odour when fragmented during surgery. Cystine is more soluble in alkaline urine and forms a soluble complex with penicillamine. Hydration, urine alkalinisation and oral penicillamine are used to prevent cystine stones.

Struvite stones

Stones caused by urinary infections are composed of magnesium ammonium phosphate commonly termed 'struvite' after the discoverer of the compound. Struvite stones occur only in the presence of urinary infection with urease-producing bacteria; the most common of these are *Proteus*, *Pseudomonas* and *Staphylococcus* spp. Urease, which is not normally present in the urine, hydrolyses urinary urea to produce ammonium. The resulting alkalinisation of the urine promotes the formation of carbonate ions from carbon dioxide and water and of phosphate ions from hydrogen phosphate. These combine with physiological amounts of magnesium to form calcium ammonium phosphate.

Struvite stones occur in population prone to recurrent urinary infections such as the elderly, women, diabetics and patients with urinary tract abnormalities and those with spinal cord injury. It is even more important than normal to completely clear these stones during surgery as residual fragments may perpetuate infection and regrow rapidly.

Calcium phosphate stones

Distal renal tubular acidosis, or type 1 renal tubular acidosis, is caused by abnormal distal tubule and collecting duct function resulting in a failure to excrete excess acid into the urine. The condition may be hereditary or acquired and presents with vomiting, diarrhoea and failure to thrive in children or metabolic acidosis and nephrolithiasis in adults.

The failure to excrete the acid load causes metabolic acidosis with bone demineralisation and secondary hyperparathyroidism and hypercalciuria and profound hypocitraturia (citrate is a urinary stone inhibitor).

The raised urine pH in conjunction with hyperparathyroidism reduces renal phosphate reabsorption. When combined with hypercalciuria, this favours the formation of calcium phosphate stones.

Evaluation of the stone former

Biochemical investigation

What is the cause of the stone, and can it be prevented? The patient who presents with their acute stone-related medical episode should first have a full history taken with the aim of identifying previous stone-related episodes and the conditions that may predispose to stone formation.

The first-time stone former should be evaluated with urine dipstick and culture to diagnose infection that is commonly present in stone formers and for serum electrolytes, particularly if the patient is vomiting, urea and creatinine to enable an estimate of renal function (eGFR) and calcium as this might be the only chance to diagnose hypercalcaemia.

Urine dipstick assessment of pH may give further information regarding possible stone composition. Any stone that is passed or retrieved surgically should be analysed by X-ray crystallography. The chances of a first-time stone former experiencing a second stone-related clinical episode is approximately 30% within 5 years and 50% within 10 years.

The recurrent stone former should undergo 16 or 24 h urine collections for more detailed metabolic analysis. Two collections are required, one with an acid preservative and the other without, as uric acid precipitates in acid solutions. Only an average value can be obtained from these collections, and it is likely that peaks and troughs of urine supersaturation occur throughout the day with stone-forming activity occurring during peaks. It is not feasible or cost effective to perform a metabolic evaluation.

Imaging

Non-contrast computerised tomography (CT) is highly sensitive for stones and the imaging modality of choice. The rare exception to this is stones caused by indinavir administration for retroviral disease, which may not be seen on CT. It is sometimes difficult to determine whether pelvic calcification is a ureteric stone or calcified thrombus in a vein (phlebolith) and contrast administration to provide a urographic phase may be required.

Most stones (90%) are also visible on plain X-ray. Non-calcium-containing stones are less so. Stones made of uric acid are completely radio-lucent, but they do cast an acoustic shadow on ultrasound scan and show up in a CT scan. Stones made of cystine are faintly radio-opaque because of their sulphur content and are always easily located with ultrasound or CT scan. Struvite stones are variably radio-opaque.

It is usually advisable to perform a plain X-ray when a stone is found on CT for use during follow-up. If an X-ray is not performed, the clinician will not be able to use X-ray to determine if the stone has passed or been successfully removed surgically as the radiolucency of the stone will be unknown for every first-time stone former.

Treatment of urinary tract calculi

It is important to consider both the patient and stone factors when considering treatment for renal calculi. For example, an asymptomatic renal stone that has not changed in years may be left alone in an unfit elderly patient with multiple comorbidities, whereas the same stone should

 KEYPOINTS

First-time stone formers—consider partial metabolic evaluation with risk stratification:

- Serum electrolytes, creatinine, calcium, uric acid and phosphorus
- Stone analysis
- Urine analysis including pH
- A 24 h urine collection volume and electrolytes

Complete metabolic evaluation—is reserved for the recurrent stone former or the high-risk stone former (e.g. children, solitary kidney, positive family history and high-risk occupations such as pilots).

be removed in an airline pilot who will not be allowed to fly until he is stone-free.

Stones in the pelvicalyceal system

Renal stones under 5 mm in diameter may pass spontaneously without severe symptoms, and provided that the patient understands the risk of ureteric obstruction, urinary infection, pain or insidious increase in stone size, asymptomatic stones of this size can be monitored.

If the stone is symptomatic and thought to be causing pain, which is often difficult to ascertain with certainty, or urinary infections, assessment of the patient should take place with a view to removing it.

Stones larger than 5 mm should generally be removed if the patient factors are favourable because the stone is less likely to pass spontaneously and the risk of the complications above is greater. The least invasive method of stone removal is extracorporeal shock wave lithotripsy (ESWL), and this is a suitable first-line treatment for stones up to approximately 1 cm in diameter.

Renal calculi that are refractory to or cannot be treated by ESWL due to failure or contraindications and larger stones can be treated by ureterorenoscopy and laser fragmentation. Good stone clearance rates using laser ureterorenoscopy for stones up to 2 cm in size have been reported, and the trend is towards more minimally invasive surgical techniques. Stones larger than this are generally treated by percutaneous nephrolithotomy (PCNL).

In practice the treatment of choice will be dictated by a full discussion of the options between the surgeon and the patient and influenced by the stone burden, location and radiodensity, the renal anatomy and the equipment availability and the experience and preference of the surgeon.

Staghorn stones (usually struvite) are stones that occupy both the renal pelvis and at least one calyx. They may fill the entire pelvicalyceal system (Figure 6.8) and may require multimodality treatment. The body of the stone is usually removed using the lithoclast probe, while the calyceal portions are broken up using laser through a flexible nephroscope or ureteroscope during

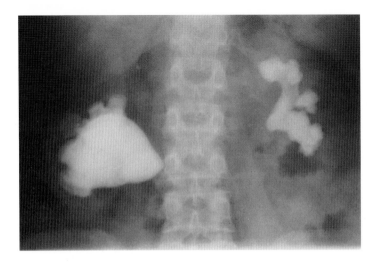

Figure 6.8 Staghorn stones may fill the entire collecting system.

PCNL. Sometimes several procedures and ESWL are required to achieve stone clearance.

Stones in the ureter

Medical management

The management of ureteric stones is influenced by patient and stone factors. Renal colic is managed by NSAID analgesia in the first instance; in this context NSAIDS are as effective as opiates in producing pain relief and, in addition to their analgesic effects, reduce pain by inhibiting prostaglandin-medicated ureteric peristalsis. Care must be taken in patients with reduced renal function, as in this situation prostaglandins are important in maintaining renal perfusion. Clinical features of a stone in the ureter are demonstrated in Figure 6.9.

The chance of a ureteric stone passing is proportional to the width of the stone. For stones less than 5 mm in width, the chance of spontaneous passage is approximately 90% within 3 weeks. Stones more than 8 mm in width are only about 20% likely to pass spontaneously over 1 year. The administration of an alpha-adrenoreceptor blocker increases these rates slightly by reducing ureteric wall tension.

Indications for surgical intervention for a ureteric stone are *failure of stone progression*

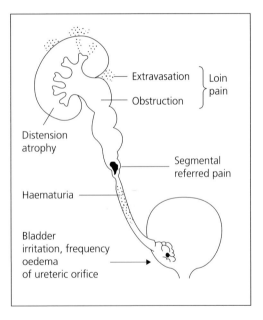

Figure 6.9 Clinical features of a stone in the ureter.

or uncontrolled pain, solitary kidney and the presence of infection.

Surgical management

In the acute situation pain and obstruction can be alleviated by the endoscopic or percutaneous insertion of a double-J ureteric stent

(Figure 6.10). This temporises the situation but also increases the need for endoscopic elective stone removal as the stone is less likely to pass spontaneously alongside the stent. Ureteric stents cause the ureter to dilate slightly facilitating subsequent surgery.

Ureteric stents can be extremely uncomfortable and if not removed promptly become encrusted in stone-forming patients resulting in a far worse clinical situation and more complicated operative procedure to remove them.

An alternative to stent insertion is primary stone removal. This is performed by either ESWL (Figure 6.11) or ureteroscopy. This is clearly preferable to temporary stent insertion; however, it requires substantial resources.

Extracorporeal lithotripsy to ureteric stones is less effective when a stent is *in situ* as the stent absorbs the shock waves, and the treatment of choice for elective removal of ureteric stones is ureteroscopy, rigid or flexible instrumentation (Figure 6.12) and laser ureterolithotomy. Some surgeons perform laparoscopic ureterolithotomy for very large ureteric stones. It is considered less invasive and is based on the anatomical approach previously adopted in open approach.

Stones in the bladder

Renal stones that are small enough to pass spontaneously are generally voided with few symptoms. Stones that form in the urinary bladder are caused by infected concentrated, stagnant urine and are composed of struvite, uric acid and calcium oxalate. Bladder stones generally occur in association with bladder outflow obstruction, neurogenic bladder dysfunction, bladder diverticula and chronic urinary tract infection. It is also

 KEYPOINT

Indications for intervention for a ureteric stone

1 Failure of progression
2 Uncontrolled pain
3 Solitary kidney
4 Presence of infection

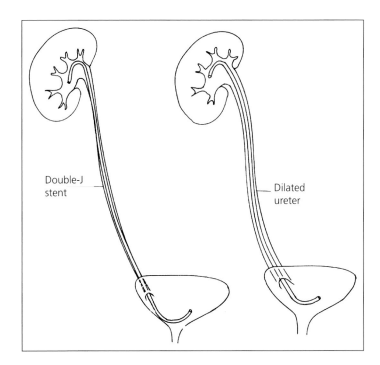

Figure 6.10 A double-J stent helps the ureter to dilate.

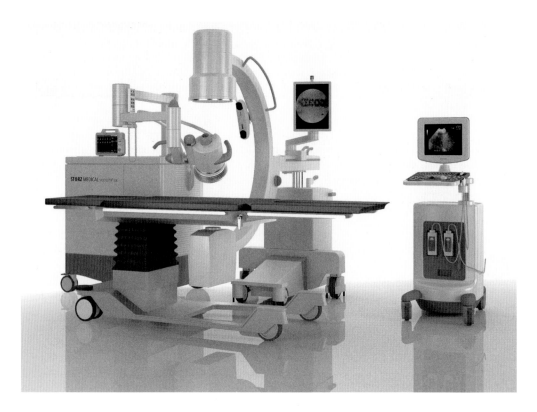

Figure 6.11 Extracorporeal shock wave lithotripsy. Reproduced with permission from KARL STORZ – Endoskope, Germany.

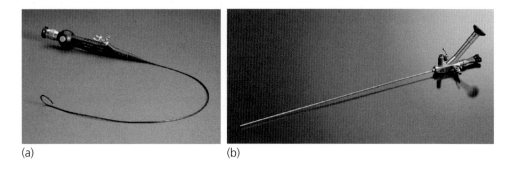

(a)   (b)

Figure 6.12 Ureteroscope: (a) flexible and (b) rigid. Reproduced with permission from KARL STORZ – Endoskope, Germany.

common for stones to form around the bladder foreign bodies such as a forgotten ureteric stent, a misplaced suture or eroded incontinence tape and possibly also a stone that has passed from the upper urinary but has not been voided. Bladder stones also commonly form in augmented bladders, partly due to stasis and also mucous production from the bowel augmentation acting as a nidus for stone formation.

Bladder stones vary greatly in size and shape and number. They may be asymptomatic, found incidentally during the investigation of lower

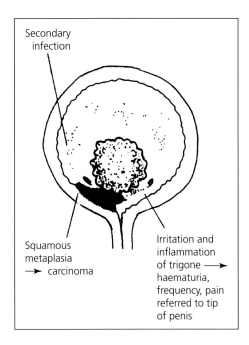

Figure 6.13 Clinical features of a stone in the bladder.

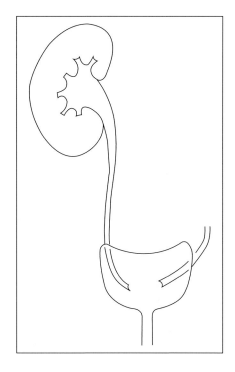

Figure 6.14 Steinstrasse – collection of fragments held up in the lower ureter after ESWL.

urinary tract symptoms or present with dysuria, haematuria or bladder pain (Figure 6.13). As they often consist mainly of urate, bladder stones may be radiolucent. Bladder stones that form due to outflow obstruction are seldom voided and may grow to a large size.

Methods for removing stones

1. **EWSL**
   - Extracorporeal generation of high-energy shock waves focused onto the stone imaged by ultrasound or X-ray.
   - Shock waves are generated by electrohydraulic spark plug or an array of piezoelectric (electrically induced conformational change in a susceptible crystal) or electromagnetic mechanisms and focused using a parabolic or ellipsoid deflector, or lens.
   - Stone fragments left to pass therefore analysis variable; impacted fragments are known as steinstrasse or street of stones (Figure 6.14).
   - Variable outcomes depending on machine, static or mobile, patient and stone factors.
   - Contraindications: pregnancy, aneurysm, aortic calcification, coagulopathies and CKD.
   - Produces temporary reduction in GFR and renal contusion.
   - Day case procedure requiring analgesia but no anaesthetic and high success rates in units with in-house lithotripters with appropriate patient selection.

2. **PCNL**
   - Replaced open stone removal (nephrolithotomy), which is now obsolete.
   - Percutaneous insertion of tract into renal collecting system under image guidance and fragmentation and removal of stones through this tract using ultrasound, mechanical lithoclast (Figure 6.15) or laser energy.
   - Optimal position of tract placement through relatively avascular Brodel's zone at poster lateral aspect of kidney; this is adjacent to lower pole posterior calyx.
   - Patient can be supine or prone.
   - In patient procedure under GA.

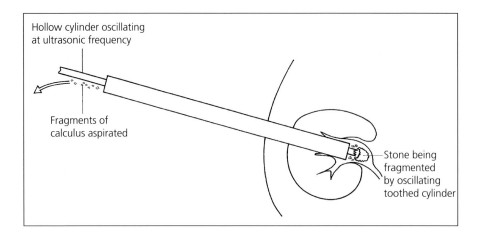

Hollow cylinder oscillating
at ultrasonic frequency

Fragments of
calculus aspirated

Stone being
fragmented
by oscillating
toothed cylinder

Figure 6.15 Percutaneous nephrolithotomy.

- Main risks: bleeding, failure to secure tract and loss of kidney.

3. Ureteroscopy and laser lithotripsy
- Endoscopic insertion of a flexible uretero-scope into the renal collecting system.
- Ureteroscopes comprise channel for laser fibre and irrigation and light source.
- Laser fragmentation and basket extraction of stone.
- Complications: failure, need for second operation, need for temporary ureteric stent afterwards, ureteric injury and stricture.
- Used for lithotripsy refractory and larger renal and upper ureteric stones.
- Day case procedure under GA.
- In expert hands increasingly used for larger stones up to 2 cm previously treated by PCNL.

4. Stones in the bladder
Bladder stones less than 5–6 cm in diameter should be removed endoscopically. Cystoli-tholapaxy is an operation in which the stone is crushed or fragmented. Using an old Mauermayer stone punch crusher (Figure 6.16a) is now rarely used and super-seded by visual lithotrite (Figure 6.16b). Ultrasound lithoclast or laser modality via optical transurethral route is preferred (Figure 6.17). Huge bladder stones could still be removed using an open surgical approach termed cystolithotomy.

Prevention of recurrent urinary stones

Medical therapy

Targeted medical therapy is effective in pre-venting recurrent stone formation in selected cases. Hypercalciuria refractory to increased fluid intake may be treated with a thiazide diu-retic, which corrects renal calcium leak by stimu-lating renal tubular calcium reabsorption.

Allopurinol decreases uric acid production and is indicated for hyperuricaemia that is resistant to increasing fluid intake and urine alkalinisation. In enteric hyperoxaluria increas-ing dietary calcium may bind intestinal oxalate and reduce its absorption; citrates are used for renal tubular acidosis and hypocitraturia.

Dietary advice

General advice for stone formers to reduce the risk of further episodes is to maintain a high-fluid, low-salt and animal protein diet and to drink citrus fruit juice. Fluid intake should be at least 2 L/day with the aim of keeping the urine so dilute that it is colourless, and this is the most important factor in reducing stone recurrence.

Salt should be used only sparingly during cooking and not added to food; the total daily

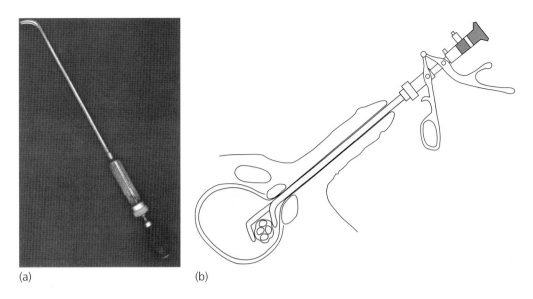

(a)   (b)

Figure 6.16 Lithotrites: (a) classical lithotrite and (b) visual lithotrite.

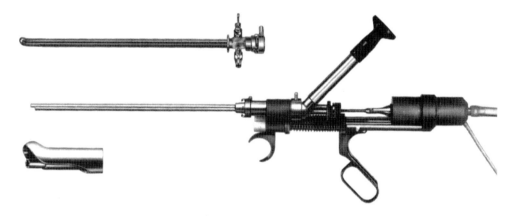

Figure 6.17 Visual ultrasonic lithotripsy. Reproduced with permission from KARL STORZ – Endoskope, Germany.

salt intake including that already in foods should be under one teaspoon. In patients with hyperoxaluria high intake of oxalate-containing foods should be identified and moderated, as should animal protein as it raises urinary calcium, oxalate and uric acid levels.

A daily intake of citrus fruit juices should be encouraged, as they increase urine citrus levels; lemon juice is preferred as orange juice may also increase urine oxalate. Exercise and weight loss should also be advised. Dietary calcium is not usually contributory to stone formation, and in fact reduced calcium intake may increase enteric oxalate absorption as oxalate normally complexes with calcium in the gut and is excreted. Oral calcium intake should therefore be normal; vitamin D and calcium supplements should be avoided, however.

KEYPOINTS

- Stones develop in supersaturated urine. Various patient and environmental factors contribute to this.

- Both patient and stone factors must be considered when deciding the treatment of patients with urinary stones.

- Ureteric stones may be treated expectantly, medically or by temporising ureteric stent. Surgical removal is by ureteroscopy or extracorporeal lithotripsy.

- Small renal stones may be treated conservatively; treatment of larger stones may be by extracorporeal or endoscopic lithotripsy or percutaneous removal depending on stone and patient factors. Evaluation of the stone former should be performed and general dietary advice always given. In some cases medication may be useful.

7

Kidney neoplasms

General management of urological disorders is based on building knowledge in basic anatomy, physiology and pathological changes. Orientation of the organs is greatly affected by the structures around it. Intimate knowledge of anatomy is a must for the practising urologist, radiological diagnostic assessments and planning successful interventions and outcomes. With advances from the days of open surgery to non-invasive techniques – laparoscopy, robotics and more to come – the basic grounding in surgical anatomy is a must.

Surgical anatomy and renal surgery

Posterior relations

The kidneys are well protected, tucked in on either side of the spine. Behind each kidney is the lung, constantly moving up and down, so the inferior border of the kidney may lie anywhere between the second and fourth lumbar transverse processes. The other posterior relations of the kidney are the 12th rib, diaphragm and psoas and quadratus lumborum muscles (Figure 7.1).

The ilio-inguinal and hypogastric nerves cross the quadratus lumborum muscle and are often injured in approaching the kidney from the loin.

Anterior relations: Left

The tail of the pancreas and the spleen lies in front of the left kidney and is easily injured at operation. The duodeno-jejunal flexure and descending colon also lie just in front of the left kidney, so indigestion or bowel distension is common when there is inflammation or obstruction of the kidney, and cancer of the kidney easily invades the adjacent bowel (Figure 7.2).

Anterior relations: Right

The ascending colon is the second part of the duodenum and common bile duct. It is not surprising that 'indigestion' often accompanies disorders of the right kidney (Figure 7.3).

Blood supply of the kidney

Renal arteries

Between them the kidneys receive one-fifth of the entire cardiac output. Usually there is one renal artery on each side, with five segmental branches arranged like the digits of the hand (Figure 7.4). Each segmental branch supplies its own geographical zone of the parenchyma. They are end

Urology Lecture Notes, Seventh Edition. Amir V. Kaisary, Andrew Ballaro and Katharine Pigott.
© 2016 John Wiley & Sons, Ltd. Published 2016 by John Wiley & Sons, Ltd.

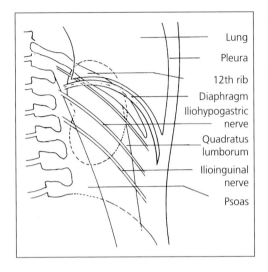

Lung

Pleura

12th rib

Diaphragm

Iliohypogastric
nerve

Quadratus
lumborum

Ilioinguinal
nerve

Psoas

Figure 7.1 Posterior anatomical relations of the kidney.

arteries and there are no anastomoses between them (Figure 7.5). The zones supplied by the segmental arteries do not match the arrangement of pyramids and calyces. In open operations any incision into the renal parenchyma is made between the main segmental arteries, which can be located with a Doppler probe. Each segmental artery divides into smaller arcuate arteries that run in the boundary between the cortex and medulla, giving off branches that run up and down parallel with the collecting tubules, as well as giving an afferent artery to each glomerulus (Figure 7.6). The afferent artery enters the glomerulus near the junction of the loop of Henle with the distal convoluted tubule: the juxtaglomerular apparatus is located here; its cells contain dark granules of the precursor of renin. The juxtaglomerular apparatus monitors the pressure in the afferent arteriole.

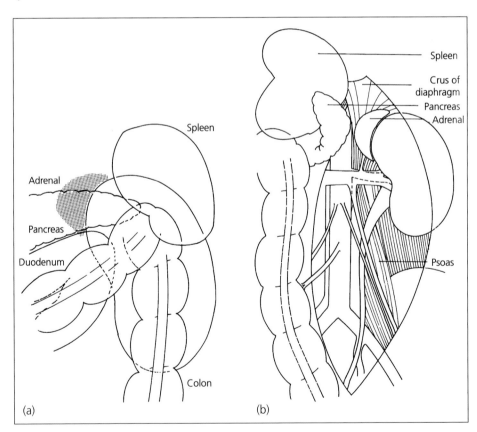

Spleen

Adrenal

Pancreas

Duodenum

Spleen

Colon

(a)

Spleen

Crus of
diaphragm

Pancreas

Adrenal

Psoas

(b)

Figure 7.2 (a) Anatomical relations of the left kidney. (b) Left kidney and surrounding structures displayed at operation by reflecting the colon, spleen and tail of pancreas medially.

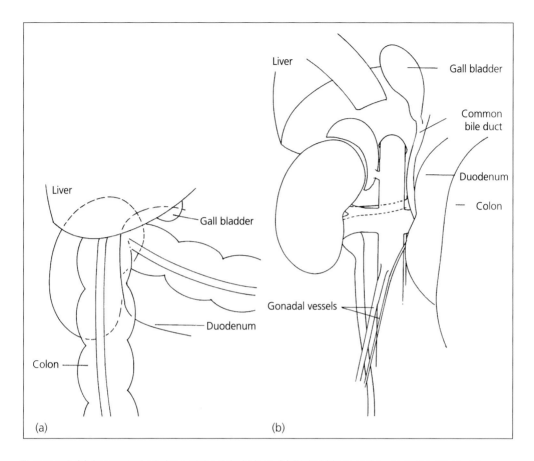

Liver

Gall bladder

Common bile duct

Duodenum

Colon

Gonadal vessels

Liver

Gall bladder

Duodenum

Colon

(a)

(b)

Figure 7.3 (a) Anatomical relations of the right kidney. (b) Right kidney and surrounding structures displayed at operation by reflecting the colon and duodenum medially.

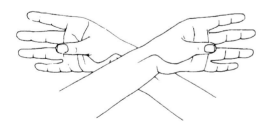

Figure 7.4 Arrangement of the branches of the renal arteries.

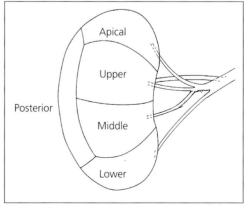

Apical

Upper

Posterior

Middle

Lower

Figure 7.5 Each segmental artery supplies its own geographical territory.

Renal veins

Unlike the segmental branches of the renal arteries, the veins communicate freely with each other (Figure 7.7). Several veins can be ligated

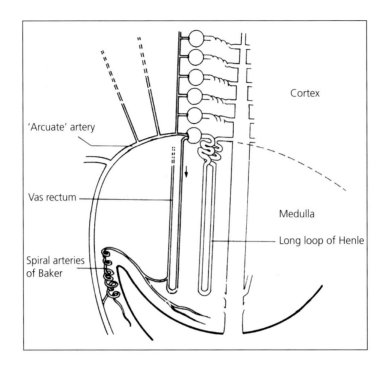

Figure 7.6 The blood supply of the renal papilla.

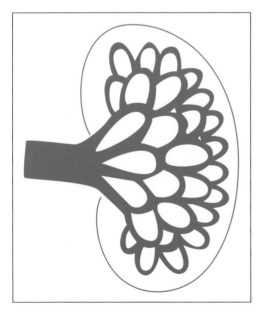

Figure 7.7 The veins of the kidney communicate with each other.

without infarcting the kidney. The main left renal vein often splits into two, one part running in front of the aorta, the other behind, posing a trap for the surgeon who is unaware of this anomaly. The left renal vein is about 5 cm long; the right is close to the inferior vena cava, another reason why the left kidney is preferred in live donor transplantation.

The collecting system

The thin cubical epithelium of the papilla is perforated with the collecting ducts of Bellini, but the rest of the pelvis and calyx is lined by urothelium like that of the bladder and ureters. The urothelium is surrounded by a wall of smooth muscle cells linked by jigsaw connections, nexuses, which transmit the wave of contraction from one muscle cell to another without the need for any nerve supply, so a transplanted kidney continues to pump out urine perfectly well. The calyces are separated from the renal parenchyma by a packing of sinus fat that is

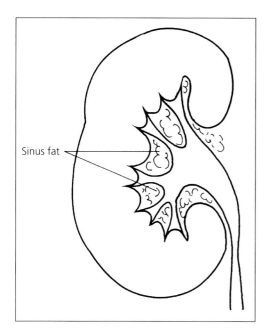

Figure 7.8 The calyces are surrounded by sinus fat that is fluid at body temperature and allows them to move freely.

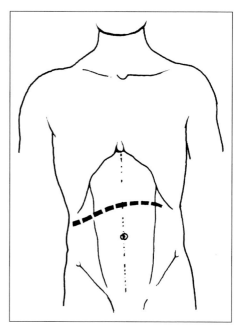

Figure 7.9 Anterior trans-abdominal approach to the right kidney through a transverse incision.

fluid at body temperature and allows them to contract freely (Figure 7.8).

Surgical approaches to the kidney

Conventional open surgery

With a large cancer of the kidney, safety demands perfect exposure to control the renal artery and vein. The choice of either a transverse or midline incision is determined by the build of the patient (Figures 7.9 and 7.10). The ascending colon, hepatic flexure and duodenum are reflected medially to give safe access to the right renal vessels (Figure 7.11). On the left side reflection of the splenic flexure, the descending colon and duodeno-jejunal flexure will give safe access to the left renal vessels (Figure 7.12).

Various approaches include the 12th rib approach (Figure 7.13), vertical lumbotomy (Figure 7.14) and thoraco-abdominal incision.

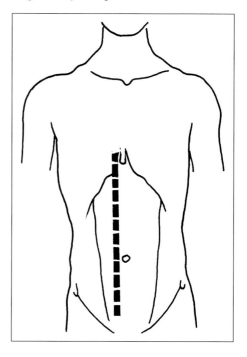

Figure 7.10 Trans-abdominal approach through vertical incision in a long thin patient.

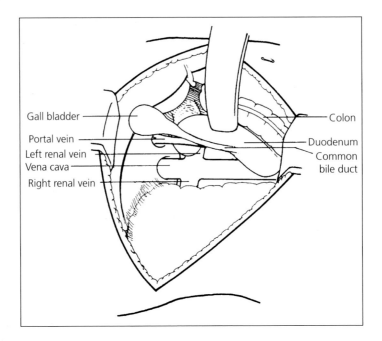

Figure 7.11 Operative exposure of right kidney: colon and duodenum reflected.

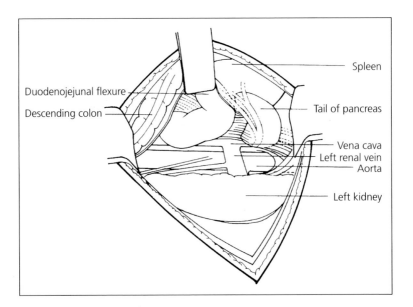

Figure 7.12 Operative exposure of left kidney: spleen, colon and duodenum reflected.

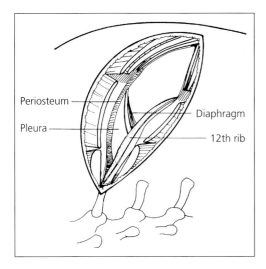

Figure 7.13 Twelfth rib bed approach to the right kidney.

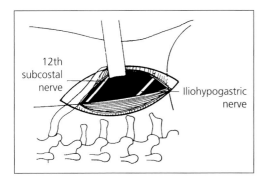

Figure 7.14 Vertical lumbotomy approach to the right kidney.

Minimal access surgery (laparoscopy–robotic)

Extra peritoneal

A balloon is passed through a cannula introduced into the perirenal fat. It is blown up to separate the peritoneum, duodenum and colon from the kidney and kept blown up long enough for bleeding to stop. When it is deflated, it leaves an empty space into which laparoscopic instruments may be introduced to carry out various operations on the kidney.

Trans peritoneal

Carbon dioxide is introduced into the peritoneal cavity with a small cannula, and then a number of 'ports' are made through which large cannulae are pushed into the gas-filled space. Through these other instruments are passed to reflect the colon and duodenum off the front of the kidney and allow the planned operation to take place.

Complications after renal surgery

The surgical relations of the kidney explain most of the common post-operative complications:

1. Pain: There is always post-operative pain on breathing and coughing. Post-operative pain can inhibit coughing and lead to atelectasis and infection in the empty lung segments. This is more common when the pleura has been opened or if part of the rib has had to be removed.
2. Pneumothorax: This may require aspiration or underwater drainage.
3. Ileus: Oedema or haematoma behind the bowel may lead to a period of abdominal distension and paralytic ileus.

Wilms' tumour (nephroblastoma)

Wilms' tumour, or nephroblastoma, accounts for 10% of all childhood cancers and is seen in 1:13 000 children and is the most common primary malignant renal tumour of childhood. The majority of Wilms' tumours arise from somatic mutations restricted to tumour tissue. WT gene is present on the X chromosome (X chromosome in males and active chromosome X in females). Approximately 10% of children with this tumour have congenital anomalies. In 5–10% the tumour is bilateral or multicentric. Familial cases are present in 1–2% only.

Chromosomal gross deletions at chromosome 11p13 are present in type WT1. Loss of heterozygosity at chromosome 11p15 is found in type WT2.

Familial WT1 and WT2 tumour genes are located at 17q12–q21 (WT1) and 19q13.4 (WT2). Other chromosomal abnormalities are being studied.

There are two distinct pathological entities – *favourable* and *unfavourable* – according to the amount of undifferentiated tissue that is present.

Clinical features

'A big lump in a wasted baby'. A mother bathing her baby notices a lump: this is the classical presentation (Figure 7.15), but these tumours may present with pain and haematuria, as well as hypertension, fever and a raised red or white cell count. Ultrasound is the first investigation, followed by computerised tomography (CT) scanning, even if this may require a general anaesthetic. The UICC system of staging is represented in Figure 7.16 and Table 7.1. In practice, the differential diagnosis is from *neuroblastoma*, which usually has speckled calcification and displaces the kidney downwards.

Management

Today, thanks to a combination of radical surgery and chemotherapy, one can expect 96% 4-year survival in stage I disease, and even in stage III

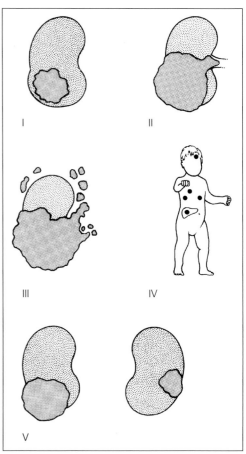

Figure 7.16 Stages of Wilms' tumour.

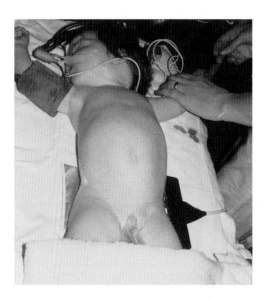

Figure 7.15 Wilms' tumour – a big lump in a wasted baby.

disease, as long as the histology is 'favourable', the survival is greater than 87%. But to achieve these results requires expert management by a dedicated team. Every child with a Wilms' tumour deserves to be referred to a specialised centre regularly auditing its results in trials of the latest protocols. It is not for the occasional surgeon in a small hospital. One such protocol calls for a 5-day course of actinomycin D followed by laparotomy at which the renal vessels are tied before the tumour is handled and the opposite kidney is carefully examined. The kidney is then removed radically, with a wide margin. Postoperatively vincristine is given. Radiotherapy is *not* necessary in stage I tumours. It is always given in stage III.

Table 7.1 Staging system of the Children's Oncology Group Stage

Stage I	Tumour confined to the kidney
	Completely resected
	No residual tumour
Stage II	Extra-capsular tumour penetration
	Completely resected
	Renal sinus extension
	Extra renal vessels harbour tumour thrombus/infiltration
Stage III	Tumour incomplete removal
	Residual tumour confined to the abdomen
	Lymph node involvement
	Peritoneal spilling
Stage IV	Haematogenous spread: lung, liver, bone, etc.
Stage V	Bilateral renal involvement at diagnosis

Renal cell cancer (hypernephroma)

Global cancer statistics indicated that renal cell carcinoma represents 2–3% of all cancers with an age-standardised rate incidence of 5.8 and mortality of 1.4/100 000. It is rare before puberty and seems to be less common in females. More and more new tumours were being found by ultrasound scanning of patients who have been on long-term renal dialysis. Ultrasound scanning and computerised tomography are frequently carried out for various medical ailments. It is associated with the *von Hippel–Lindau syndrome*: that is angiomas in the cerebellum and retina and cysts in the liver and pancreas. Aetiological factors seem to include lifestyle factors such as smoking, obesity and hypertension. It may be associated with cadmium pollution.

Presentation

The classic triad of flank pain, gross haematuria and palpable abdominal mass is now rare, probably 6–10% (Figure 7.17). Renal cell carcinoma

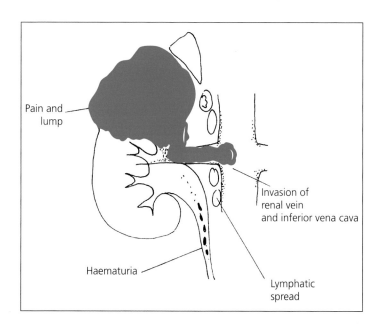

Figure 7.17 Clinical features of renal cell carcinoma.

is detected incidentally in more than 50% of cases diagnosed as they are asymptomatic. Paraneoplastic syndromes are found in approximately 30% of symptomatic renal carcinoma cases (Table 7.2).

Investigations

Ultrasound shows a mass in the kidney that contains echoes. Strict ultrasound criteria for simple cysts have been identified. Bosniak classification divides renal cystic lesions into four categories

Table 7.2 Neoplastic hormone syndromes in renal cell cancer

Pyrogen	Loss of weight, pyrexia, night sweats, raised ESR
Erythropoietin	Erythrocytosis without increase in platelets
Marrow toxin	Anaemia
Renin	Hypertension
Parathyroid hormone	Hypercalcaemia
Stauffer's factor	Hepatosplenomegaly
Glucagon	Diarrhoea, enteropathy
Tumour proteins	Glomerulonephritis
Amyloid	Amyloid in the contralateral kidney
Unknown factor	Paraneoplastic motor neurone disease

that are distinct in terms of the likelihood of malignancy (Table 7.3). The intravenous urography (IVU) and CT scan show a mass distorting the collecting system (Figure 7.18) but may not be able to distinguish between a collection of cysts and cancer. With a very large tumour, one needs to know whether the vena cava has been invaded: here spiral magnetic resonance imaging (MRI) is more accurate than either CT or a cavogram (Figure 7.19). Many tumours are detected only when a distant metastasis is biopsied and the unmistakable histological picture of a renal cell cancer is found (Figure 7.20).

Staging

The Union for International Cancer Control (UICC) system TNM based on the findings on CT scanning is shown in Table 7.4 (Figure 7.21).

Treatment

Small tumours

Many tumours are now detected incidentally in the course of ultrasound and CT scanning (Figure 7.22).

Partial nephrectomy

Removal of the tumour leaving a safe clear margin of healthy tissue. After exposing the kidney, the renal artery is secured. The cancer is then removed

Table 7.3 Bosniak renal cyst classification system

Category	Wall	Septa	Calcification	Solid component	Measures water density	Enhance
I	Hairline thin	No	No	No	Yes – uniformly	No
II	Hairline thin	Few (<1 mm thick)	Yes – fine thickened	No	Yes	No
IIF[a]	Smooth thickening	Multiple	Yes – thick and nodular	No	Some parts may	No
III	Thickened or irregular	Yes (>1 mm thick)	Yes – thick and irregular	No	Some parts may	Yes
IV	Thickened or irregular	Yes	Yes	Yes	Some parts may	Yes

[a] These lesions are poorly defined but possess features requiring follow-up.

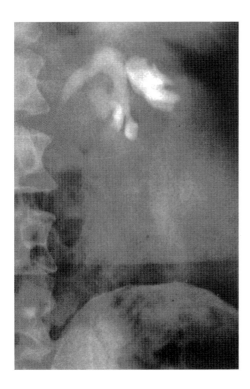

Figure 7.18 IVU showing the left renal pelvis grossly distorted by huge soft tissue mass arising from the lower pole.

with a clear margin, checked by frozen section if necessary. Every vessel is then suture ligated to secure complete haemostasis. In selected cases this operation can be done laparoscopically or robotically assisted.

Thermal ablative techniques

Renal cryosurgery and radiofrequency ablation (RFA) emerged as an alternative nephron-sparing treatment. They can be applied percutaneously or laparoscopically. They promise reduced morbidity and quicker recovery and the experience with both modalities is increasingly gaining grounds with regard to efficacy, but long-term results and outcomes are still being scrutinised. Strict criteria of selection of cases and application are being monitored.

New exciting technologies that include high-intensity focused ultrasound (HIFU) and image-guided radiotherapy (CyberKnife) are under development and might gain a place in management of small renal tumours in the future. Microwave thermotherapy and laser interstitial thermal therapy are available but should be considered investigational until prospective long-term studies are available.

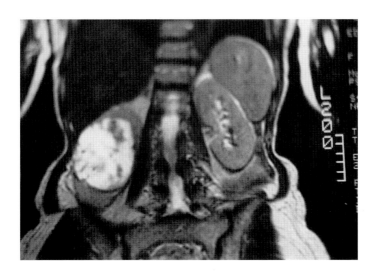

Figure 7.19 MRI image showing renal cell carcinoma in the right kidney.

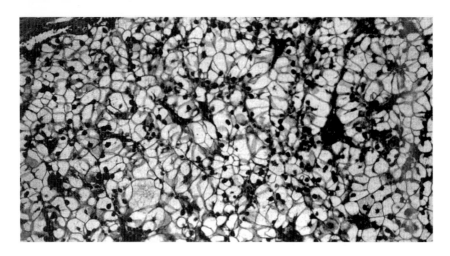

Figure 7.20 Typical clear-celled renal cell carcinoma of the kidney.

Table 7.4 **International TNM system of staging for renal cell carcinoma**

T: Primary tumour

TX	Primary tumour cannot be assessed
T0	No evidence of primary tumour
T1	Tumour ≤7.0 cm and confined to the kidney
T1a	Tumour ≤4.0 cm and confined to the kidney
T1b	Tumour >4.0 cm and ≤7.0 cm and confined to the kidney
T2	Tumour >7.0 cm and confined to the kidney
T2a	Tumour >7.0 cm and ≤10.0 cm and confined to the kidney
T2b	Tumour >10.0 cm and confined to the kidney
T3	Tumour extends into major veins or perinephric tissues
	Not in ipsilateral adrenal gland
	Not beyond the fascia of Gerota
T3a	Tumour grossly extends into the renal vein or branches
	Tumour invades perirenal and/or renal sinus fat
	Not beyond the fascia of Gerota
T3b	Tumour grossly extends into the vena cava below the diaphragm
T3c	Tumour grossly extends into the vena cava above the diaphragm
	Or invades the wall of the vena cava
T4	Tumour invades beyond the fascia of Gerota including extension
	Into the ipsilateral adrenal gland

N: Regional lymph nodes

NX	Regional lymph nodes cannot be assessed
N0	No regional lymph nodes metastasis
N1	Metastasis in a single regional lymph node
N2	Metastasis in more than 1 regional lymph node

M: Distant metastases

MX	Distant metastasis cannot be assessed

Table 7.4 (*Continued*)

M0	No distant metastasis
M1	Distant metastasis present
Stages	
Stage I	T1 N0 M0
Stage II	T2 N0 M0
Stage III	T1 or T2 N1 M0
	T3 any N M0
Stage IV	T4 any N M0
	Any T any N M1

Modified from Edge, S., Byrd, D.R., Compton, C.C., Fritz, A.G., Greene, F.L., and Trotti, A. (eds) (2010) *AJCC cancer staging manual*, 7th ed. Springer, New York.

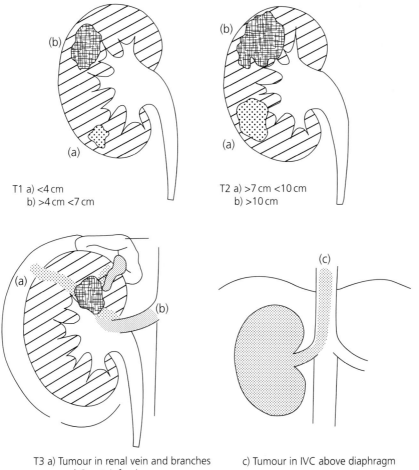

T1 a) <4 cm
    b) >4 cm <7 cm

T2 a) >7 cm <10 cm
    b) >10 cm

T3 a) Tumour in renal vein and branches
    and Gerota's fascia

b) Tumour into IVC below diaphragm

c) Tumour in IVC above diaphragm

Figure 7.21 Stages of renal cell carcinoma.

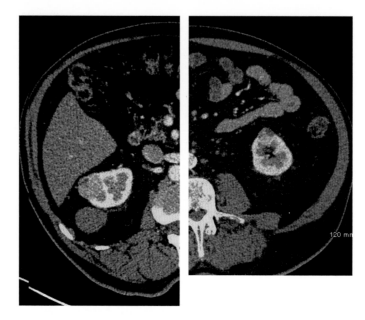

Figure 7.22 Bilateral small renal cell carcinoma tumours.

Large tumours: Radical nephrectomy

Open surgical approach has been through a generous incision (either vertical or transverse – according to the build of the patient) (Figure 7.23). Increasingly, hand-assisted laparoscopic and robotic-assisted approaches have gained preferences subject to the expertise of the operating surgeon and facilities availability. The anatomical details are more or less the same.

The colon and duodenum are reflected from the front of the kidney. The renal artery is ligated. Then the vein is divided between ligatures, and an intact block of tissue is then removed containing the kidney, all the surrounding fat inside Gerota's fascia and the lymph nodes along the side of the aorta (on the left) or the vena cava (on the right). When a tumour is found growing into the renal vein, after taping the cava, lumbar veins and opposite renal veins, the vena cava is clamped and the lump of tumour is removed cleanly.

When preoperative investigations have shown that the tumour has extended along the inferior vena cava into the heart, the abdominal incision is prolonged through the sternum. The patient is put on cardiac bypass. The vena cava is secured below and above the liver and the tumour extension is removed. Worthwhile survival has been reported following this intervention.

The choice between partial and total nephrectomy, either performed in an open fashion, laparoscopically or robotically assisted, is an ongoing topic for debate. Patients with a solitary kidney, severe renal insufficiency or bilateral renal masses are candidates for partial nephrectomy if possible as more radical surgery would render them dependent on dialysis. Suitability for partial nephrectomy depends on the size and position of the tumour and the experience of the surgeon. The disadvantages of partial nephrectomy include tumour recurrence in the remaining part of the kidney and the potential complications and morbidity of the procedure. Frozen section pathological examination of the tumour margin seems to be unreliable and its routine use cannot be supported.

Pathology

A radical nephrectomy specimen is seen in Figure 7.24a and b. Histological examination of the excised specimen major subtypes is

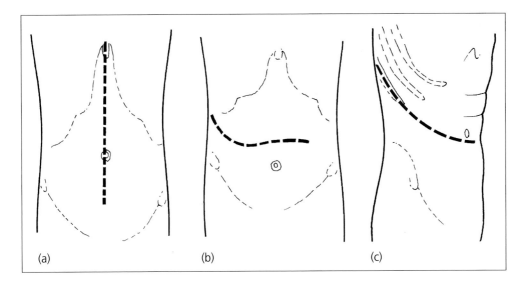

Figure 7.23 Incisions for radical nephrectomy chosen according to the site and size of the tumour and build of the patient: (a) midline, (b) transverse anterior and (c) trans-costal (12th rib).

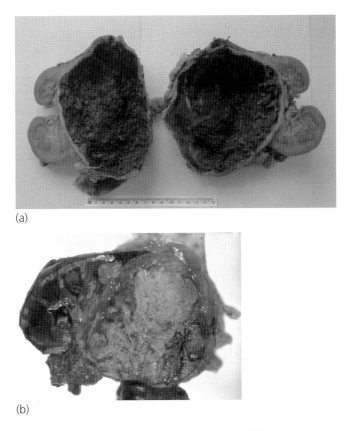

Figure 7.24 Radical nephrectomy specimen showing: (a) cystic and (b) solid tumours.

Table 7.5 Major histological subtypes

Histology	Pattern	Associated genetic changes
Clear cell 80–90%	Clear cytoplasm Growth: may be solid, tubular and cystic	Specific deletion of chromosome 3p and mutation of VHL gene Possible duplication of chromosome band 5q22 Possible deletion of chromosome 6q, 8p, 9p and 14q
Papillary 10–15%	Small cells with scanty cytoplasm Growth: predominantly papillary Type 1 small cells and pale cytoplasm Type 2 large cells and eosinophilic cytoplasm	Trisomies of chromosomes 3q, 7, 8, 12, 16 and 17 Loss of the Y chromosome
Chromophobe 4–5%	Pale or eosinophilic granular cytoplasm Growth: solid sheets	Combination of loss of chromosomes 1, 2, 6, 10, 13 and 17

described in Table 7.5. This allows stage grouping as seen in Table 7.3.

Grade

Typical clear-celled renal cell carcinoma of the kidney shows a number of nuclear varied features that lead to a number of grading systems addressing this issue. Fuhrman's system has been most generally adopted. It is now recognised as an important independent prognostic factor. It is based on such features as nuclear size and shape and the presence or absence of prominent nuclei (Table 7.6).

Prognosis

If the cancer is confined to the kidney, nephrectomy alone is followed by over 80% 5-year survival. The outlook is worse when the lymph nodes are involved or the fat and vena cava are invaded. Sometimes, miraculously, distant metastases go away once the primary tumour has been removed, suggesting that there might be a powerful natural immune system against renal cell cancer although good survival is only seen in otherwise fit patients whose tumours are relatively well differentiated. Solitary lung secondary has been labelled as a 'cannon ball' (Figure 7.25).

Table 7.6 Fuhrman grading system

Grade 1	Nuclear shape	Round, uniform
	Nucleoli	None
Grade 2	Nuclear shape	Slightly irregular
	Nucleoli	Visible at high power × 400 magnification
Grade 3	Nuclear shape	Very irregular outlines
	Nucleoli	Prominent visible at × 100 magnification
Grade 4	Nuclear shape	Bizarre and multilobed spindle-shaped cells
	Nucleoli	Prominent

A single large metastatic lesion has been considered for lobectomy in selected patients particularly after radical nephrectomy. Analysis of prognostic factors using the Leibovich scoring system (Table 7.7) has increased our predictive capability. Nomograms are being developed over the years for estimating the probability of outcomes based on patients' characters, details of

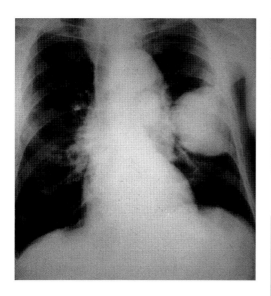

Figure 7.25 Chest X-ray demonstrating a solitary lung lesion 'cannon ball'.

Table 7.8 Estimated metastasis-free survival

Group	Scores	Year 5 (%)	Year 10 (%)
Low risk	0–2	97.1	92.5
Intermediate risk	3–5	73.8	64.3
High risk	6 or more	31.2	23.6

 KEYPOINTS

- Surveillance following radical, partial or ablative therapies for renal cell carcinoma should be adopted based on the disease risk elements identified.
- US/CT/MRI scan utilisation should be followed per individual patient based on the risk factors identified.

Table 7.7 Leibovich score

Pathological factor	Score
pT category of primary tumour	
pT1a	0
pT1b	2
pT2	3
pT3-4	4
Regional lymph node status	
pNx or pN0	0
pN1 or pN2	2
Tumour size	
<10 cm	0
>10 cm	1
Nuclear grade	
1 or 2	0
3(= Fuhrman 3)	1
4(= Fuhrman 4)	3
Histological tumour necrosis	
No	0
Yes	1

pathology results, tumour stage and increasingly new genetic tools. Estimated metastasis-free survival based on the risk groups is presented in Table 7.8.

The median survival for patients with metastatic disease has improved significantly for 9 months to 2 years because of the introduction of targeted treatments.

Management of metastatic disease: Systemic therapy

Selected patients with solitary or a limited number of distant metastases can achieve prolonged survival with nephrectomy and surgical resection of the metastases. Even patients with brain metastases had similar results. The likelihood of achieving therapeutic benefit with this approach appears enhanced in patients with a long disease-free interval between the initial nephrectomy and the development of metastatic disease.

Radiotherapy

Radiotherapy to the tumour bed following nephrectomy leads to no survival advantage in patients with adenocarcinoma of the kidney and is associated with increased morbidity. It can however have a useful role in palliating patients with symptoms from brain and bone metastases.

Chemotherapy

Chemotherapy is generally ineffective in treating advanced adenocarcinoma of the kidney. The most active drugs such as the vinca alkaloids have response rates of less than 10%.

Immunotherapy

Your body's immune system is responsible for protecting you from viruses, bacteria and cancer cells. Immunotherapy, sometimes called biological therapy, is a form of treatment that boosts the body's own immune defences. It is one of the standard treatment options for kidney cancer patients with advanced metastatic disease.

Well-documented, but very rare, cases of spontaneous regressions in kidney cancer patients with metastatic disease suggest that the immune system can play an important role in the control and potential treatment of this disease.

Interferon alpha and interleukin 2 have been shown to induce an objective response with interferon alpha having a modest impact on survival in highly selective patients. The overall objective response rates for both agents are about 15–20%. The most significant aspect of interleukin 2 is that response rates are durable in about 5%.

Targeted therapy

Targeted therapy refers to drugs that inhibit or interfere with specific molecular pathways shown to be important in cancer cell growth. The aim of targeted therapy is to kill cancer cells while sparing normal cells (unlike chemotherapy, which often kills normal rapidly dividing cells).

Side effects from targeted therapies are generally more manageable compared to chemotherapy. Furthermore they have demonstrated impressive activity against kidney cancer.

For malignant tumours to expand and metastasise, they must be able to form new blood vessels by a process called angiogenesis. Tumours overproduce 'growth factors' that stimulate the development of new blood vessels to supply oxygen and nutrition. These include 'vascular endothelial growth factor' (VEGF) and 'platelet-derived growth factor' (PDGF). These growth factors activate certain tyrosine kinases, proteins inside cancer cells that are important in cell functions, including the development of new blood vessels. This allows tumours to grow and to metastasise to other parts of the body.

The role of targeted therapy with anti-angiogenic agents is to stop blood vessels from forming in tumours, causing the tumour to starve, stop growing or shrink.

1. Monoclonal antibodies: Bevacizumab is a biologic antibody designed to interfere with the blood supply to a tumour by directly binding to the VEGF protein to prevent interactions with receptors on blood vessel cells. It does not bind to receptors on normal or cancer cells. The tumour blood supply is thought to be critical to a tumour's ability to grow and metastasise.
2. Tyrosine kinase inhibitors: Oral tyrosine kinase inhibitors available include sunitinib, pazopanib and sorafenib.

Response rates for these drugs approach 40% and those patients who respond do appear to have responses that are sustained. Treatment toxicity on the whole is mild. However, as the treatment targets VEGF receptors, gastrointestinal bleeding and perforation may occur.

Mammalian target of rapamycin (mTOR) inhibitors:

These drugs block the mammalian target of rapamycin, a serine/threonine protein kinase, that regulates cell growth and division and survival and are used in the management of advanced renal cell cancer. These include temsirolimus and everolimus.

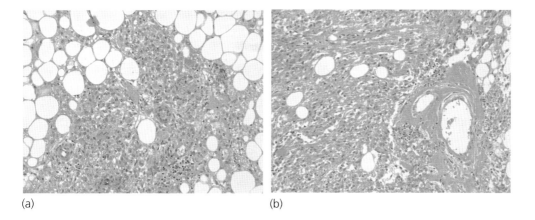

(a)   (b)

Figure 7.26 Angiomyolipoma is composed of a variety of abnormal vessels, smooth muscle cells and fat-containing cells.

Other renal tumours

- *Oncocytomas*
  Benign tumours about 3–7% of all renal tumours. Imaging characteristics are difficult to differentiate between oncocytomas and renal cell carcinoma. Histological diagnosis is a must. 'Watchful waiting' is only considered if histological diagnosis is verified.
- *Angiomyolipoma*
  Angiomyolipomas are benign tumours composed of varying amounts of abnormal blood vessels, smooth muscle cells and fat-containing cells (Figure 7.26). Most often they occur in females more than males and can increase in size with age. They are incidentally identified through imaging studies investigating other problems. Its content of fat gives it an unmistakable appearance in the CT scan. MRI is considered the preferred modality for identification and surveillance of these lesions. Renal angiomyolipomas can be associated with tuberous sclerosis complex (TSC), which is an autosomal dominant genetic condition. Mutation in TSC1 or TSC2, which regulates cellular growth and function, could lead to the development of benign tumours in a variety of organs including the kidneys. These lesions might stop growing spontaneously or may continue to grow and become eventually symptomatic. The complications that could be encountered include rupture of the fragile blood vessels leading to haemorrhage and gradual destruction of neighbouring normal renal tissue.

- *Unclassified carcinomas*
  Detailed morphological studies and immunohistochemical and molecular techniques lead to identification of a variety of sporadic, uncommon and familial carcinomas:

1. Collecting duct carcinoma (Bellini duct carcinoma)
2. Renal medullary carcinoma
3. Sarcomatoid renal cell carcinoma
4. Multilocular cystic renal cell carcinoma
5. Mucinous tubular and spindle cell carcinoma
6. Metanephric tumours
7. Carcinoma associated with end-stage renal disease

8

The renal pelvis and ureter

Anatomy

The ureters descend from the renal pelvis anterior to the psoas muscle and the ilio-hypogastric and ilio-inguinal nerves. Halfway down, they are crossed anteriorly by the vessels of the testis or ovary, and near the lower end by the branches of the internal iliac artery and veins going to and from the uterus and bladder.

In women, the ureter is vulnerable during the operation of hysterectomy where it passes under the uterine artery and veins (Figure 8.1). If there is bleeding, the ureter is easily injured in the course of efforts to secure haemostasis.

Blood supply

The main blood supply of the ureter comes down from the inferior segmental artery of the kidney (Figure 8.2), which runs down the ureter, and is reinforced by unimportant small branches from the lumbar arteries. Towards the lower end, it is joined by an ascending branch of the superior vesical artery. If the ureter is divided near the bladder, this ascending branch is cut and the lower end of the ureter may be ischaemic.

Nerve supply

Sensory nerves from the ureter follow a segmental pattern: the upper part, like the kidney, is supplied by T10, and pain is referred to the umbilicus. Lower down pain is referred to more caudal segments (L2,3,4) until pain from the lowest part of the ureter may be referred to the vulva or tip of the penis (S2,3) (Figure 8.3).

Peristalsis

The ureter is lined by urothelium on a thin layer of submucosa (Figure 8.4) outside of which the smooth muscle cells are connected with each other so that excitation passes along the muscle without the need for nerves or ganglia (Figure 8.5). Peristalsis in the ureter can be provoked by pinching or irritation. As a result, the denervated ureter of a transplant functions perfectly well.

Inflammation of the ureter

Acute and Chronic

Acute ureteritis may explain much of the pain in the groin, which patients so often describe during acute urinary infection. It is rarely investigated or documented and always recovers completely with time and antibiotics.

Urology Lecture Notes, Seventh Edition. Amir V. Kaisary, Andrew Ballaro and Katharine Pigott.
© 2016 John Wiley & Sons, Ltd. Published 2016 by John Wiley & Sons, Ltd.

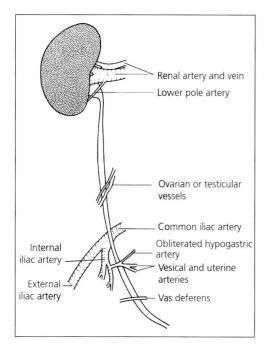

Renal artery and vein
Lower pole artery

Ovarian or testicular vessels

Common iliac artery
Obliterated hypogastric artery
Vesical and uterine arteries
Vas deferens

Internal iliac artery
External iliac artery

Figure 8.1 Anatomical relations of the right ureter.

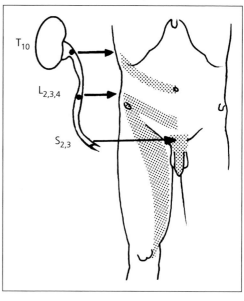

T_{10}

$L_{2,3,4}$

$S_{2,3}$

Figure 8.3 Pain from a stone in the ureter is referred to relevant dermatome.

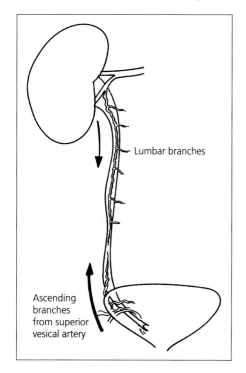

Lumbar branches

Ascending branches from superior vesical artery

Figure 8.2 Blood supply of the ureter.

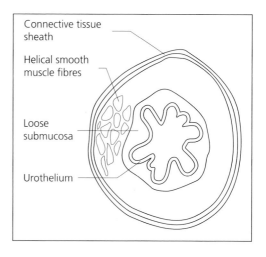

Connective tissue sheath

Helical smooth muscle fibres

Loose submucosa

Urothelium

Figure 8.4 Transverse section of the ureter.

- **Non-specific**
  Ureteritis cystica
  Following a prolonged urinary infection, the intravenous urogram (IVU) or ureterogram may show multiple rounded filling defects in

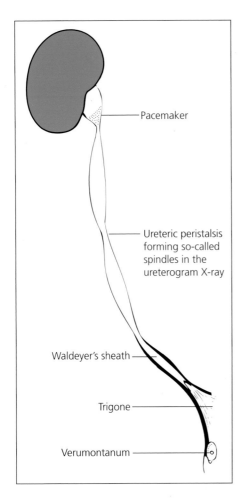

Figure 8.5 Peristalsis in the ureter.

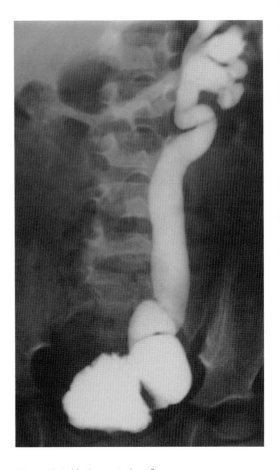

Figure 8.6 Vesicoureteric reflux.

the ureter and renal pelvis. These are caused by a particular kind of chronic inflammation of the urothelium – ureteritis cystica – where little nests of urothelium get buried and swell up to form tiny cysts. It resolves completely when the underlying infection has been cured.

- **Specific**
  1. *Tuberculosis*
     The ureter is often involved in tuberculosis as discussed in Chapter 5.
  2. *Schistosomiasis*
     The wall of the ureter is always involved in schistosomiasis. Pairs of *Schistosoma* flukes nest in the submucosal veins and lay eggs

that provoke chronic inflammation, turning the ureter into a stiff, inert tube that is dilated, obstructed and often calcified. Schistosomiasis is discussed in more detail in Chapter 11.

Megaureter

- This is a common and important entity in children. It causes confusion because it is often assumed that whenever a dilated ureter is discovered, there must necessarily be obstruction.
- ***Reflux***: Most megaureters are caused by reflux (Figure 8.6).
- ***Congenital stenosis***: At the lower end of the ureter: a narrowing, from an unknown cause, occurs at the lower end of the ureter, giving rise to obstruction upstream (Figure 8.7).

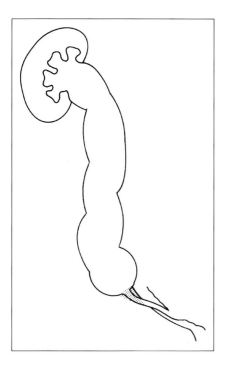

Figure 8.7 Obstructed ureter caused by stenosis at the lower end.

- *Idiopathic*: In a number of boys, the ureters are found to be huge, but there is no reflux and no narrowing at the lower end. One plausible suggestion is that at some time in foetal life, there was a posterior urethral valve, which gave rise to gross obstruction and dilatation of the ureters, and then the valve ruptured spontaneously, leaving the child with large ureters without any apparent reason for them.

Vesicoureteric reflux

Aetiology

Many children are born with a defective valve mechanism at the entry of the ureters into the bladder. The cause of this failure is muscular weakness of the trigone and lower ureter, and this is related to the development of the ureteric bud and early joining of the mesonephric duct with the urogenital sinus causing it to acquire deficient surrounding mesenchyme.

Reflux nephropathy

Reflux nephropathy occurs both in the presence of vesicoureteric reflux in an otherwise normal bladder when the urine is infected and also in the absence of infection when the bladder is obstructed and the urine is under higher pressure due to bladder outflow obstruction. The degree of renal damage caused is determined by the morphology and shape of the renal papillae. Compound renal papillae have several collecting ducts opening on to the same orifice that is as a result ovoid and refluxing as opposed to single ducts of non-refluxing papillae that are slit-like and close off under pressure. Infected urine, and that under high pressure, is forced into the parenchyma through the compound papillae causing acute inflammation of the renal parenchyma, which is followed by typical deeply pitted scars of reflux nephropathy that become more pronounced as the rest of the kidney continues to grow. Compound papillae are usually found at the upper and lower poles of the kidney so it is here that the scarring of reflux nephropathy is mostly marked (Figure 8.8).

Diagnosis and management

The diagnosis is made by a micturating cystogram, or radionuclide scan cystogram. Ultrasound is also used. Three grades of reflux are recognised (Figure 8.9). In grades I and II, where the reflux is not severe, the urine can usually be kept sterile with a small daily dose of an antimicrobial such as trimethoprim, and it is safe to wait for the valve to mature and become competent.

In grade III, where the reflux is gross, it may be impossible to keep the urine sterile, or there is repeated breakthrough infection, and it may be better to perform an operation to prevent reflux. The most simple of these is to inject a small amount of collagen paste through a cystoscope under the mucosa of the ureteric orifice to change its opening into a crescent (Figure 8.10). When the ureters are vastly dilated, it may be necessary to reimplant the ureter through a long tunnel between the urothelium and muscle of the wall of the bladder (Figure 8.11).

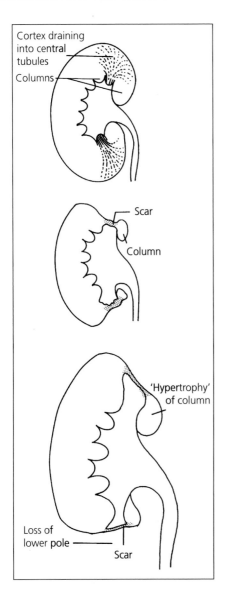

Figure 8.8 Formation of the pitted scars of reflux nephropathy.

Ureteric obstruction

Obstructive uropathy

Obstruction to the flow of urine from the kidney may occur at any point between the pelviureteric junction (PUJ) and the external urethral meatus and is termed obstructive uropathy. The obstruction usually results in the radiologically detectable distension of the renal pelvis and calyces termed hydronephrosis. Hydronephrosis, however, is not pathognomonic of obstructive uropathy as obstructive uropathy can occur without pelvic distension and hydronephrosis can occur without obstruction, for example, in high diuretic states with a capacious extrarenal pelvis.

Obstructive nephropathy

Obstructive nephropathy refers to the anatomical or functional renal damage as a result of obstruction. The effects of obstructive uropathy on renal function and the patient as a whole are influenced by whether the obstruction is unilateral or bilateral, acute or chronic, the degree of obstruction and the underlying condition of the affected kidney.

Obstruction to the ureter generates a tri-phasic haemodynamic response, which alters renal blood flow and glomerular filtration rate. This is mediated by prostaglandins and nitrous oxide acting on first afferent subsequently efferent glomerular arterioles. This response differs in unilateral and bilateral obstruction, the difference being that in unilateral obstruction the contralateral kidney, provided that it is healthy, takes over the functions of the obstructed kidney resulting in normalisation of intrarenal pressures.

Prolonged obstructive uropathy leads to progressive tubular atrophy, interstitial fibrosis and permanent loss of renal function. The degree to which renal function is permanently lost is influenced by the duration and degree of obstruction. In dogs, full recovery of renal function may occur after 7 days of unilateral complete ureteric obstruction within 14 days. Approximately two-thirds of function returns after 14 days of obstruction; however, this recovery takes several weeks to mature, and after 6 weeks of ureteric obstruction, the kidney is irreversibly lost. In humans the effect of obstruction is likely to be similar. The degree of recovery of renal function is influenced by the age of the patient and the baseline renal function, with older kidneys and those with pre-existing impairment recovering less. In the presence of

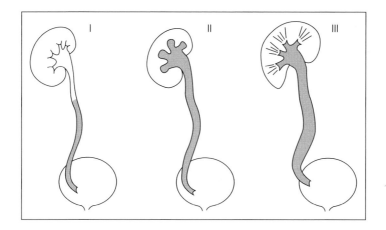

Figure 8.9 Three grades of reflux.

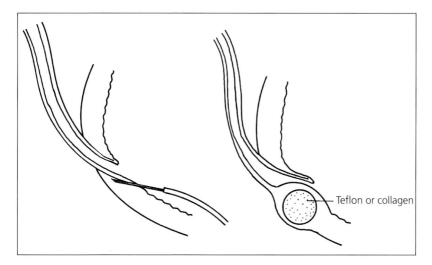

Teflon or collagen

Figure 8.10 A blob of Teflon paste or collagen is injected under the urothelium of the ureteric orifice.

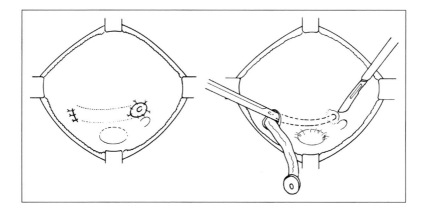

Figure 8.11 Reimplantation of the ureter using Cohen's method.

pyonephrosis, irreversible and progressive renal damage occurs immediately.

Relief of obstruction: Post-obstructive diuresis

The relief of bilateral ureteric obstruction, which is most commonly a result of bladder outflow obstruction with high-pressure chronic retention, or obstruction of a solitary kidney, is accompanied by a post-obstructive diuresis. This may result in large volumes of urine being passed and may suggest that intravenous saline replacement is required. In the majority of cases, however, the diuresis is a physiological response to the volume and solute overload that has built up during the period of obstruction. Provided the patient is able to drink water freely, the diuresis requires no active treatment other than fluid balance and serum electrolyte monitoring, and the diuresis will self-limit when homeostasis is restored.

Occasionally a pathological diuresis may occur due to impaired renal handling of water or solutes due to damage sustained during the obstruction. A saline diuresis is caused by derangement of the renal medullary concentration gradient, which impairs sodium reabsorption. A water diuresis is caused by impaired responsiveness of receptors to antidiuretic hormone. In these conditions, close monitoring, appropriate fluid balance correction and occasionally intensive care input are required. It is important to identify these patients promptly. It is therefore recommended that all patients who pass more than 200 mL/h of urine for 2 consecutive hours after relief of bilateral or solitary kidney obstruction have the urine osmolality determined.

Diagnosis of ureteric obstruction

The degree of pain produced by ureteric obstruction is variable and dependent on the speed and duration of the obstruction. Sudden complete obstruction of the ureter, such as caused by an impacting stone, causes characteristic renal colic as described in previous chapters. Insidious obstruction, however, may be asymptomatic with an end-stage grossly dilated kidney discovered incidentally after many years. It is likely that the degree of pain produced is also influenced by the coaptation properties of the renal pelvis and ureter.

Provided that the contralateral kidney has normal function, unilateral obstruction does not cause a significant rise in serum creatinine levels or urine output, although GFR falls; in patients with normal functioning kidneys, the serum creatinine does not rise until GFR falls to approximately a quarter. Bilateral complete ureteric obstruction will clearly cause anuria and rapidly rising serum creatinine levels.

Obstructive uropathy is often diagnosed radiologically, and ultrasound is a sensitive non-invasive method of detecting hydronephrosis. It is important, however, to recognise the limitations of hydronephrosis as a marker for obstruction. Ultrasound can often determine whether the dilatation is limited to the renal pelvis in which case the site of the obstruction is likely to be the PUJ (Figure 8.12), or includes the ureter. Once hydronephrosis has been identified, the cause, if not clinically evident, should be sought using cross-sectional imaging by computerised tomography or magnetic resonance imaging. This will show the precise level of obstruction in the ureter or distally and usually the cause. Isotope renography may be used to detect functional obstruction to urine flow from the kidney and to confirm obstruction in a dilated system (Figure 8.13).

Management of ureteric obstruction

Management of obstructive uropathy should be tailored to the patient. It is not always necessary to de-obstruct an obstructed kidney; a good example of this is the terminally ill patient with ureteric obstruction due to extrinsic compression by a tumour. In such a patient relief of the obstruction may not prolong life and will cause distress, reducing the quality of that remaining. Usually, however, relief of the obstruction is required. The methods employed to do this are influenced by patient and disease factors.

Temporary decompression may be achieved by percutaneous insertion of a nephrostomy tube

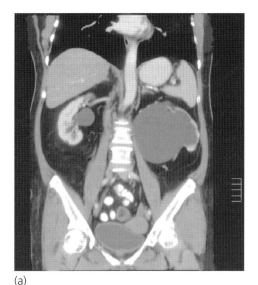

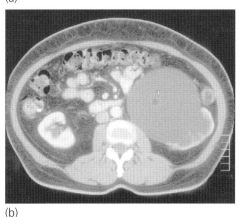

(a)

(b)

Figure 8.12 Hydronephrosis from obstruction of the pelviureteric junction: (a) longitudinal and (b) transverse.

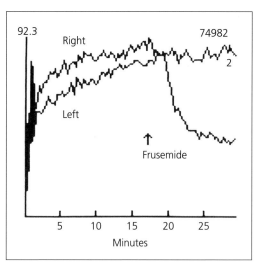

Figure 8.13 DTPA renogram showing retention of isotope in the left kidney in spite of frusemide.

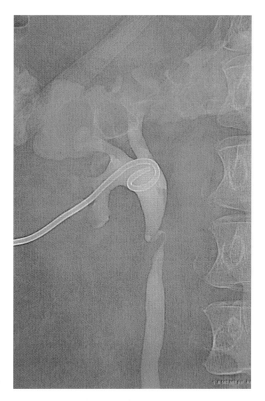

Figure 8.14 Right nephrostomy.

into the renal collecting system (Figure 8.14) and either antegrade or retrograde insertion of a double-J ureteric stent. This reduces pain and allows time for planning a definitive procedure, which will depend on the cause of the obstruction.

If the obstruction has been prolonged, a considerable degree of renal function may have been lost. This will usually be apparent from the history and imaging, with the kidney grossly dilated and with a thin cortex. In this event, DMSA scan should be obtained several weeks after de-obstruction, and if this shows that the kidney is contributing less than 10–15% of the total and would therefore be unable to support prolonged survival without renal support in the event that the contralateral kidney was lost, nephrectomy should be considered. The sequelae of a non-functioning kidney are stone formation, pain and uncontrollable hypertension, and these are all indications for nephrectomy.

Causes of ureteric obstruction

In some conditions such as a ureteric stone, the cause of the obstruction can be readily dealt with endoscopically, as described in Chapter 6. The management of luminal and extra-luminal obstruction may be more complex depending on the cause.

PUJ obstruction

PUJ obstruction may be congenital or acquired. The most common cause of congenital PUJ obstruction is anatomical compression by crossing blood vessels passing anteriorly from the aorta and vena cava to the lower pole of the kidney (Figure 8.15). The presence of an aperistaltic segment of the upper ureter may also impair urine drainage, and progressive asymmetric dilatation of the renal pelvis may cause its rotation relative to the ureter and add to the obstruction by kinking the upper ureter.

Congenital PUJ obstruction may present at any stage of life, although the condition is increasingly being diagnosed and treated in the perinatal period. In adults, conservative management with serial follow-up MAG3 renogram may be appropriate. Indications for operative intervention are limited to pain, evidence of progressive impairment of function of the involved kidney or the development of stones or recurrent infections. Clinically significant recovery of lost renal function does not occur after treatment.

Treatment of PUJ obstruction is, most appropriately, with dismembered pyeloplasty (Figure 8.16). This can be performed laparoscopically and robotic assistance reduces the technical difficulty of the procedure. The ureter is transected below the PUJ, spatulated and reconstructed anterior to the crossing vessels. While it is sometimes necessary to ligate the crossing renal vein during the procedure, it is important not to damage the lower pole artery as it is an end artery. Endoscopic incision of the PUJ and prolonged JJ ureteric stent placement may also be used in selected cases but have a higher failure rate. Failure of PUJ surgery condemns the patient to recurrent endoscopic procedures, permanent stenting or nephrectomy, and careful consideration should be given to this on a patient-by-patient basis.

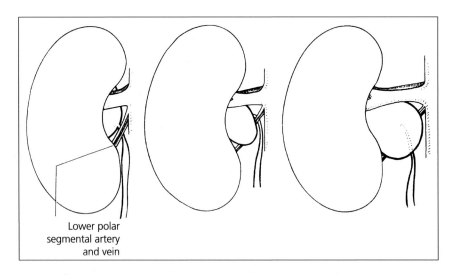

Lower polar
segmental artery
and vein

Figure 8.15 The obstructed renal pelvis often bulges out between the two lower pole segmental arteries.

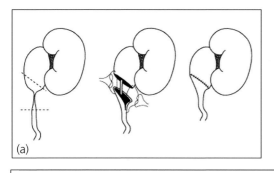

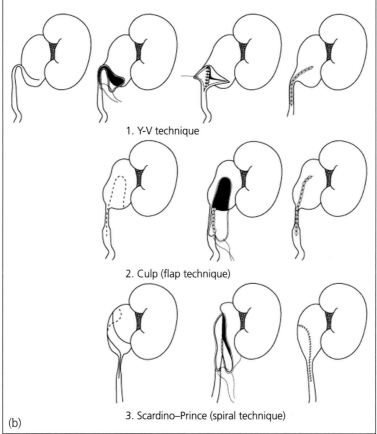

Figure 8.16 Open pyeloplasty: (a) dismembered pyeloplasty and (b) flap pyeloplasty.

Retroperitoneal disease

A wide variety of diseases involving the retroperitoneal structures may cause extrinsic compression of the ureter and obstructive nephropathy. The most common of these are malignant tumours of the retroperitoneal lymph nodes or colon and fibrosis resulting from either inflammatory aneurysms, surgery to structures adjacent to the ureter such as colon or major blood vessels or in association with various drugs and infections.

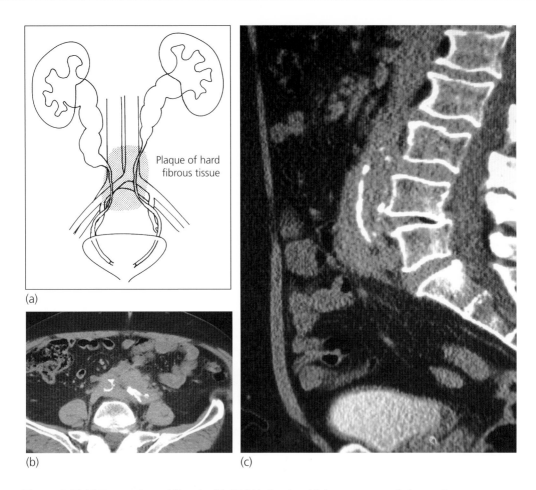

(a)

(b)

(c)

Figure 8.17 (a) Retroperitoneal fibrosis. (b) CT IVU showing thick mass upper abdomen: transverse. (c) CT IVU showing thick mass upper abdomen: longitudinal.

Idiopathic retroperitoneal fibrosis is characterised by backache, fever and weight loss. The ureter is encased in a stiff plaque of fibrous tissue and becomes obstructed (Figure 8.17, b and c). The fibrous plaque may involve the great vessels and extend up to the mediastinum. Treatment of retroperitoneal ureteric compression is aimed at the cause of the compression. Primary medical management of retroperitoneal fibrosis has been steroid therapy. If clinically indicated, the ureter is de-obstructed temporarily by insertion of a ureteric stent until the obstruction is relieved and renal function is stabilised, in some cases permanent ureteric stenting. Surgical ureterolysis aiming at intraperitonealisation or omental wrapping of the ureters (Figure 8.18) may be performed successfully adopting both open and laparoscopic techniques.

Retrocaval ureter

Very rarely the post-cardinal veins of the embryo fail to become obliterated, and the ureter has to wind round behind the inferior vena cava. The radiological appearance is

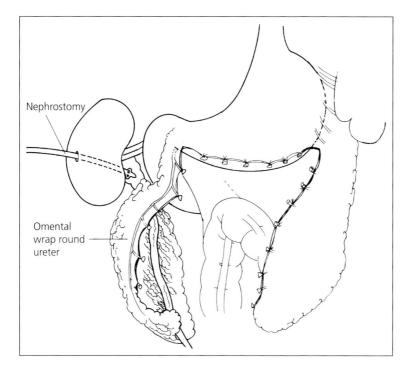

Nephrostomy

Omental
wrap round
ureter

Figure 8.18 Wrapping the ureter in omentum prevents recurrence of retroperitoneal fibrosis.

unmistakable (Figure 8.19). There is no need to meddle with the little bit of ureter behind the vena cava. The lower end is detached and anastomosed to the dilated upper part just as in any other hydronephrosis.

Ureteric stricture

The most common causes of ureteric strictures are iatrogenic as a result of ureteroscopy or gynaecological surgery. A less common cause is pelvic radiotherapy. Modern radiotherapy is closely targeted to the organ or tumour with peripheral damage limited, the fields of the cervical radiotherapy of 20 years ago however were considerably larger and involved structures adjacent to the target organ. The endarteritis obliterans and tissue damage from radiotherapy may progress for many years after the actual treatment and so can the stricture.

Ureteric strictures most commonly occur at the junction of the lower third and middle third at the pelvic brim (the boundary of the middle third and upper third is at the level of the lower border of the kidney). At this point the ureter deflects into the pelvis and therefore presents a greater surface area to the radiotherapy beam. At this point in the ureter, there is also a vascular watershed, with blood supply superiorly coming medially from the aorta and below laterally from the iliac vessels along the pelvic sidewall. This relatively under-perfused area is therefore more susceptible to ischaemia particularly when combined with the small vessel damage associated with radiotherapy. A further reason why the ureter is vulnerable at the pelvic brim is that the bend can be difficult to negotiate endoscopically and is the most common site for iatrogenic injury.

Management of ureteric stricture may be short- or long-term stents, ureteric dilatation

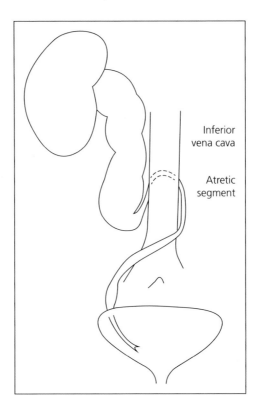

Figure 8.19 Retrocaval ureter.

 KEYPOINTS

- Obstructive nephropathy refers to the structural and functional effects of obstructive uropathy.
- Hydronephrosis is reliably detected on ultrasound; however, it is not pathognomonic for obstruction.
- The effect on the obstructed kidney depends on the degree of obstruction, the state of the kidney and the age of the patient.
- Kidney function is permanently lost after a week of obstruction and the whole kidney is lost after 6 weeks in experimental models.

and segmental resection of the stricture or ureteric reconstruction. Ureteric reconstruction techniques vary according to the state of the tissues, anatomy and cause of the stricture and its position. For lower third ureteric strictures, it is usually possible to reimplant the healthy ureter proximal to the stricture into a bladder with or without surgically extending it using the Boari flap technique (Figure 8.20); the anastomosis is stabilised against the posterior retroperitoneum by the psoas hitch procedure.

Ureteric injury

- *Accidental trauma*
  Closed injuries of the ureter are very rare. Open injuries caused by a knife or bullet are easily overlooked at the time the wound is explored and may only be noticed afterwards when urine leaks from the wound.
- *Iatrogenic trauma*
  The ureter is at risk in any operation in the pelvis, especially hysterectomy. The ureter is most prone to be injured where it is crossed by the uterine arteries and veins, but it can also be

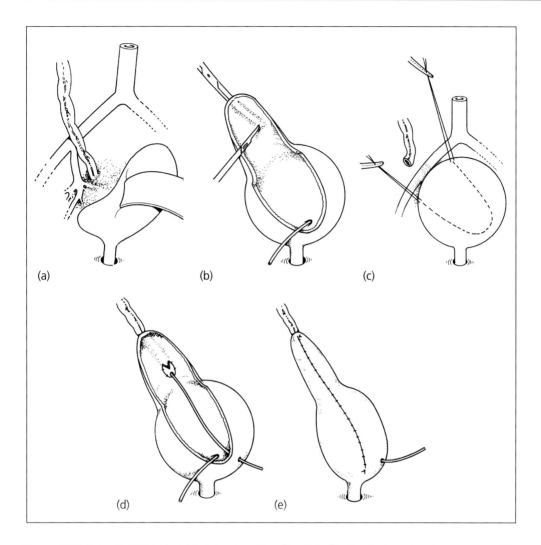

Figure 8.20 Reimplantation of an injured ureter with a Boari bladder flap (a, b, c, d and e are sequential surgery steps).

caught a little higher up by a suture used to close the peritoneum. There are three distinct clinical scenarios:

- **Injury noticed at operation**

  If the ureter is healthy, it may be repaired by end-to-end anastomosis using absorbable sutures and a stent left in.

- **Immediate post-operative symptoms**

  1. ***Loin pain and fever***: More often the injury to the ureter is not noticed during the operation. The patient may have pain in the loin afterwards and, if the urine is infected, a fever. These are important symptoms that demand an immediate CT with urographic phase (CT IVU).

  2. ***Anuria***: If both ureters have been obstructed at the time of injury, the patient will be anuric. In practice, the problem arises in just the kind of operation where there is likely to have been considerable loss of blood, and it is reasonable to think that shock has caused renal failure from under perfusion. When there is any doubt, a CT should be performed: if there is obstruction there will be a delayed nephrogram.

- **Late leak of urine**

  Sadly, the pain in the loin is often put down to normal post-operative discomfort. After 7–10 days, fluid begins to escape from the vagina (in the case of vaginal hysterectomy).

  The first and most urgent task is to confirm that the fluid is urine. This is easy: have it sent to the laboratory for an urgent creatinine measurement. If the creatinine is greater than that in the blood, the fluid contains urine.

  The second step is to image the lesion with a CT IVU. This will usually show some obstruction and occasionally will show extravasation of the contrast into the vagina or soft tissues (Figure 8.21). The sooner the diagnosis is confirmed and the injured ureter is repaired, the better (and the easier to do).

  A bulb-ended catheter is placed in the ureter and contrast is injected to give a *ureterogram*. This will show extravasation or a block. It ought to be performed on the other side as well since the injury is often bilateral (Figure 8.22).

- **Repair of the ureter**

  The previous incision is reopened. The ureter is traced down to the site of injury, divided where it is healthy and implanted into a U-shaped (Boari) flap made from the wall of the bladder, with a tunnel to prevent reflux.

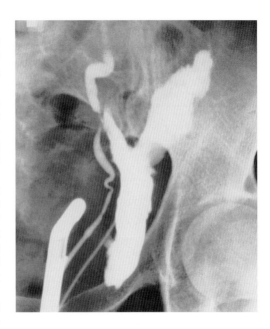

Figure 8.22 Retrograde ureterogram showing contrast leaking out from the ureter.

Carcinoma of the ureter

Since the ureter is lined with urothelium, it can form all the types of transitional cell cancer that are seen in the renal pelvis and bladder. They present with haematuria or pain from obstruction to the ureter (Figure 8.23). Urothelial cancer is strongly associated with smoking. Haematuria is the most important symptom: pain is late.

Pathology

Urothelial cancer in the *upper* tract, like that in the bladder, is classified in three grades, 1, 2 and 3. Metaplasia of the transitional epithelium gives rise to squamous cell cancers and adenocarcinomas, both of which are usually poorly differentiated. The tumours spread directly into the muscle of the pelvis and the renal parenchyma as well as into the surrounding fat. They can seed further down the urinary tract and they metastasise via lymph nodes rather than veins.

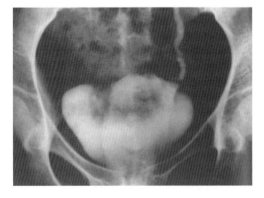

Figure 8.21 IVU in uretero-vesical fistula following hysterectomy: contrast medium outlines the vagina. The ureter is a little obstructed.

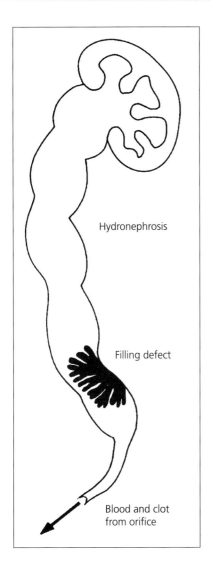

Hydronephrosis

Filling defect

Blood and clot
from orifice

Figure 8.23 Clinical features of a carcinoma of the ureter.

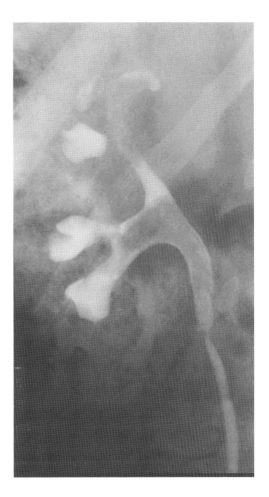

Figure 8.24 Filling defects in the renal pelvis and calyces from multifocal urothelial carcinoma of the right kidney.

Diagnosis

CT IVU can show a filling defect (Figure 8.24) in the renal pelvis. A small tumour in the ureter may be difficult to detect. It can be confirmed by an ascending ureterogram if necessary (Figure 8.25). Ureteroscopy gives a clear picture of the tumour and allows a biopsy to be taken (Figure 8.26). Malignant cells may be found in the urine on cytology if the tumour is G2 or G3. A small brush may be used to acquire cells from the tumour for cytology. A ureteric tumour at the lower end could come through the ureteric orifice into the bladder, and hydronephrosis as a result of long-standing obstruction can be clearly seen in a CT IVU study (Figure 8.27a and b). With ureteric transitional cell tumours, the stage closely correlates with the grade.

Treatment

Single G1 tumours can occasionally be removed locally, or coagulated with a laser through the ureteroscope (Figure 8.28), but unfortunately

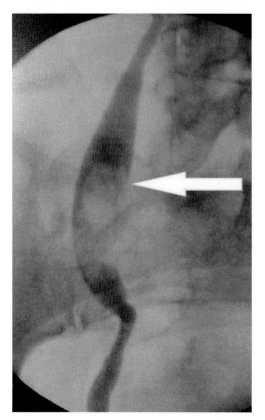

Figure 8.25 Ascending ureterography showing a filling defect suggestive of a ureteric tumour.

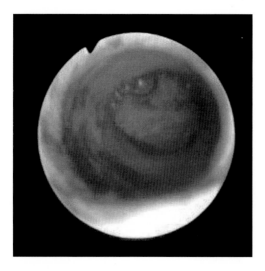

Figure 8.26 Ureteroscopy showing a ureteric tumour.

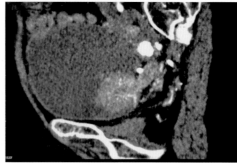

(a)

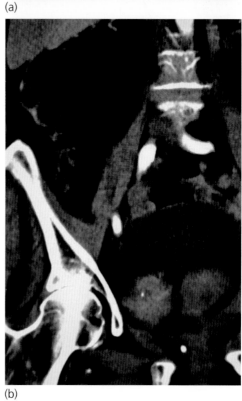

(b)

Figure 8.27 CT IVU study showing: (a) lower right ureteric tumour projecting in the bladder and (b) right hydronephrosis as a result of a long-standing obstructive right ureteric tumour.

they are usually multiple. G3 tumours have a very bad prognosis and have often invaded through the wall of the ureter by the time they are detected. Radical nephroureterectomy, *en bloc* removal of the kidney and ureter

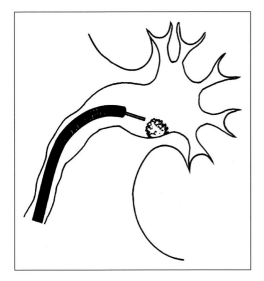

Figure 8.28 Coagulation of a small tumour in the renal pelvis with the YAG laser through a flexible ureteroscope.

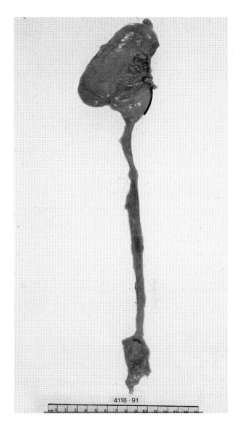

4118-91

Figure 8.29 Nephroureterectomy specimen showing tumour in the lower ureter and excision of a cuff of the bladder wall.

(Figure 8.29), is conducted by either open surgery, laparoscopy or robotically assisted. If the ureter is left behind, there is an almost inevitable chance of recurrence. In G3 tumours, adjuvant radiotherapy is often given before the nephroureterectomy, or combination chemotherapy is given afterwards.

9

The adrenal gland

Surgical anatomy and physiology

Each adrenal gland lies just medial to the upper pole of the kidney. The arteries supplying the adrenals arise from the aorta, phrenic and renal arteries and are all quite small. The right adrenal vein drains into the vena cava: it is short and easily torn. The left adrenal vein enters the left renal vein (Figure 9.1).

The adrenal gland is like a three-layer sandwich – the *cortex* – folded over a jam filling – the *medulla* (Figure 9.2). The outer layer of the cortex – the *zona glomerulosa* – secretes aldosterone. The middle layer, the *zona fasciculata*, secretes cortisol. The inner layer, *zona reticularis*, secretes androgens (Figure 9.3). The medulla plays an integral part of the autonomic nervous system. It is made of sympathetic nerve endings and *pheochromocytes* that secrete catecholamines (epinephrine, norepinephrine and dopamine).

Physiology and disorders of the adrenal cortex

Zona glomerulosa tumours (Conn's syndrome)

These may be single or multiple and may occur on both sides. They are usually benign. Excess secretion of aldosterone leads to retention of sodium causing hypertension and loss of potassium causing weakness. The diagnosis is made by the combination of hypertension, unexplained low plasma hypokalaemia, high level of aldosterone and low level of renin. It is confirmed by giving spironolactone that reverses the picture. The patient can often be controlled with spironolactone, but its side effects, for example, enlargement of the breasts, indigestion and impotence, may be unbearable and the patient may prefer an operation. Open surgery, laparoscopic or robotic-assisted modalities can be offered depending on the surgeon's expertise in the technique chosen. If a single adenoma is found, the entire adrenal is removed: if both adrenals are involved with multiple adenomas, both are removed and adrenal replacement with hydrocortisone is required afterwards.

Zona fasciculata tumours (Cushing's syndrome)

Excess cortisol results in the patient having a buffalo hump at the back of the neck, hirsutism, a red face, subcutaneous haemorrhages, cutaneous striae, hypertension, diabetes and osteoporosis that may lead to pathological fractures (Figure 9.4).

KEYPOINTS

- The only zone that contains the enzyme aldosterone synthase (CYP11B2). As a result, it is the sole source of aldosterone.
- Aldosterone levels are primarily regulated by angiotensin II. This is through the renin–angiotensin–aldosterone system and directly by serum potassium levels.

Urology Lecture Notes, Seventh Edition. Amir V. Kaisary, Andrew Ballaro and Katharine Pigott.
© 2016 John Wiley & Sons, Ltd. Published 2016 by John Wiley & Sons, Ltd.

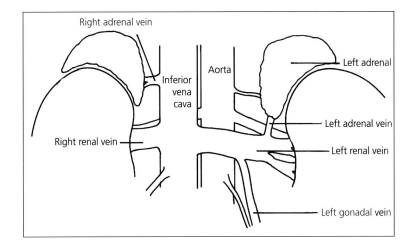

Figure 9.1 Anatomical relations of the adrenal gland.

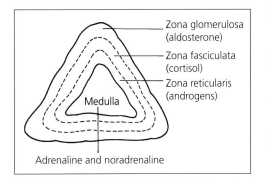

Figure 9.2 The folded sandwich arrangement of the adrenal.

There may be a single cortisol-secreting tumour, or there may be bilateral hyperplasia. In turn, hyperplasia is sometimes caused by a basophil adenoma of the pituitary that is secreting adrenocorticotrophic hormone (ACTH). Very rarely the ACTH may be secreted by another tumour, for example, carcinoma of the bronchus.

The diagnosis of Cushing's syndrome is confirmed by a dexamethasone suppression test. If there is a primary adrenal tumour, the ACTH will be undetectable.

If a CT/MRI scan reveals a primary adrenal tumour, it is removed. If there is hyperplasia of both adrenals, a pituitary tumour must be excluded, and if none is found, then both adrenals are removed and adrenal replacement is given afterwards.

Zona reticulosa tumours (virilisation)

Isolated androgen-secreting tumours causing virilisation are rare, but an excess of androgens is often secreted by malignant adrenal tumours that are also producing cortisol. In children this causes increased growth, hirsutism, enlarged genitalia, a deep voice and, in girls, early onset of menses. In adults there may be acne, hirsutism and disturbance of menstruation.

 KEYPOINTS

- Zonal expression of 17α-hydroxylase, 21α-hydroxylase and 11β-hydroxylase enzymes makes it the source of cortisol, the glucocorticoid secreted.
- Its function is tightly controlled by ACTH secreted by the anterior pituitary.

 KEYPOINTS

- Zonal presence of 17α-hydroxylase and 17,20-lyase results in production of dehydroepiandrosterone.
- Manipulation of adrenal androgen is increasingly a viable target strategy for castrate-resistant advanced prostate cancer.

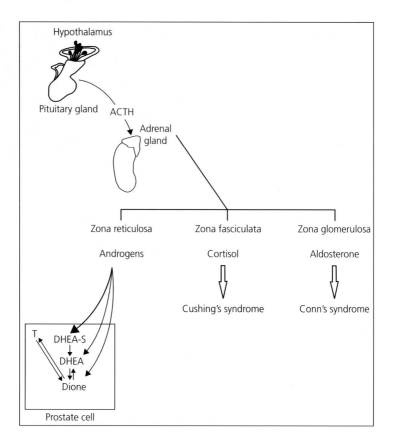

Figure 9.3 Adrenal cortex layers and secretions.

Adrenal tumours

Tumours can arise from any part of the adrenal and may or may not secrete the appropriate hormone.

Non-functioning tumours (incidentalomas)

These are usually detected by accident in the course of an ultrasound or computerised tomography (CT) scan (Figure 9.5). Rarely may they be the first presentation of metastases or primary adrenal cancer. Size is the usual but rather over simple guide to malignancy, that is, tumours less than 3 cm diameter are mostly benign and those more than 6 cm diameter are usually malignant. Each

 KEYPOINTS

- Low attenuation on unenhanced CT corresponds to high intracellular lipid and is extremely specific for identification of adrenal adenoma.
- CT washout studies are considered the gold standard for adrenal imaging.

case has to be considered on its merits. Biopsy is rarely helpful and careful imaging is required.

Adrenal CT scanning protocol to assess the nature of adrenal lesions utilises the different enhancing characteristics that rely on excretion of contrast material. Images are acquired at three different enhancing stages: un-enhanced, 1 min post IV contrast and 10 min post IV contrast

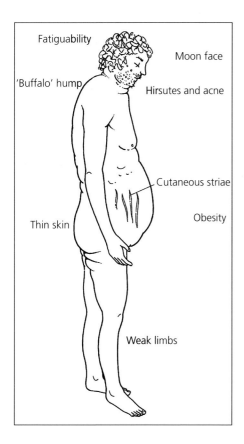

Fatiguability

Moon face

'Buffalo' hump

Hirsutes and acne

Cutaneous striae

Thin skin

Obesity

Weak limbs

Figure 9.4 Cushing's syndrome.

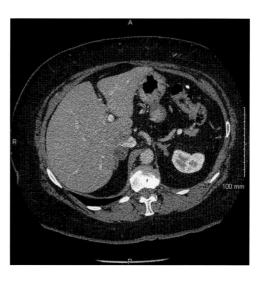

Figure 9.5 CT of the upper abdomen showing left adrenal tumour.

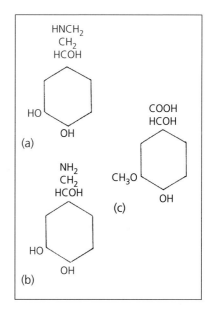

Figure 9.6 (a) Adrenaline, (b) noradrenaline and (c) 3-methoxy 4-hydroxy mandelic acid (VMA).

administration. A wash out greater than 60% probably favours a benign adenoma nature. High intracytoplasmic lipid content is unique to adenomas. Malignant lesions have disordered capillary permeability that probably results in prolonged retention of contrast given.

- **Pheochromocytoma**
  This may occur in association with inherited disorders such as the multiple endocrine neoplasia type II and von Hippel–Lindau disease. They arise either in the adrenal medulla or on the aorta at the origin of the inferior mesenteric artery and, very rarely, in the bladder. The excess of adrenaline and noradrenaline causes paroxysms of hypertension with headache, sweating, flushing, tremor and pain in the chest.
  Diagnosis is based on a 24-h collection of urine acidified with hydrochloric acid, of

metanephrines and plasma catecholamines (Figure 9.6). During this test, the patient avoids anything containing vanilla, for example, bananas, chocolate and coffee. Although these tumours are so vascular that they show up vividly in an angiogram, they are more easily located with a CT scan or MRI.

The tumour must be removed. About 10% are malignant. To protect the patient from a sudden surge of catecholamines, phenoxybenzamine is given to block the alpha receptors and propranolol to block the beta receptors preoperatively with experienced anaesthetic support. Even though these have been blocked, the tumour is handled as little as possible until the veins have all been ligated, at which moment the anaesthetist must be ready to deal with a fall in blood pressure. How the tumour is surgically approached depends on its position: tumours near the adrenal are reached through a 12th rib tip incision and those near the inferior mesenteric artery through a midline laparotomy. Again, laparo-scopic or robotic-assisted modalities can be offered depending on the surgeon's expertise in the technique chosen.

- **Neuroblastoma**

These are malignant tumours arising from nerve cell elements. They occur in toddlers, frequently with widespread metastases. The most common site of origin of the primary is in the region of the adrenal, but they can arise anywhere. They grow to an enormous size and displace the kidney downwards. They must be distinguished from Wilms' tumours. Occasionally, they secrete catecholamines and elevated levels of vanillylmandelic acid (VMA) are found in the urine. They are treated in a specialised children's hospitals by a combination of surgery and chemotherapy.

Part 3

The bladder
and urethra

10

The bladder: Structure, function and investigations

Structure

In children the bladder may be palpated easily; in adults it cannot be felt unless it is distended because it lies deep behind the symphysis pubis. The bladder in an adult will assume an ovoid shape when full. It is described to have a superior surface, or dome of the bladder, covered by peritoneum, against which lie the loops of small bowel and sigmoid colon. A long tail of urachus tethers the dome to the umbilicus: this is the vestigial remnant of the foetal allantois. Posteriorly, the bladder is separated from the rectum by the fascia of Denonvilliers, which consists of two fused layers of the peritoneum. This forms a remarkable biological barrier, which seems to hinder carcinoma of the bladder or prostate spreading into the rectum, and is a useful plane of cleavage during radical surgery on the prostate (Figure 10.1).

In the male the bladder lies superiorly the prostate gland. The bladder base is related to the seminal vesicles, ampulla of vas and terminal ureters. The bladder neck is fixed to the pelvic fasciae, and its position changes very little in relation to the bladder or rectum. In females, the bladder is related to the anterior wall of the vagina (Figure 10.2). As the bladder becomes distended, it rises, not always in the midline, and it may rarely protrude into the inguinal canal if a hernial defect is present there. As it rises out of the pelvis, the bladder peels the peritoneum from the visceral surface of the anterior abdominal wall, and hence a suprapubic cystotomy can be performed without the fear of entering into the peritoneal cavity, as long as the bladder is full.

The contractile function of the bladder is provided by the detrusor smooth muscle, the fibres of which are not arranged in layers as in the skeletal muscle and the bowel but randomly. Unlike most other viscera, the bladder has no capsule; its muscle lies against fat, connective tissue and a plexus of large pelvic veins. The detrusor muscle is lined by a thin layer of lamina propria on which lies the seven-cell layer thick urothelium (Figure 10.3).

Blood supply

The arteries of the bladder originate from the branches of the internal iliac artery of which the largest, the *superior vesicle artery*, crosses in front of the ureter (Figure 10.4). However, the bladder may be supplied by any adjacent branch of the internal iliac artery including the inferior vesicle artery that also supplies the lower part of the ureter.

Urology Lecture Notes, Seventh Edition. Amir V. Kaisary, Andrew Ballaro and Katharine Pigott.
© 2016 John Wiley & Sons, Ltd. Published 2016 by John Wiley & Sons, Ltd.

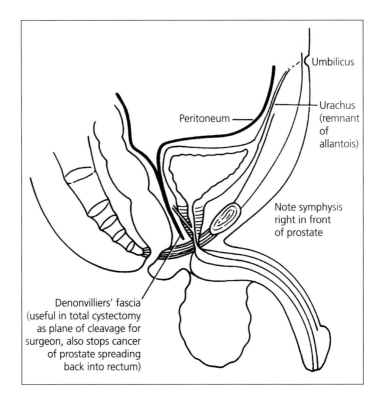

Figure 10.1 Surgical anatomy of the male bladder.

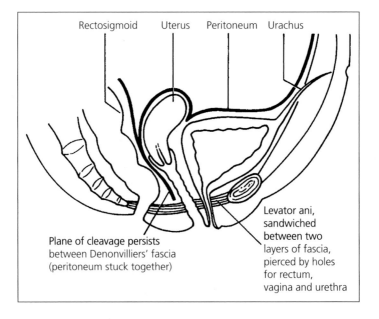

Figure 10.2 Surgical anatomy of the female bladder.

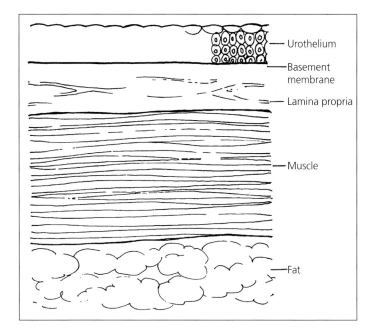

Figure 10.3 Diagram of section through wall of bladder.

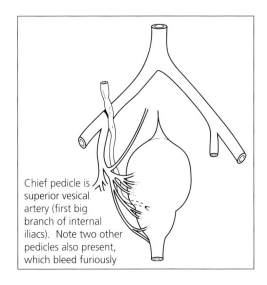

Chief pedicle is superior vesical artery (first big branch of internal iliacs). Note two other pedicles also present, which bleed furiously

Figure 10.4 Blood supply of the bladder.

The veins of the bladder drain into the internal iliac veins, but in addition, a second 'backstairs' system drains into the marrow of the pelvic bones, femora and vertebral bodies. Any increase in intra-abdominal pressure may induce blood to flow from the bladder into the bone marrow, explaining why metastases from cancer of the prostate and bladder are often found there.

The rich network of lymphatics in the deeper layers of the detrusor muscle drains into the lymph nodes of the pelvis. Like the veins, there are also direct communications with the bone marrow of the pelvis, vertebrae and femora.

Nerves of the bladder

The bladder is a fascinating organ. It is one of the few that is under both voluntary and involuntary neurological control. This gives it a unique function and accounts for the complexity of symptoms when things go wrong.

The bladder is supplied by the autonomic nervous system via both the sympathetic and parasympathetic systems. Both sets of nerves carry afferent and efferent fibres. Additionally, the external sphincter is supplied by the somatic nervous system.

Efferent

Parasympathetic system

The parasympathetic innervation originates in the ventral grey matter of the S2–4 segments of the sacral spinal cord. The fibres travel via the pelvic nerves and synapse with ganglia both in the pelvic plexus and within the detrusor muscle itself and excite the bladder causing it to contract and relax the urethral sphincter.

Sympathetic system

The cell bodies are situated in the lateral grey column between T11 and L2 segments of the spinal cord. The fibres travel via the hypogastric plexus and then the pelvic plexus to the bladder neck and internal sphincter area. The thoracolumbar sympathetic nerves inhibit the bladder and excite the bladder neck and urethra.

Somatic

Somatic motor neurons are located along the lateral border of the ventral horn of S2–4 segments in an area known as Onuf's nucleus. They form the pudendal nerve and excite the striated muscle of the external urethral sphincter and pelvic floor muscles.

Afferent

Afferent impulses from the bladder are transmitted by A-delta fibres in the pelvic parasympathetic nerves to the S2–4 segments of the spinal cord. Noxious sensation is transmitted by C fibres. Sensation of *pain* is also conveyed in sympathetic fibres that run via the presacral plexus and lumbar sympathetic ganglia to reach surprisingly high levels in the spinal cord: indeed to block all pain from the bladder, a spinal anaesthetic must reach as high as T6 (Figure 10.5).

The urinary sphincter unit

Internal sphincter

In both sexes there are two sphincteric elements. The internal sphincter at the bladder neck is a continuation of detrusor muscle and is under sympathetic control and involuntary. This actively contracts as part of the ejaculatory reflex preventing retrograde ejaculation. During bladder filling the bladder neck remains closed

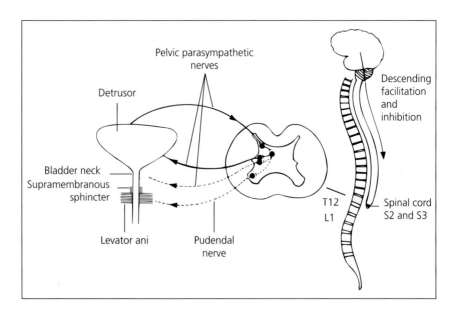

Figure 10.5 Nerve supply of the bladder.

to provide a continence mechanism and in men can maintain continence when the external sphincter is damaged.

External sphincter

In both sexes the external sphincter consists of several parts.

The membranous urethra itself has viscoelastic properties that endow sphincteric function; in addition, it contains a thin smooth muscle layer extending along its length that is under sympathetic control.

Around this is the signet ring-shaped *rhabdosphincter* that consists of slow-twitch skeletal muscle and is under voluntary control. It is situated just distal to the prostate apex around the membranous urethra in men and at the mid-urethra in women and provides the primary continence mechanism by maintaining a constant tone.

The periurethral striated muscles of the *pelvic floor* lie external to the rhabdosphincter, and sphincteric activity can be increased by voluntary contraction of the pelvic floor muscles in both sexes. In females, a hammock-like sling of endo-pelvic fascia within the pelvic floor supports the mid-urethra and plays a crucial additional role in maintaining continence when the mobile urethra is compressed against it and kinks during rises in intra-abdominal pressure.

Bladder function

The function of the urinary bladder is to store the slowly accumulating urine that is continuously produced by the kidneys and to actively void it when socially acceptable to do so. These storage and voiding functions are mutually exclusive and controlled by neural networks, which are influenced by conscious neurological activity to switch between the two states. The bladder spends over 98% of the time in storage mode; the decision to empty it is influenced by the perceived sense of bladder fullness and the social practicality of voiding, a conscious decision. The normal bladder is able to hold up to approximately 350 mL of urine without significant increase in intravesical pressure and a maximum capacity of 4–500 mL.

Neural control of micturition

Central control of micturition occurs in three distinct areas of the central nervous system; the sacral micturition centre is responsible for mediating bladder contraction, the pontine micturition centre acts as a relay and switches the bladder between storage and voiding functions, and the cerebral cortex inhibits the sacral centre and provides conscious input to the pontine centre.

Storage phase

Filling of the bladder stimulates the detrusor *stretch receptors*, which send impulses via the parasympathetic afferent A-delta fibres in the spino-thalamic tract to the pontine micturition centre, and these are then relayed to the higher centres in the brain. If it is not socially acceptable to pass urine, signals are passed back to the sacral micturition centre to inhibit the parasympathetic pathways to the detrusor and stimulate the sympathetic and pudendal pathways to contract the sphincter and bladder neck, thereby preventing involuntary bladder emptying. When the stimulatory signals from the bladder reach threshold intensity and a conscious decision to void has been made, the inhibitory signals from the cortex are withheld and the pontine micturition centre switches from storage to voiding function. The voiding reflex then takes over and is responsible for the coordinated void.

Voiding phase

In voiding mode the pontine micturition centre activates the descending reflex pathways that mediate coordinated pelvic floor and urethral sphincter relaxation via the pudendal nerve and efferent sympathetic pathways to the bladder neck and, a few seconds later, stimulate sacral parasympathetic outflow causing the detrusor muscle to contract. When the bladder has been emptied, first the pelvic floor contracts and then the bladder neck closes (Figure 10.6).

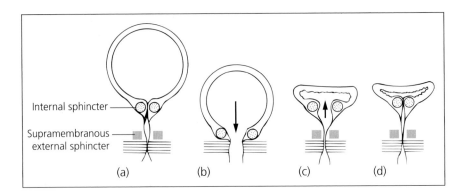

Internal sphincter

Supramembranous external sphincter

(a)   (b)   (c)   (d)

Figure 10.6 Sequence of bladder emptying: (a) full resting bladder, (b) detrusor contraction, (c) milking back and (d) bladder emptying completed.

Bladder investigations

A variety of investigations can be performed for evaluation of bladder dysfunction. These include:

- **Urinalysis**
  A dipstick test of the urine will pick up a number of abnormalities including blood, proteins, nitrites and leucocytes, which might identify urine infection as a cause for voiding dysfunction. It can also pick up glucose, which usually indicates poorly controlled diabetes.
- **Frequency/volume chart**
  A frequency volume chart or bladder dairy is very helpful to quantify the capacity of bladder and evaluate the frequency and nocturia. It also gives insight into fluid intake. This forms the basis for urodynamic studies later on.
- **Flow rate and ultrasound of bladder with and estimation of post-void residue**
  The urinary flow rate is a measure of the quantity of urine excreted over time. The patient voids into a uroflowmetry device and a graph of urine flow of volume per unit time is produced. Analysis of the maximum and average flow rate, the total time and volume of the void and the shape of the flow curve can give insight into the causes of voiding dysfunction. For example, a reduced maximum flow may indicate bladder outflow obstruction or detrusor weakness, a truncated curve suggests a urethral stricture, and multiple peaks may

indicate a straining pattern of voiding. A post-void ultrasound checks for residual urine and the efficacy of bladder emptying and is also part of basic urodynamic evaluation.

In addition to imaging modalities described in Chapter 2, two bladder specific investigations are commonly used in everyday urological practice: pressure-flow urodynamics, which enables investigation of bladder function, and cystoscopy, which allows direct inspection of the bladder lumen. There are in addition uncommonly used investigations sometimes required during evaluation of the neurogenic bladder including urethral pressure profile and pelvic floor electromyography.

Urodynamics

Although some information regarding the bladder storage and voiding functions can be inferred from pre- and post-micturition ultrasound images and urine flow rates, information concerning activity of the detrusor muscle itself can only be attained by cystometry. Urine flow rate is a function of both the detrusor contraction and the bladder outflow resistance; the same flow might be produced by a patient with an obstructed but forcefully contracting bladder as one with a weak but unobstructed bladder and one with no bladder contraction at all but who voids by abdominal straining. The cystometrogram is an invasive test used to quantify objectively the function of the bladder in isolation from other factors. It is an important test in patients with neurogenic bladders and in those with mixed stress and urge incontinence and may also be used to determine the presence of bladder outflow obstruction in patients with mixed storage and voiding lower urinary tract symptoms.

Cystometry

Through a fine catheter, saline at body temperature is slowly run into the bladder while the bladder pressure (Pves) is continually recorded through a second lumen (Figure 10.7). A further catheter is placed inside the rectum and measures the intra-abdominal pressure (Pabd). This is digitally subtracted from the intravesical measurement to give the true detrusor pressure (Pdet) (Figure 10.8). The measurements are made continuously while the bladder is filled and while the patient passes urine into an electronic *flow*

meter, a device that automatically records the flow rate (Qmax) and the volume of urine that has been collected (Vcomp) (Figure 10.9). The flow rate is then equated with the detrusor pressure and compared with a nomogram from which it can be determined whether the bladder is obstructed or not. In addition, analysis of the filling pressures can be used to determine the presence of the involuntary bladder contractions that are characteristic of overactive bladder.

Voiding cysto-urethrography

Standard cystometry can be combined with a video X-ray recording of the *cystogram*, by using dilute contrast medium instead of saline instilled into the bladder. This imaging allows analysis of the bladder neck opening and closing, identification of vesicoureteric reflux during voiding and detrusor sphincter dysynergia (see Chapter 12).

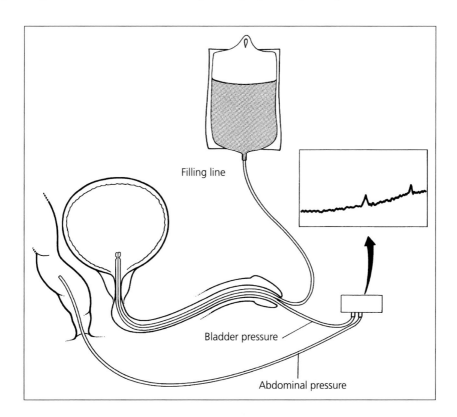

Filling line

Bladder pressure

Abdominal pressure

Figure 10.7 Cystometry.

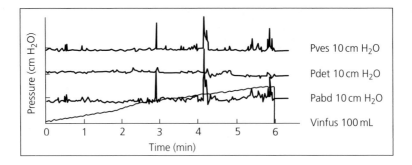

Figure 10.8 Cystometrogram.

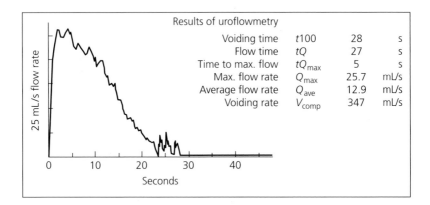

Figure 10.9 Normal uroflow measurement.

Cystoscopy

Flexible cystoscopy

Fine glass fibres are flexible. If made of completely clear optical glass, the light entering one end will undergo total internal refraction and leave from the other (Figure 10.10). A fibre-optic cable comprises a large number of these fibres and when fitted to an appropriate lens and deflecting mechanism can be introduced into any orifice of the body and manipulated within the body to investigate disease and will transmit an image in a series of tiny dots like ground glass (Figure 10.11).

The modern flexible cystoscope has channels for irrigation, for light and for passing flexible instruments such as biopsy forceps, laser fibres or a diathermy electrode. Passing the cystoscope is uncomfortable but usually painless. It is gently

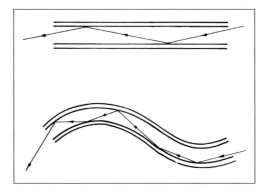

Figure 10.10 Total internal reflection along a glass fibre.

advanced along the urethra under vision as water is slowly run in. After examining the urethra, sphincter, prostatic urethra and bladder neck, the inside of the bladder is carefully

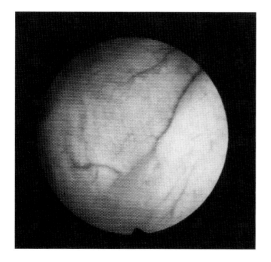

Figure 10.11 Image obtained through flexible cystoscope.

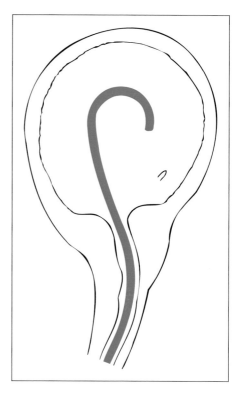

Figure 10.12 The flexible cystoscope can give a view of the trigone and bladder neck.

inspected. By bending the cystoscope back on itself, the bladder neck and prostate can be viewed from the inside (Figure 10.12). Flexible cystoscopy is usually performed in the out-patient clinic/day surgery units and under local anaesthetic using lignocaine gel instilled into the urethra, which is very convenient for the majority of patients and is cost effective.

Rigid cystoscopy

The image seen through the rigid cystoscope is much clearer than that of the flexible instrument, and the instrument channel allows a large variety of instruments to be used inside the bladder (Figure 10.13). Biopsies can be taken, tumour resected, stones crushed and ureters catheterised and examined. It is less comfortable for the patient than the flexible cystoscopy, and general anaesthetic is required. The patient is placed in the lithotomy position (Figure 10.14).

Technological advances are continuously ongoing to improve the characteristics of the instruments to achieve superior visualisation. There has been an introduction of improved camera system with 3D system for improved vision. Using the camera allows projection of the view on large screens, which is valuable in teaching members of staff. It also allows photography and video recording for record keeping and exchange of information.

Electromyography

The activity of the striated muscle of the levator ani can be recorded from small needle electrodes inserted into the muscle. This is not a routine investigation and calls for considerable experience in its use and interpretation. It is sometimes useful during evaluation of the neurogenic bladder (Figure 10.15).

Urethral pressure profile

The pressure inside the lumen of the urethra can be measured with a catheter that is withdrawn at a constant rate along the urethra. The pressure is

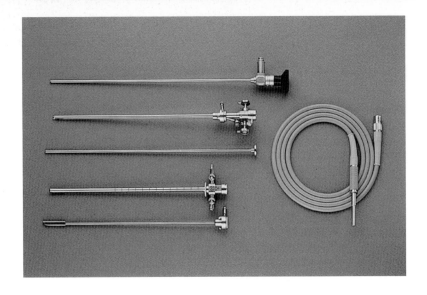

Figure 10.13 Variety of instruments used in modern cystoscopy.

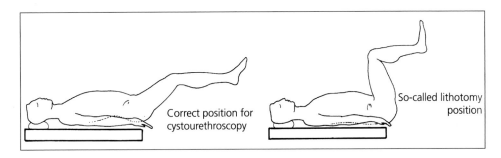

Correct position for cystourethroscopy

So-called lithotomy position

Figure 10.14 Correct position for cystoscopy.

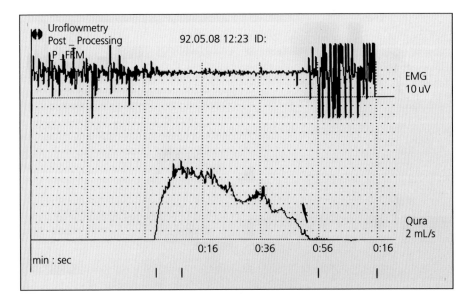

Figure 10.15 Electromyogram from external sphincter during voiding.

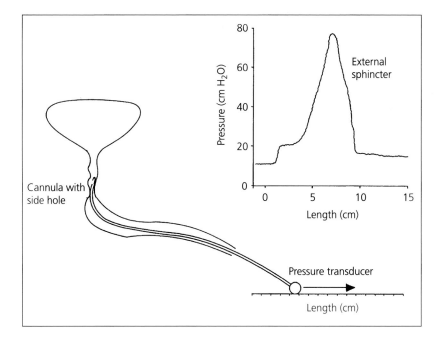

Figure 10.16 Urethral pressure profile.

drawn on a graph, which measures the pressure along the urethra, giving the urethral pressure profile. This is not a routine investigation but is of help in some cases of urinary retention when failure of sphincter function is suspected (Figure 10.16).

11

Bladder infections and inflammation

Lower urinary tract infection

Lower urinary tract infection is the inflammatory response of the urothelium to bacterial invasion and is normally associated with the presence of bacteria (bacteriuria) and inflammatory cells in the urine. The urine is normally sterile and bacteria ascend from the rectal flora. In health there exists a delicate balance between bacterial virulence host defence mechanisms, and any factor that tips this balance in favour of the bacteria may result in infection.

Bacteriuria does not always result in infection and, as an isolated entity, may be asymptomatic. This is illustrated in patients with long-term catheters in whom catheters and urine both rapidly become colonised.

Simple cystitis

Cystitis is the clinical symptom complex of dysuria, urinary frequency, urgency and suprapubic pain. The condition reflects inflammation of the bladder and occurs most commonly as a result of bacterial infection. Inflammation can also result from non-infective causes, the most common of these bladder foreign bodies such as stones or tumours, and inflammation from diseases of surrounding organs such as bowel inflammation and gynaecological infections (Figure 11.1). Drugs such as cyclophosphamide may also cause acute cystitis.

As with upper urinary tract infections, the term 'uncomplicated' refers to an infection in a healthy patient with a structurally normal urinary tract, as opposed to a 'complicated' infection when some host structural or immunological factor increasing the chance of infection is present, or the bacteria exhibit antimicrobial resistance.

In females, acute bacterial cystitis is common and usually innocent. Investigation and prophylactic treatment is required for recurrent infections. Haematuria occurs with the infection in as many as 10% of cases in otherwise healthy woman; this condition is termed haemorrhagic cystitis and should generally be investigated.

In males, bacterial cystitis is more likely to be complicated and may signify an important underlying disorder. It therefore requires investigation with at least urinary tract ultrasound and usually cystoscopy.

Treatment

Uncomplicated bacterial cystitis should be treated for 3 days. A 7-day course of appropriate antimicrobial therapy is recommended in patients who have had symptoms for 1 week or more, those with complicating factors, and in men. Recurrent urinary tract infections due to new infections from bacteria outside the

Urology Lecture Notes, Seventh Edition. Amir V. Kaisary, Andrew Ballaro and Katharine Pigott.
© 2016 John Wiley & Sons, Ltd. Published 2016 by John Wiley & Sons, Ltd.

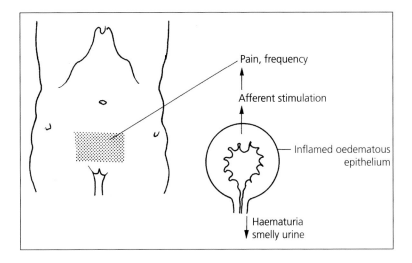

Figure 11.1 Clinical features of cystitis.

urinary tract should be distinguished from causes of bacterial persistence. If no cause is found, host defences may be enhanced by long-term prophylactic antibiotics changing every 3–6 months to reduce the development of bacterial resistance.

Pathogenesis

- Bacterial virulence

  Most urinary tract infections are caused by facultative anaerobes originating from the bowel flora. **Escherichia coli** is by far the most common causing 85% of community-acquired and 50% of nosocomial infections. *Proteus*, *Klebsiella*, coliforms form the remainder. Bacterial virulence factors enhance the pathogenicity of *E. coli* species and enable the bacteria to adhere to vaginal mucosal cells and bladder urothelium and migrate to the bladder where they promote the inflammatory response.

- Host defences

  Variations in the receptiveness of vaginal epithelial cells to bacterial colonisation play an important role particularly in the pathogenesis of recurrent urinary tract infections in women; this trait appears to be partly genetically inherited and is also influenced by the oestrogen status of the woman. The bladder only stays clean if it is emptied regularly

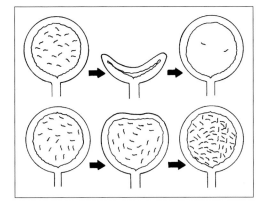

Figure 11.2 The chief defence of the bladder against infection to keep itself regularly emptied out completely.

(Figure 11.2), and any factor that causes incomplete bladder emptying predisposes to infection. These include bladder outflow obstruction, impaired bladder emptying due to detrusor failure or neuropathy and vesicoureteric reflux. Structural abnormalities in the bladder such as stones and tumour may act as a nidus for bacteria to adhere to and evade defence mechanisms. Diabetes may cause infections by several mechanisms; these include glycosuria and bladder dysfunction.

The prevalence of bacteriuria in pregnant women is approximately 5% and of these 25% will suffer pyelonephritis. The clinical severity of this may be enhanced by the temporary high pressures in the upper tracts that occur as a result of increased urine production and compression of the ureter. Prophylactic antibiotics are therefore indicated.

Chronic cystitis

There are several bladder abnormalities that are usually diagnosed on cystoscopy and biopsy that may be classified as chronic cystitis:

- **Follicular cystitis**: Here repeated infections give rise to collections of lymphocytes under the urothelium that can be recognised as pale specks on cystoscopy (Figure 11.3).
- **Cystitis cystica**: This occurs in response to inflammation, groups of cells in the urothelium coalesce to form von Brunn's nests. The central area of the von Brunn's nest degenerates forming little cysts under the mucosa that look like little bubbles on cystoscopy.
- **Cystitis glandularis**: This is similar to cystitis cystica, but the buried cysts of the urothelium undergo metaplasia, secrete mucus and turn into intestinal mucosa – adenomatous metaplasia – which may be the precursor of adenocarcinoma (Figure 11.4).
- **Malacoplakia**: A variation on this is malacoplakia, which forms collections of soft brown lumps in the urothelium that are easily mistaken for cancer.
- **Squamous metaplasia**: Persistent infection, especially when associated with a stricture or schistosomiasis, causes the urothelium to undergo squamous metaplasia. This is very sinister because it often progresses to squamous cell cancer.
- **Alkaline encrusted cystitis**: Infection with *Proteus mirabilis* can lead to a peculiarly disabling condition in which chronic inflammation accompanied by calcification involves the entire wall of the bladder, converting it into a rigid sphere. Cystoscopy shows stony encrustation all over the wall of the bladder. The urine reeks of ammonia.

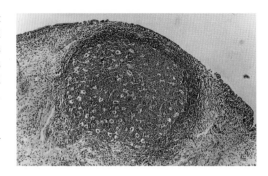

Figure 11.3 Cystitis follicularis.

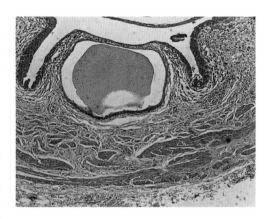

Figure 11.4 Cystitis cystica.

Interstitial cystitis

Interstitial cystitis is a clinical syndrome characterised by urinary frequency and urgency and bladder pain. The cause of this strange condition is still unknown. It occurs more often in middle-aged women and only unusually in men and is a diagnosis of exclusion, that is, can be used when all other causes for the patient's symptoms have been excluded. These include all other causes of bacterial, chemical and radiation cystitis. Interstitial cystitis is associated with abnormalities of the urothelium on cystoscopy; these include the presence of small punctate bleeding points after bladder distension and ulcers (Hunner's ulcer).

The bladder capacity is normally low, less than 150 mL, and biopsy shows chronic inflammation of the urothelium and the underlying submucosa. It has been suggested (but not proved) that an excess of mast cells are present. There is a subgroup of patient in whom there appears to be a defect in the bladder surface glycosaminoglycan layer, with increased urothelial permeability. Some patients respond well to bladder instillations with drugs such as dimethyl sulfoxide (DMSO) and hyaluronic acid directed at restoring this barrier function.

Some patients are improved if the bladder is stretched; others are better if the 'ulcer' is diathermised. The condition usually recurs; rarely the only remedy may be to remove the entire bladder, replacing it with some form of cystoplasty.

Schistosomiasis (bilharziasis)

The trematode flukes *Schistosoma haematobium*, *S. mansoni* and *S. japonicum* are flatworms with a life cycle that involves one stage in a mollusc and another in a vertebrate. The adult flukes are about 5 mm in length and live inside human veins (Figure 11.5). The male enfolds the female in a long slit down his belly – hence the name *schisto* (split) and *soma* (body). They were discovered in the portal vein of children by the German pathologist Theodor Bilharz when he was working in Cairo – hence the alternative name bilharziasis. The females lay eggs with terminal spines that vary according to the species (Figure 11.6).

The adult flukes migrate to the submucosal veins of the bladder where they lay eggs. These, by virtue of the spines, bore their way through the urothelium causing haematuria, bladder ulceration and polyp formation. The dead eggs calcify in the submucosal layers and can be seen on cystoscopy to glisten liken grains of sand under the urothelium. The urothelium undergoes squamous metaplasia in response to the chronic inflammation and eventually may form squamous cell cancer.

A plain X-ray shows the outline of the bladder, lower ureters and vasa deferentia, traced by the millions of dead calcified ova (Figure 11.7). Low-power microscopy of the urine shows the ova.

If the patient urinates into a slow-moving river or irrigation channel, the eggs hatch into the *miracidia* that are attracted to freshwater snails, which they invade. They divide inside the body of the snail and form sporocysts that burst to liberate thousands of minute flukes – *cercariae*. These penetrate the skin of any unwary human whose hand or foot happens to be in the water at the right time. It only takes a few seconds for them to enter the skin (Figure 11.8).

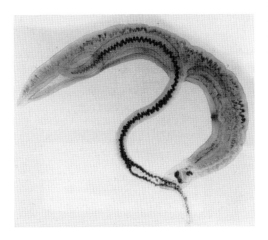

Figure 11.5 *Schistosoma haematobium*: pair of adult worms removed from a vein schistosomes (about 1 cm long).

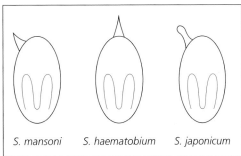

S. mansoni   S. haematobium   S. japonicum

Figure 11.6 Bilharzia ova.

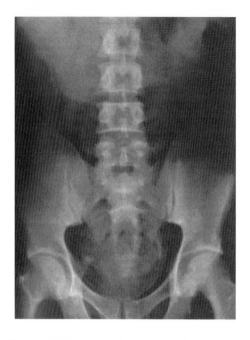

Figure 11.7 Plain X-ray in schistosomiasis showing clarification in the bladder.

Under the skin, the cercariae cause an itching rash – swimmer's itch. Later they reach the circulation through the lymphatics and cause a systemic illness – *Katayama fever*. Finally, adult flukes settle in little veins, which may be anywhere in the body including the brain and spinal cord, and reach the portal circulation and then the bladder. In small children large masses congregate and obstruct the portal vein.

Schistosomiasis is second only to malaria as a cause of disease, and its eradication depends on the provision of clean water and effective disposal of sewage.

Treatment

It is futile to treat infestation if the patient at once returns to work in an infected paddy field. Treatment consists of a single dose of praziquantel that may be repeated after 1 month. Surgical resection of polyps and ulcers may be necessary, and the squamous cell cancer may require

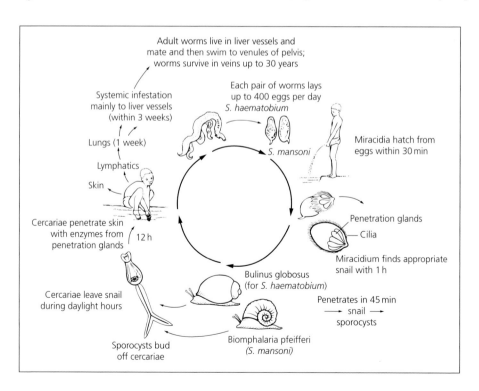

Figure 11.8 Life cycle of *Schistosoma haematobium*.

cystectomy. Obstruction, dilatation and stone formation in the ureters may require appropriate surgery.

Radiation cystitis

Radiation cystitis is a complication of radiotherapy to pelvic tumours. The radiation causes the death of rapidly dividing cells, such as those of the bladder mucosa, and an *endarteritis obliterans* resulting in hypoxia, necrosis and fibrosis of bladder tissue (see Chapter 20). This may lead to ulceration and urothelial damage exposing the submucosa to the caustic effects of urine and perpetuating the chronic inflammation. The condition may present within a year of the radiotherapy with symptoms ranging from mild voiding lower urinary tract symptoms to severe bladder pain and intractable haematuria. Symptoms are usually progressive and in the worse cases may lead to a fibrotic, small capacity and chronically painful bleeding bladder requiring cystectomy.

12

Disorders of bladder function

Disorders of bladder function may affect urine storage or voiding and generate storage or voiding type lower urinary tract symptoms, respectively. The causes may be neurogenic or non-neurogenic.

Overactive bladder syndrome

The overactive bladder syndrome (OAB) is a symptomatic diagnosis defined as urinary urgency with or without urge incontinence usually with frequency and nocturia.

> **Urinary urgency** is the complaint of a sudden compelling desire to pass urine that is difficult to defer.
> **Urge incontinence** is the complaint of involuntary leakage of urine accompanied by or immediately preceded by urgency.
> **Urinary frequency** is the complaint of passing urine too often during the day.

Nocturia is the complaint of having to wake at night one or more times to pass urine.

The OAB syndrome is extremely common, probably affecting up to 10% of the population, and consumes a large proportion of healthcare budgets. It is assumed to be due to *detrusor overactivity*, which is the presence of involuntary detrusor contractions detected during the filling phase of a cystometrogram. However, involuntary detrusor contractions are commonly seen during urodynamic investigation of asymptomatic patients, and OAB symptoms often occur in the absence of demonstrable detrusor contractions. Whether or not these are caused by focal bladder activity of an amplitude too low to be detected is unknown. Sensory disturbances of the bladder due to cancer and stones may cause OAB in the absence of detrusor overactivity due to excitation and possibly sensitisation of bladder afferent nerves.

Detrusor overactivity

Detrusor overactivity may be caused by disruption of the bladder's neurological control when it is termed *neurogenic detrusor overactivity*. Non-neurogenic causes of detrusor overactivity include sensory stimulation and bladder changes that occur in response to bladder outflow obstruction. When there is no identifiable cause, detrusor overactivity is termed *idiopathic*.

There are two types of overactive detrusor contraction:

1. *Phasic* contractions characterised by low-amplitude, frequent and probably focal detrusor contractions that usually cause urgency and may cause urge incontinence

Urology Lecture Notes, Seventh Edition. Amir V. Kaisary, Andrew Ballaro and Katharine Pigott.
© 2016 John Wiley & Sons, Ltd. Published 2016 by John Wiley & Sons, Ltd.

2. *Terminal* contractions that occur when the bladder is full and usually result in involuntary bladder emptying

Idiopathic detrusor overactivity

Several mechanisms for idiopathic detrusor overactivity have been proposed; most supportive evidence exists for a detrusor myopathy involving increased spontaneous detrusor activity and its abnormal propagation throughout the bladder and changes in parasympathetic neuromuscular transmission. These changes may be associated with the bladder ultrastructural changes that occur in response to age or hormonal influences.

Management

Conservative

The initial management includes fluid evaluation with cutting back on caffeinated beverages and fizzy drinks, as these may stimulate the detrusor muscle directly. It also includes life style changes and pelvic floor exercises.

Bladder training involves teaching the patient to void at fixed intervals with the intention that the bladder is emptied before the onset of urgency or incontinence. These intervals are then gradually increased.

Pharmacological

The smooth muscle of the detrusor is activated by cholinergic neurotransmission. The smooth muscles of the sphincters are alpha-adrenergic (Figure 12.1).

Anticholinergics (oxybutynin, tolterodine, solifenacin and fesoterodine) are the mainstay in the treatment of OAB. They are effective in about 50–70% cases. However, they give side effects mainly dryness of the mouth, blurring of the vision and constipation, and many patients stop them in less than a year.

Beta-adrenergic agonists (mirabegron) are the newly developed medication for the control of OAB symptoms. Instead of blocking the release of acetylcholine, this medication acts on beta-receptors and leads to relaxation of the detrusor muscle.

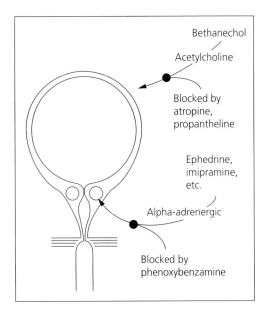

Figure 12.1 Action of drugs on the bladder.

Interventional

Botulinum toxin A therapy

Botulinum toxin A therapy has now been recognised as an established therapy for the treatment of OAB symptoms secondary to both neurogenic and idiopathic bladders. It is performed under local anaesthesia as a day case. One hundred units are injected mixed with 20 mL of normal saline at 20 sites in the bladder sparing the trigone (Figure 12.2). The effects are temporary lasting on an average of 9 months. The main drawback is the need for self-catheterisation in about 10% of patients.

Sacral neuromodulation

Neuromodulation is the process in which the influence of activity in one neural pathway modulates the pre-existing activity in another pathway through synaptic interactions. A small device is surgically implanted in the buttocks about the size of a stopwatch (Figure 12.3). This stimulates the appropriate nerves by using mild or moderate electrical impulses. This can help restore coordination between brain, pelvic floor, bladder or bowel and sphincter muscles. The procedure is performed in two stages. The first is the test

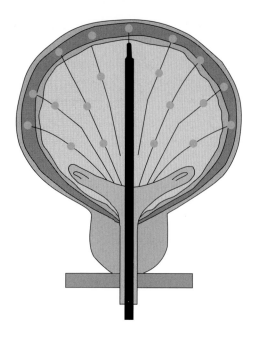

Figure 12.2 Schematic diagram of botulinum toxin A injections into the bladder.

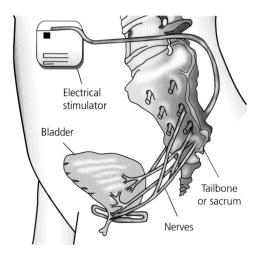

Electrical stimulator

Bladder

Tailbone or sacrum

Nerves

Figure 12.3 A sacral neurostimulator.

implant and if successful the permanent implant is performed with the wire at the S3 nerve roots and the transmitter box in the buttock area. The battery life is 7 years. The success rate for test implant is 70%, while for permanent it is close to 80%. It is a minimally invasive procedure.

Neurogenic detrusor overactivity and neurogenic bladder dysfunction in general

Disruption of the bladder's neural control may occur at any point along its axis. The effects on bladder function and symptoms are varied and subject to plasticity and include both detrusor overactivity and detrusor failure but as a simplified model can be predicted according to the location of the insult.

Lesions above the brain stem

Neurologic lesions above the brainstem that affect micturition usually cause detrusor overactivity with coordinated sphincter function. Dementia is often associated with incontinence in the elderly; this is multifactorial but contributed to loss of conscious inhibitory influences on the pontine micturition centre (see the following text). Cerebrovascular accidents and tumours involving the frontal cortex also cause storage symptoms and incontinence by the same mechanism.

Brain stem lesions

The effect of Parkinson's disease on bladder control mechanisms is complex and varied. Patients usually present with storage lower urinary tract symptoms including urge incontinence; however, they are often elderly men in whom bladder outflow obstruction is also common, and this should be excluded first. In the presence of severe lower urinary tract and only mild Parkinsonian symptoms, multiple system atrophy (MSA) should be suspected instead of Parkinson's disease. This is a motor neurone degenerative disease and causes a denervated weak bladder that is also overactive and a denervated weak urinary sphincter resulting in incontinence.

Investigation of patients with lower urinary tract symptoms and suspected Parkinson's disease or MSA should include urodynamics. If there is convincing evidence of bladder outflow obstruction, outflow tract surgery will help; however, results are unpredictable and, particularly in the case of MSA, may worsen the situation by decreasing bladder outflow tract resistance proximal to a weakened sphincter, thereby exacerbating urge incontinence.

Lesions of the spinal cord

Spinal cord trauma

After spinal cord trauma there is a period of *spinal shock* during which the bladder becomes acontractile. It empties by overflowing, and this short-lived phase is managed by catheterisation. After a few weeks the bladder begins to show signs of activity, and the end-stage clinical picture begins to emerge. This can vary enormously; however, it can be predicted to some extent and simplified according to the location of the spinal lesion.

Supra-sacral cord trauma

Normal voiding depends upon coordinated nervous activity being transmitted from the pons to the sacral micturition centre through the spinal cord, mediating relaxation of the sphincter and contraction of the detrusor at the same time. Disruption of the spinal cord results in coordination between these two actions being lost and also separates the sacral micturition centre from central inhibitory signals. This results in neurogenic detrusor overactivity and involuntary bladder contractions against a closed sphincter without sensation (Figure 12.4); this is termed *detrusor sphincter dysynergia* (DSD). The intravesical pressure rises and the bladder becomes trabeculated and loses compliance and obstructive uropathy usually

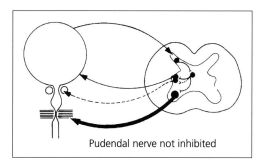

Pudendal nerve not inhibited

Figure 12.4 Failure of the external sphincter to relax when the detrusor contracts.

results. Incontinence may result from detrusor overactivity, but the sphincter dysfunction may also cause urinary retention.

Long-term management options for supra-sacral cord injury

Management of the supra-sacral spinal cord injury is directed at protecting the upper tracts from the effects of a high-pressure bladder and DSD and minimising incontinence. There are a number of treatment options available. The choice of these depends on the physical ability of the patient and his/her desires and needs and should be discussed in a multidisciplinary setting. These include:

1. ***Intermittent self-catheterisation***: The patient learns to pass a catheter regularly to keep the bladder empty. Unfortunately, with some high spinal cord lesions, the detrusor may contract spontaneously even when the bladder is almost empty, so that the patient is wet, and a dangerously high pressure may still be generated inside the bladder. All options are coupled with anticholinergic medications to decrease bladder pressures.

2. ***Sphincterotomy***: The three parts of the sphincter in the male may be divided surgically, in the hope that the bladder will empty at a less than dangerously high pressure. Sometimes sphincterotomy of the bladder neck is enough to allow the patient to remain dry. More often it is necessary to divide the supramembranous and external sphincters as well.

3. ***Botulinum toxin type A therapy***: Botulinum toxin A therapy is now licensed for use in neurogenic detrusor overactivity patients. A dose of 200 U is mixed with 30 mL of saline and injected at 30 sites sparing trigone. The results are excellent and repeated injections are equally effective.

4. ***Augmentation (clam) cystoplasty***: When there is a very high pressure inside the bladder, an operation may be performed that opens it (like a clam), and a patch of detubularised ileum is isolated, sewn into the gap (Figure 12.5). When the detrusor contracts, the patch of bowel balloons out and the pressure

does not rise. This protects the kidneys. In some cases, with the assistance of a partial sphincterotomy, continence can be preserved. In others, the patient may still have to empty the bladder by intermittent clean self-catheterisation.

5. ***Nerve root division and stimulation***: The afferent nerve roots to S2 and S3 may be divided, and the efferent nerve roots may be fitted with stimulators that enable the bladder to contract at will (Figure 12.6).

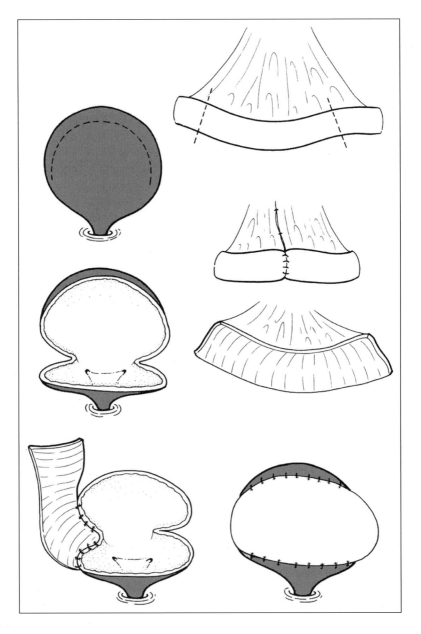

Figure 12.5 Clam cystoplasty.

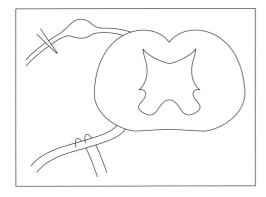

Figure 12.6 Nerve root division and stimulation.

6. ***Urinary diversion***: Unfortunately many patients, particularly those with weakness of the upper limbs, or who are confined to a wheelchair, are not able to practise intermittent clean self-catheterisation. For them an ileal conduit or a form of continent diversion may be the most appropriate solution.

7. ***Suprapubic catheters (SPC)***: Those patients who cannot self-catheterise and do want to undergo sphincterotomy can have SPC. This can lead to problems of its own including infections, blockages, need for regular changes and a small risk of developing malignancy. However, it is easy to use and patients generally find it quite convenient.

Non-traumatic supra-sacral cord lesions

A variety of neurological conditions affect the spinal cord and may disrupt normal bladder function. The most common of these is multiple sclerosis. This is a progressive, relapsing and remitting autoimmune inflammatory disease of the central nervous system characterised by demyelination and spinal cord plaque deposition. The neurological consequences are diverse; the most common bladder abnormality seen is neurogenic detrusor overactivity. Even in advanced disease, DSD and upper tract obstruction are not usually a feature, and management is directed at symptom control.

Sacral spinal cord trauma

Patients with injuries to the spinal cord or nerve roots below the S2 level generally develop detrusor areflexia (failure of contraction). The parasympathetic fibres from the cord synapse at ganglia within the detrusor muscle itself, so the bladder is decentralised with the loss of autonomic reflexes but not completely denervated. The sphincter may maintain tone but may lose voluntary control. The bladder is atonic and the sensation of fullness associated with bladder filling is lost. It leaks when full with no sensation. Obstructive nephropathy does not occur, nor generally does detrusor overactivity, and the bladder may still be voluntarily emptied either by straining (Valsalva) or manual extravesical pressure (Figure 12.7).

To show whether the sacral nerves are intact, there are three useful tests:

1. ***The bulbospongiosus reflex***: Pinch the glans penis and feel for a contraction of the bulbospongiosus muscle (Figure 12.8).
2. ***Cystometrogram***: The return of detrusor contractions means that the reflux arc must be intact.
3. ***Electromyography of the levator ani***: When the S2 and S3 segments are destroyed, there are no action potentials in the levator ani.

Long-term management options for sacral cord injury

Management of the sacral cord injury is directed at restoring continence and socially acceptable bladder emptying:

1. ***Suprapubic compression***: This may raise the pressure inside the bladder, and many patients can void using this technique. Emptying may be incomplete, however, and infection can develop in the residual urine.
2. ***Intermittent self-catheterisation***: The patient learns to pass a catheter regularly to keep the bladder empty.
3. ***SPC***: For patients who don't want to utilise the first two options and cannot empty the bladders, an SPC can be fitted. However, this can cause problems including blockages, stone formation and recurrent urinary tract infections.

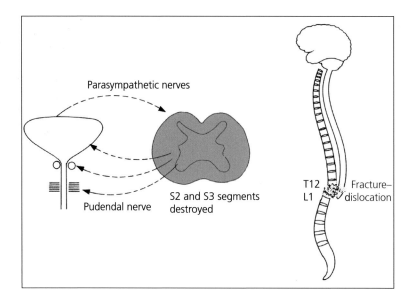

Figure 12.7 Destruction of the S2 and S3 segments, for example, by fracture.

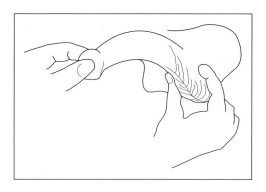

Figure 12.8 Bulbospongiosus reflex.

Importantly, patients have to be warned of a small but definite risk of developing cancer due to chronic irritation.

4. ***Artificial urinary sphincter (AUS)***: If urinary leakage due to sphincter weakness is a problem, then these patients can be fitted with an AUS. However, the results in spinal cord injury patients are not as good as after post-prostatectomy incontinence. There is an increased risk of the sphincter eroding due to the patient sitting on the wheelchair leading to constant pressure on the cuff.

Cauda equina syndrome

In addition to trauma, the cauda equina may be involved in a number of pathological processes causing a combination of slow progressive loss of bladder sensation and overflow incontinence. The most common cause is compression by a central prolapse of a lumbar intervertebral disc typically the T12–L1 disc, as the sacral segments of the cord are at the level of the L1 and 2 vertebral bodies. In addition to bladder symptoms, there is severe lower back pain radiating along the affected nerve root distributions, 'saddle' paraesthesia in the perianal area of the S2–4

Summary box: Spinal cord trauma

Initially there is spinal shock during which there is no bladder or activity and overflow incontinence.

Supra-sacral lesions generally cause detrusor overactivity with sphincter dysynergia.

Sacral cord and peripheral nerve lesions generally cause detrusor areflexia with various types of sphincter dysfunction, usually with some tone but loss of voluntary control.

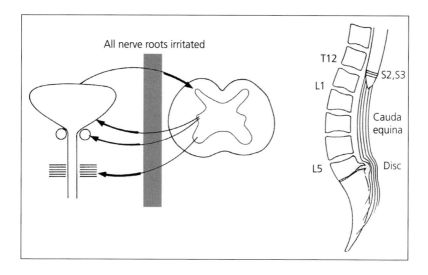

All nerve roots irritated

T12

S2,S3

L1

Cauda equina

L5

Disc

Figure 12.9 Cauda equina lesion irritating afferent and efferent limbs of the reflex arc.

dermatomes and lower limb motor weakness and sensory disturbance to the lateral aspect of both feet. This is a neurosurgical emergency as permanent neurological dysfunction may be prevented by prompt relief of the compression (Figure 12.9).

Lesions of pelvic nerves

The pelvic parasympathetic nerves may be torn in *fractures* of the pelvis and damaged in the course of *radical surgery* for cancer. The incidence of bladder dysfunction after operations for low rectal tumours is as high as 15%, and parasympathetic nerves may be damaged during dissection and also by traction injury during exposure of the rectum as they run close to the rectum. Damage to these nerves causes loss of bladder sensation, painless urinary retention and a poor urinary stream. Damage to the nerves to the urethral sphincter may occur during radical prostatectomy and results in various degrees of incontinence.

Generally, the results of lesions of the bladder's peripheral nerves are similar to that of sacral cord injury with detrusor areflexia and a weak sphincter that is difficult to relax voluntarily.

Diabetic cystopathy

Diabetic cystopathy occurs as a result of neuropathy of both the bladder's sensory and motor innervation. It is a feature of advanced diabetes and there is nearly always evidence of a generalised sensory neuropathy. There is a slow and progressive loss of bladder sensation and contractility resulting in failure of bladder emptying and low-pressure chronic urinary retention. Overactive bladder contractions may also occur, probably due to direct bladder effects of the large residual urine volume and its complications.

Non-neurogenic detrusor overactivity

Bladder dysfunction associated with obstruction

Whether the cause is neuropathic failure of the urinary sphincters to relax in harmony with the contraction of the detrusor (DSD), obstruction by enlargement of the prostate or a stricture of the urethra, the detrusor may respond to chronic obstruction in two contrasting ways. Which response occurs may be determined by the degree and speed of onset of the obstruction and the underlying state of the detrusor muscle, which in turn is related to its age:

- ***Detrusor overactivity***: The detrusor may respond to the demand for a stronger contraction by an increase in the size and strength of its smooth muscle fibres and a coarsening of the connective tissue matrix in which they arranged – this causes bladder trabeculation (Figure 12.10). The urothelium begins to bulge out through the gaps in the matrix forming saccules, which eventually balloon outside the bladder as diverticula. During this phase of compensatory hypertrophy, overactive detrusor contractions occur generating high intravesical pressures and sometimes lead to incontinence of urine.

Detrusor overactivity caused by obstruction in adults resolves about half of the time after relief of the obstruction within 6 months. Until then it may be expressed as incontinence. The mechanism of obstruction-related detrusor overactivity is thought to be increased excitability of detrusor cells caused by a functional denervation due to detrusor structural changes.

- ***Detrusor failure***: In some patients with bladder outflow obstruction, the detrusor muscle fibres do not hypertrophy and strengthen but fail instead of emptying the bladder completely; this slowly permits the quantity of residual urine after voiding to increase causing chronic urinary retention. The time comes when detrusor contractions disappear entirely. The urinary flow is reduced

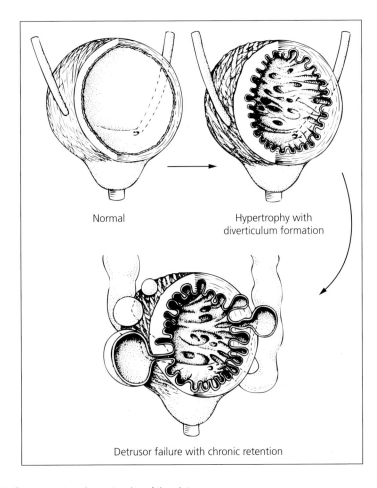

Normal

Hypertrophy with diverticulum formation

Detrusor failure with chronic retention

Figure 12.10 Compensatory hypertrophy of the detrusor.

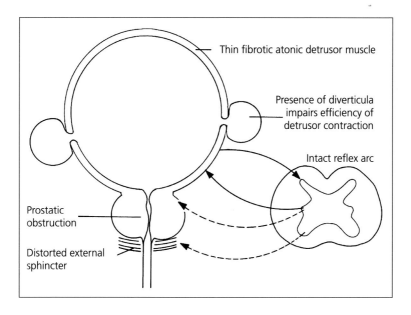

Figure 12.11 Detrusor failure.

to a trickle, and then the pressure in the bladder can only be increased by abdominal straining or coughing. Before long the huge floppy bladder dribbles without control – *retention with overflow* (Figure 12.11). Such a bladder never recovers its normal function even with prolonged drainage and removal of the obstruction. The residual urine easily becomes infected. Stones may develop.

Excess bladder sensory stimulation

Anything that stimulates the lining of the bladder may increase afferent nerve activity and lead to overactive detrusor contractions before the bladder is full (Figure 12.12), for example, a stone, infection or carcinoma. At its worst the patient may be unable to inhibit this contraction, and there is *urge incontinence*. Urodynamic studies will show uninhibited detrusor contractions, a normal flow rate, normal sphincters but a small voided volume.

Excessive central facilitation

Every examination candidate knows that anxiety can cause frequency (Figure 12.13). In major anxiety states, frequency and even urge incontinence

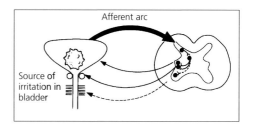

Figure 12.12 Overstimulation of the afferent arm of the micturition reflex.

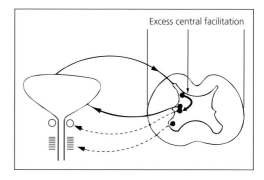

Figure 12.13 Excessive central facilitation.

are common and can make life intolerable. As a general rule this type of frequency only occurs in the daytime, in contrast to the frequency caused by irritation of the urothelium.

Non-neurogenic neurogenic bladder (Hinman syndrome)

This is a condition characterised by functional bladder outlet obstruction. It presents in late childhood or adulthood with urinary urgency and urge incontinence with hesitancy and having to strain to void. It is thought to arise in childhood from psychosocial disorders and half of patients have a history of family violence. It is thought that during toilet training, affected children voluntarily contract the external sphincter to prevent incontinence, and this results in sphincter hypertrophy and bladder changes as a result of the obstruction. These bladder changes include hypertrophy and trabeculation with obstruction of the ureters at the uretero-vesical junction and obstructive uropathy and nephropathy. The clinical picture therefore can mimic neurogenic overactive bladder.

 KEYPOINTS

Overactive bladder and detrusor overactivity
Overactive bladder syndrome is a symptomatic diagnosis and may or may not be associated with detrusor overactivity.
Detrusor overactivity is an urodynamic diagnosis based on the presence of involuntary detrusor contractions.
Detrusor overactivity may be due to **neurogenic**, **non-neurogenic** or unknown causes when it is termed **idiopathic**.
Neurogenic detrusor overactivity is caused by disruption of the bladder's neurological control, generally supra-sacral lesions.
Idiopathic detrusor overactivity is very common and accounts for a large proportion of healthcare budgets.
Non-neurogenic detrusor overactivity may be caused by direct bladder stimulation, sensitisation of sensory bladder nerves and structural changes resulting from anatomical and functional outflow obstruction.

Incontinence

Incontinence is the complaint of any involuntary loss of urine (see Chapter 1). The causes are summarised below.

Causes of incontinence

1. Continuous:
   Complete sphincter disruption
   Vesico- or uretero-vaginal fistula
   Ectopic ureter insertion if present from birth
2. Intermittent:
   Urge incontinence
   Detrusor overactivity
   Impaired detrusor compliance (e.g. radiation cystitis)
3. Stress incontinence:
   Intrinsic sphincter deficiency
   Failure of urethral support mechanisms

The cause of urge incontinence is generally detrusor overactivity. Stress urinary incontinence is caused by deficiency of either the sphincter mechanisms or the urethral support mechanisms.

Stress urinary incontinence

Males

In men, stress urinary incontinence is caused by damage to the urinary sphincter mechanism; this occurs due to direct trauma or neurological injury:

- *Prostatectomy*: The bladder neck is removed as a deliberate art of the operation of transurethral resection for benign enlargement of the prostate and radical prostatectomy for cancer. Sometimes the supramembranous component of the external sphincter is cut by accident during transurethral resection (Figure 12.14).
- *Fractured pelvis*: The sphincters may be injured if the bladder neck is lacerated by a fracture of the pelvis, or if the fracture ruptures the presacral sympathetic nerves.
- *Cancer of the prostate*: Prostatic cancer may infiltrate the sphincters causing them to lie permanently stiff and half-open.

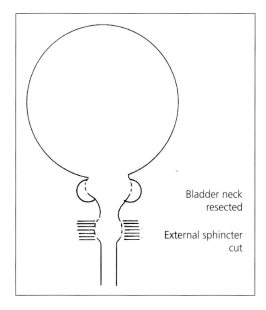

Figure 12.14 Incontinence following division of both sphincters.

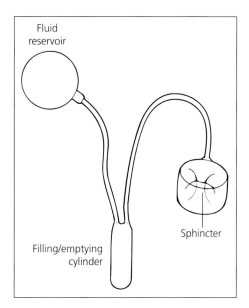

Figure 12.15 Brantley–Scott artificial sphincter.

Treatment of genuine stress incontinence in males

1. **Pelvic floor exercises** – When the lesion is minor, the external sphincter may be strengthened by active exercise.
2. **Indwelling catheters** – In an unfit patient a catheter might keep the patient dry although it can bring problems of its own, that is, blockages, stone formation and urine infections.
3. **Penile sheaths** – Some patients might use the contained continent technique with the use of penile sheath and an attached catheter. It does not have problems of an indwelling catheter but might slip off the penis. Occasionally, it is difficult to fit a sheath due to problems with penile length.
4. **AUS** – However, the most definite way of restoring urinary continence is by the artificial sphincter. A thin silicone balloon shaped like a doughnut is placed round the urethra and connected to a reservoir that can be emptied or filled by a bulb placed under the skin where the patient can compress it. It has been shown to work well over the years although there can be problems with mechanical fail-

ure, infection and erosion into the urethra (Figure 12.15).
5. **Male slings** – These have been gaining popularity in recent years as minimally invasive options for treatment of mild to moderate incontinence in male patients. The initial results are encouraging, but patient selection is the key to success (Figure 12.16).
6. **Bulking agents** – In men with partially functioning sphincters, a number of bulking agents, such as Macroplastique, can be injected into the submucosal layer of the urethra at the sphincter area to increase its size and efficacy (Figure 12.17).

Females

In women there is a short length of urethra above the levator ani shelf, and the urethra rests on a hammock-like musculofascial layer (Chapter 10). When she coughs, the abdominal pressure compresses the urethra against this supporting structure helping to prevent the sharp rises in intravesical pressure causing urine loss. This urethral support mechanism can be damaged by a

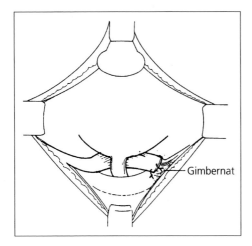

Figure 12.16 Male sling operation.

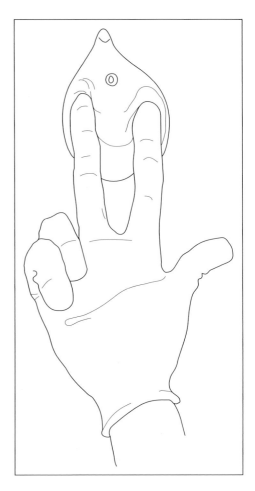

Figure 12.18 Marshall's test.

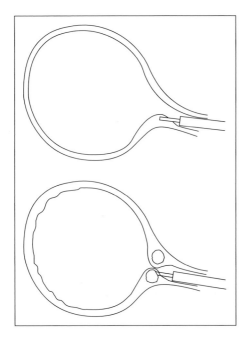

Figure 12.17 Injections of Teflon or collagen paste around the bladder neck.

number of conditions including pelvic radiotherapy and surgery; the most prevalent insult however is childbirth and vaginal delivery.

In addition to causing injury to the fascial support layer of the pelvic floor, vaginal delivery, particularly a prolonged second stage of labour, may cause pressure damage to the pelvic nerves innervating the pelvic floor musculature and external striated sphincter resulting in intrinsic sphincter deficiency.

Clinical examination

In genuine stress incontinence (GSI) there is a leakage of urine when the patient coughs on urodynamics. This can be prevented by lifting up the anterior wall of the vagina with a finger on either side of the urethra (Bonney's or Marshall's test). The test should be done with the patient standing upright (Figure 12.18).

Urodynamics

Because a similar escape of urine is seen in idiopathic detrusor overactivity, these patients need urodynamic testing to rule it out before they are accepted as having GSI.

Treatment of GSI in females

Pelvic floor physiotherapy

This aims to strengthen the pelvic floor musculature and restore urethral support mechanisms. It is effective in most women with mild stress incontinence and should be the first treatment option in all but the completely incontinent patient.

Pharmacological treatments

Duloxetine inhibits the reuptake of noradrenaline and serotonin and has been used to treat stress incontinence; the mechanism is the enhancement of the pudendal nerve activity at the Onuf's nucleus in the sacral spinal cord.

Surgical procedures

1. *Bulking agents*: Various substances have been injected around the bladder neck to give bulk to the tissue around the bladder neck and sphincter. A suspension of Teflon was the first but was given up when it was discovered that the material goes into the brain of experimental animals. Collagen paste and suspensions of the patient's own fat have been used but now abandoned as the results are unsatisfactory. Currently, silicone-based materials are used with some success in cases unfit for other types of procedures.
2. *Burch colposuspension*: This is the classical and most reliable procedure, which has been 'invented' by several surgeons. Essentially, stitches are placed into the vaginal wall on either side of the urethra and then through the pectineal fascia recreating the vesico-urethral angle (Figure 12.19). This procedure has stood the test of time, and most new procedures are evaluated against this standard.
3. *Sling operations*: Stamey sutures were introduced in the past aiming at lifting the bladder neck and support it via inserting the sutures in the vaginal cornu (Figure 12.20). A plethora of

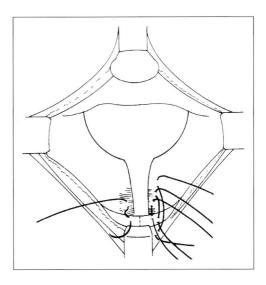

Figure 12.19 Burch colposuspension.

modifications have since then been introduced utilising either synthetic mesh or autologous material to lift up the bladder neck. The most commonly performed sling procedures for incontinence are now the tension-free vaginal tape (TVT) and the tension-free obturator tape (TOT). As a minimally invasive procedure, it is popular and the medium-term results are good. Sometimes synthetic mesh may erode through the urethra or bladder and acts as a nidus for stone formation and has to be removed.

4. *AUS*: In women this is reserved for patients with demonstrated intrinsic sphincter deficiency.

Incontinence associated with extremes of age

This is a common problem that can put a lot of pressure on families and carers.

Children

Babies, like puppies and kittens, have to learn to inhibit the reflex emptying of the full bladder until socially convenient. In some children this learning process is delayed resulting in daytime incontinence.

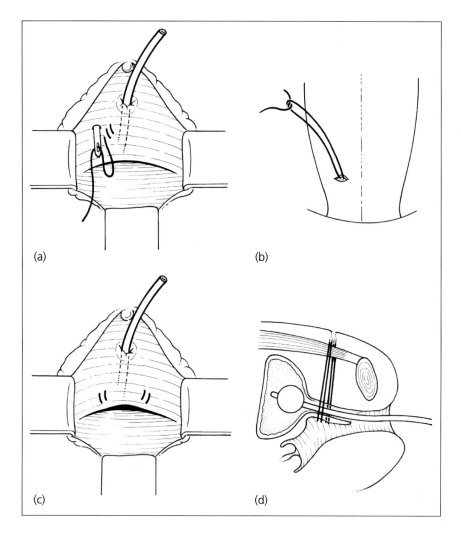

(a)

(b)

(c)

(d)

Figure 12.20 Stamey sutures (a, b, c and d are sequential surgery steps).

Nocturnal enuresis

Many children who wet the bed seem to sleep unusually deeply. In practice it is difficult to know how far to investigate an otherwise normal child, since bed-wetting is considered normal up to the age of 5 or 6, and every year thereafter the percentage of children that continue to bed wet declines by around 15%. Pathological bed-wetting has a multifactorial aetiology including detrusor overactivity and sleep arousal disorder.

The urine should always be tested to exclude infection. Treatment exploits three principles:

1. A small dose of pituitary antidiuretic hormone is given (desmopressin 5–20 µg at bedtime).
2. Imipramine may work by lightening sleep, or by soothing the detrusor.
3. A buzzer that sounds when soaked with urine may establish a conditioned reflex provided the child is woken up and taken to the lavatory.

Elderly

Incontinence in the institutionalised elderly is multifactorial. In addition to the effect of dementia on voluntary inhibition of the micturition reflex, contractility of the detrusor deteriorates with age resulting in chronic urinary retention. The ageing bladder also develops specific ultrastructural abnormalities leading to detrusor overactivity, and it is therefore common to see elderly patients with urinary urgency and urge incontinence with large residual urine volumes in the absence of bladder outflow obstruction. Chronic urinary retention may predispose to recurrent urinary tract infections and stone formation, which in turn may cause incontinence by direct bladder stimulation. Incontinence may also be exacerbated by poor mobility and constipation.

The management of the incontinent elderly person is therefore complex and difficult, particularly if the patient is a poor historian, and management involves identifying and treating reversible underlying causes and containing

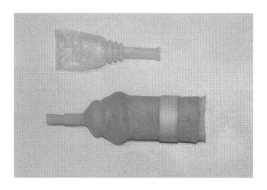

Figure 12.21 Condom urinal.

the leakage in as socially acceptable and comfortable way as possible. For men a condom urinal may keep him dry and comfortable (Figure 12.21).

13

Bladder cancer

Bladder cancer accounts for 3% of all new cancer diagnosis and 3% of cancer deaths in the United Kingdom. It is nearly three times more common in men than in women; however women suffer a worse prognosis, and the incidence and mortality increase with age. Because the bladder is lined entirely by transitional cell urothelium, its neoplasms are nearly always transitional cell carcinomas, but if urothelium undergoes metaplasia into squamous or glandular epithelium (as happens with prolonged irritation or infection), then squamous cell cancer and adenocarcinoma can occur. Secondary cancer is sometimes seen from direct invasion from a primary tumour in the colon, rectum or uterus.

In 1894 Rehn noticed that workers in the aniline dye industry were developing an unduly large number of cancers of the bladder. Hueper subsequently showed that the cause was neither aniline nor the finished dyestuffs, but a group of intermediate nitrophenols (Figure 13.1) of which the most dangerous were β-naphthylamine and benzidine. These substances were also present in tobacco smoke and other industries including rubber moulding and the coal gas industry. Men and women thought to be at risk, for example, who worked in the chemical and rubber industry before the carcinogens were eliminated, have their urine screened annually for malignant cells. All these industries have now eliminated these chemicals from their factories, but tobacco smoking continues to be the major hazard. In other parts of the world, the prolonged irritation of the urothelium by schistosomiasis continues to be a major cause of squamous cell carcinoma, added to by tobacco smoking. A diet rich in fruits and vegetables seems to be protective against bladder cancer formation.

Clinical features

Symptoms

- *Painless haematuria*. More than 80% of patients with bladder cancer present with haematuria (Figure 13.2), which is the reason why every patient with haematuria should undergo cystoscopy. The remaining 20% may have other symptoms; bladder cancer is quite often found incidentally on abdominal imaging.
- *'Cystitis' with sterile pyuria*. The urothelium around a bladder tumour is often inflamed, and the patient may have frequency and pain on voiding, just like bacterial ordinary cystitis. The clue is to find pus cells in the urine on microscopy, but no microorganisms in culture that is termed sterile pyuria and may indicate urothelial cancer and also tuberculosis.
- *Lower urinary tract symptoms*. Most bladder cancers occur in the elderly, in whom lower

Urology Lecture Notes, Seventh Edition. Amir V. Kaisary, Andrew Ballaro and Katharine Pigott.
© 2016 John Wiley & Sons, Ltd. Published 2016 by John Wiley & Sons, Ltd.

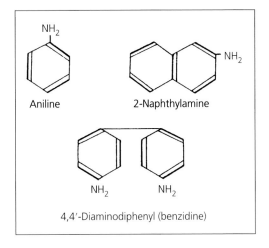

Figure 13.1 Aniline and its carcinogenic relatives.

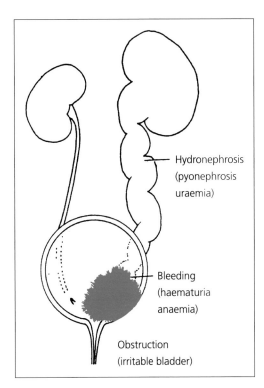

Figure 13.2 Clinical features of bladder cancer.

urinary tract symptoms are common. Bladder cancer may itself cause bladder storage symptoms, and their presence in the absence of voiding symptoms, or their persistence

after other causes are treated, should prompt investigation with a flexible cystoscopy. It is partially for this reason that all men presenting with lower urinary tract symptoms should undergo urine dipstick testing.

- *Anaemia.* Continued loss of blood in the urine may uncommonly bring a patient to the doctor with anaemia; they usually present with haematuria first however.
- *Urinary infection.* Infection occurring for no obvious reason in an elderly patient, particularly a heavy smoker, should be regarded with suspicion: it may be arising in the necrotic superficial part of a solid tumour.
- *Pain.* This usually means that the cancer has invaded outside the bladder.

Physical signs

There are usually none, except in the rare tumour that arises from the urachus (this is an adenocarcinoma), when a mass may be felt between the symphysis and the umbilicus. Otherwise if a mass can be felt, it signifies gross extravesical extension of the cancer. As with any advanced pelvic malignancy, a large bladder tumour can present with lower limb oedema due to venous and lymphatic obstruction.

Investigations

- Imaging required to investigate haematuria is discussed in Chapter 2.
- **Urine cytology**
  The cytological diagnosis of cancer depends on recognising large multinucleated malignant cells in the urine (Figure 13.3). Automated *flow cytometry* measures the nuclear/cytoplasm ratio in large numbers of cells, thus avoiding observer error. If the tumour is grade 1 (well differentiated), the cells may go unrecognised unless by chance a broken-off frond of a papillary tumour is discovered. Higher-grade tumours are more readily detected using urine cytology, and the investigation is useful in the diagnosis of carcinoma *in situ* (CIS).
- **Cystoscopy**
  Flexible cystoscopy is quick and painless and does not require admission to hospital.

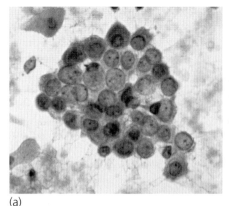

(a)

Cluster of urothelial cells exhibiting nuclei with micro-nucleoli and a high nuclear-to-cytoplasmic ratio. The nuclei are open with pale granular DNA. Appearances are severe ly atypical (×80).

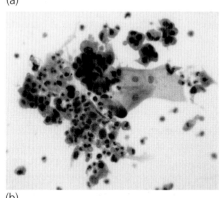

(b)

Clusters of poorly differentiated urothelial carcinoma cells surrounded by acute and chronic inflammatory cells together with red blood cells. The malignant cells are small, contain dense compact nuclei with high nuclear-to-cytoplasmic ratio and exhibit poor cohesion. Comparison is made with adjacent benign urothelial cells (×40).

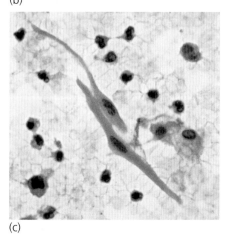

(c)

Urine cytology in which there are two atypical keratinizing spindle-shaped 'fibre' cells with small condensed nuclei and coarsely granular chromatin characteristic of keratinising squamous carcinoma (×80).

Figure 13.3 Urine cytology. (a) Tumour: Cluster of urothelial cells exhibiting nuclei with micro-nucleoli and a high nuclear-to-cytoplasmic ratio. The nuclei are open with pale granular DNA. Appearances are severely atypical (×80). (b) Dysplasia: Clusters of poorly differentiated urothelial carcinoma cells surrounded by acute and chronic inflammatory cells together with red blood cells. The malignant cells are small, contain dense compact nuclei with high nuclear-to-cytoplasmic ratio and exhibit poor cohesion. Comparison is made with adjacent benign urothelial cells (×40). (c) Squamous cells: Urine cytology in which there are two atypical keratinizing spindle-shaped 'fibre' cells with small condensed nuclei and coarsely granular chromatin characteristic of keratinising squamous carcinoma (×80).

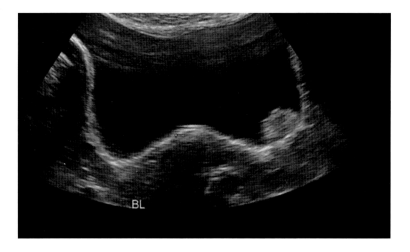

Figure 13.4 Ultrasound image showing bladder tumour.

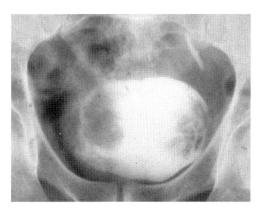

Figure 13.5 Large filling bladder cancer defects.

If a cancer has already been detected on bladder ultrasonography (Figure 13.4) or CT IVU (Figure 13.5), the flexible cystoscopy (Figure 13.6) can be bypassed and arrangements made for cystoscopy under general or regional anaesthesia. Blue light cystoscopy can performed A porphyrin dye, such as hexaminolevulinate, instilled into the bladder several hours before cystoscopy preferentially accumulates in the neoplastic tissue, emitting red fluorescence under blue light. Its use improves detection of small papillary lesions and CIS.

Tumour markers

The work-up of patients with haematuria is costly as it may require cytology, cystoscopy and intravenous urography or computerised tomography (CT). Thus, tumour markers could be useful in identifying patients who require more intensive clinical work-up for bladder cancer.

Currently available tumour markers include:

- Nuclear matrix protein test: The nuclear matrix protein 22 (NMP22) test, a double monoclonal antibody test designed to measure quantitatively the nuclear mitotic apparatus protein. This component of the nuclear matrix is overexpressed by bladder cancer and is released into the urine in increased quantity.
- ImmunoCyt test: The ImmunoCyt test detects bladder cancer markers present on exfoliated cells using a cocktail of fluorescent antibodies. When used with cytology, the ImmunoCyt test appears to improve the detection of low-grade tumours.
- UroVysion test: Multi-target fluorescence *in situ* hybridisation (FISH) detects cancer cells based on the aneuploidy of selected chromosomes. The UroVysion test employs centromere probes specific to chromosomes 3, 7, 17 and 9 to detect aneuploidy associated with bladder cancer.

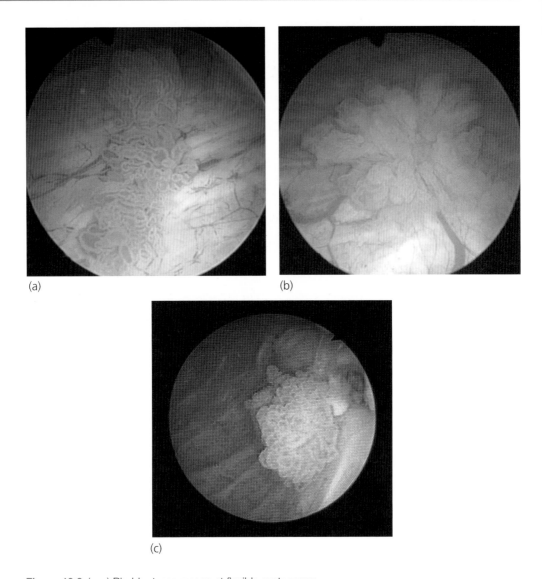

Figure 13.6 (a–c) Bladder tumour seen at flexible cystoscopy.

Role of urine markers in early detection of bladder cancer

There is a high false positive rate of all the above urine-based tests when they are used to assess patients who present with haematuria or are used in patient surveillance. The low false negative rate of these tests is their strength, leading to a high negative predictive value that effectively rules out disease in a significant proportion of patients, thereby potentially eliminating unnecessary clinical work-ups for bladder cancer.

Pathology

1. ***Transurethral cell carcinoma***
   Approximately 90% of bladder tumours in the United Kingdom are transitional cell carcinoma

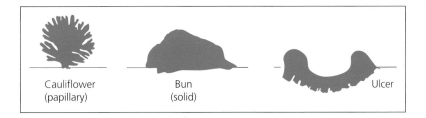

Figure 13.7 Macroscopic features of bladder cancer.

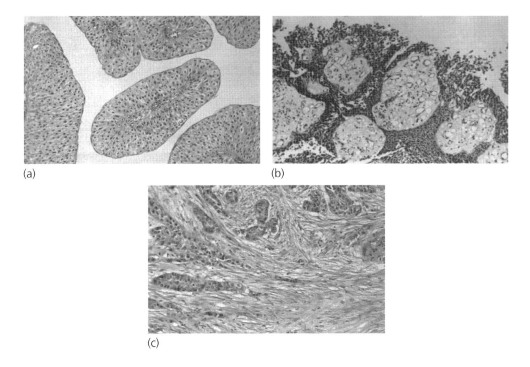

(a)

(b)

(c)

Figure 13.8 Grades of bladder cancer: (a) G1, (b) G2 and (c) G3.

of the bladder. Bladder tumours may be single or multiple and, like all cancers, can take the shape of a cauliflower, an ulcer or a solid lump (Figure 13.7). Truly benign papillomas are rare. There are three grades of malignancy (Figure 13.8).

2. *Squamous carcinoma*

 Squamous changes are often seen in patches in grade 3 transitional cell cancers and carry a bad prognosis. Pure squamous cancers arise in areas of squamous metaplasia that occur as a result of chronic bladder irritation most commonly worldwide by schistosomiasis. These tumours may have a layer of white keratin over them.

3. *Adenocarcinoma*

 The glandular metaplasia seen in chronic infection and bladder exstrophy may proceed to adenocarcinoma. Adenocarcinoma may also arise in the vestige of the foetal allantois, the urachus, as a cherry-like lump at the dome of the bladder.

Spread

- **Direct spread**
  Cancer may invade the surrounding fat and adjacent organs but never seems to cross De- nonvilliers' fascia into the rectum, although cancer of the rectum appears to have no diffi- culty crossing into the bladder.
- **Implantation**
  Bladder cancer may be seeded into the urethra and possibly within the bladder during manip- ulation. It is thought that the success of post- operative mitomycin C instillation in reducing recurrence rates is due to its action on these seeding cells.
- **Lymphatic spread**
  Once a bladder cancer has invaded the detru- sor muscle, it finds there a rich plexus of lym- phatics and may spread into the lymph nodes along the internal iliac artery and aorta. There is also a direct connection between these lym- phatics and the bone marrow of the pelvis, the upper end of the femur and the lower verte- brae as discussed.
- **Systemic spread**
  Metastases are seen in the lungs, liver and brain, but they are rare when compared with other cancers of the viscera.

Staging of bladder cancer

The Union for International Cancer Control (UICC) uses the TNM system of staging, which is intended to enable different centres to compare their results (2009).

The **T** staging system takes into account the evidence on which the depth of invasion has been assessed based on imaging or the clinical assessment at the time of cystoscopy (Figure 13.9). The prefix of a lower case **p** is added to indicate histopathological confirmation.

Tx	Primary tumour not assessed
T0	No evidence of tumour
Ta	Non-invasive papillary carcinoma
Tis	Carcinoma *in situ*

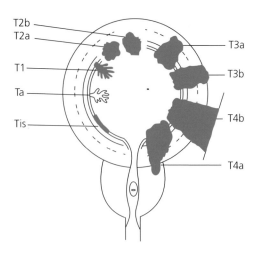

Figure 13.9 Staging of bladder cancer.

T1	Tumour invades lamina propria
T2	Tumour invades muscle: T2a superficial muscle T2b deep muscle (outer half)
T3	Tumour invades perivesical tissue: T3a microscopically T3b macroscopically
T4	T4a tumour invades prostate, seminal vesicles, uterus or vagina
	T4b tumour invades pelvic wall or abdominal wall

N staging – the assessment of lymph node involvement – is always guesswork unless the lymph nodes have been removed surgically and sent for histological examination. CT and magnetic resonance imaging (MRI) can detect the larger metastases with much less accuracy; it is thought that the extent of actual lymph node involvement is usually one lymph node group more advanced than imaging suggests, that is, if the pelvic nodes appear to be enlarged, there are probably micro metastasis in the para-aortic nodes.

Nx	Regional lymph nodes not assessed
N0	No regional lymph node metastases
N1	A single lymph node metastasis in the true pelvis
N2	Multiple lymph node metastasis in the true pelvis
N3	Metastasis in common iliac lymph nodes

M staging – the detection of visceral metastases – depends on CT, MRI and photon emission tomography (PET).

The differences in the methods used to stage bladder cancer make it necessary to be wary of comparing the results of different forms of treatment, for example, *total cystectomy* (where there is pathological evidence of depth of invasion and lymph node involvement) with *radiotherapy* or *chemotherapy*, where staging based only on biopsies and imaging tend to underestimate the stage.

M0	No distant metastasis
M1	Distant metastasis

Treatment of bladder cancer

Transurethral resection of a bladder tumour

Bladder tumours are removed endoscopically. Under anaesthesia the tumour is resected with the resectoscope (Figure 13.10), or at the very least a biopsy is obtained with the forceps (Figure 13.11). The object is to cut away the 'bush' to reveal the 'stalk' of the cancer removed down to the deeper layers of the detrusor muscle and thoroughly coagulate the bleeding. The 'bush' and the 'stalk' are sent separately to the laboratory so that the pathologist can tell how deeply the muscle is invaded. After all the bleeding has been stopped, a catheter is left in for a day or two. Possible complications include perforation of the wall of the bladder, absorption of irrigating fluid and bleeding. An adequate biopsy must include muscle from the base of the tumour to establish its depth of invasion (Figure 13.12).

Both before and after the tumour has been resected, bimanual examination should be performed to detect induration or a residual mass. If there remains a mobile mass after resection, the tumour will be muscle invasive and may be

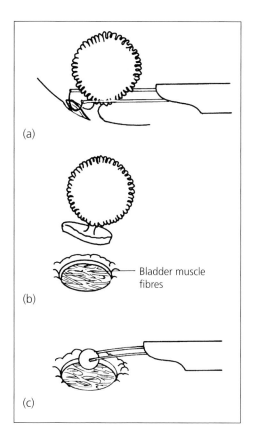

(a)

(b)

Bladder muscle fibres

(c)

Figure 13.10 Small papillary tumour removed with resectoscope loop and cauterisation of base: (a) resection, (b) resected area base and (c) cauterisation of base.

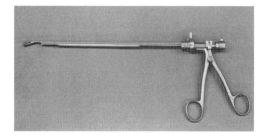

Figure 13.11 Storz cup biopsy forceps.

locally advanced (T2 or T3 staging). If there is a fixed mass, the tumour will be infiltrating the pelvic side wall (T4 staging) and probably inoperable.

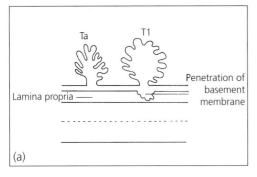

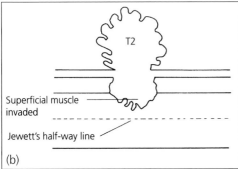

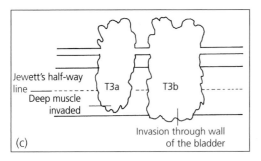

Figure 13.12 Bladder cancer T stages in relation to depth invasion: (a) Ta, T1, (b) T2 and (c) T3a, b.

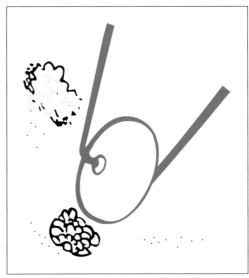

Figure 13.13 Small papillary tumour coagulated with roly-ball electrode.

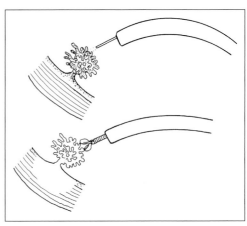

Figure 13.14 Small papillary tumour coagulated with YAG laser through flexible cystoscope.

Ta and T1 urothelial cancer

These tumours are initially removed by the resectoscope at the time of the initial assessment. If two or three have been resected with an adequate base of muscle, the remainder may be coagulated with the diathermy ball (Figure 13.13). The same coagulation can be obtained using the neodymium–yttrium/aluminium/garnet (YAG) laser (Figure 13.14). Patients are all carefully followed up at regular intervals by cytology and flexible cystoscopy. Recurrences are treated by transurethral resection or coagulation.

Bladder carcinoma *in situ*

CIS is the presence of malignantly transformed cells that have not breached the basement membrane. Unlike CIS of most other organs, CIS of the bladder is a highly aggressive and potentially life-threatening malignancy. Bladder CIS may present as isolated primary disease and occur with superficial or muscle invasive bladder tumours or after primary tumour reaction, in which case it represents disease progression. CIS is the earliest manifestation of invasive bladder cancer and may involve the urothelium in a focal or diffuse manner. When diffuse, it typically causes cystitis and storage lower urinary tract symptoms, and most patients exhibit positive urine cytology. On cystoscopy there is no tumour, and therefore nothing to resect, but the bladder may look a little inflamed. It may be very difficult to see and cannot reliably be eradicated endoscopically. Bladder CIS shows up well with blue light cystoscopy. Biopsies of the urothelium confirm the diagnosis (Figure 13.15).

Bladder CIS is cured by intravesical bacillus Calmette–Guérin (BCG) therapy in approximately

50% of patients, and this response is maintained long term and improved with maintenance therapy. When it reoccurs or fails to respond, radical cystectomy is the only cure, as CIS does not respond to radiotherapy. Early cystectomy instead of BCG therapy should be discussed with patients as there is an argument that the delay in treatment that occurs in patients who do not respond to BCG may be fatal. Even with cystectomy 5% of patients die of metastatic disease.

Adjuvant intravesical therapy in superficial bladder cancer

Instillation of a single dose of the chemotherapeutic antibiotic mitomycin C following resection is always given to reduce the chance of tumour recurrence. It probably works by

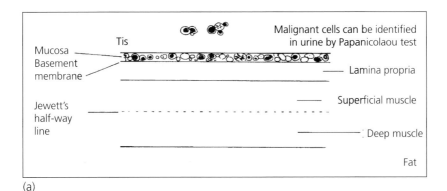

(a)

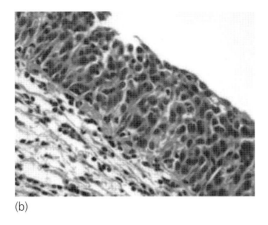

(b)

Figure 13.15 (a and b) Flat carcinoma *in situ*.

Table 13.1 EORTC risk tables for stage Ta T1 bladder cancer

Prior recurrence rate	Number of tumours	Tumour diameter
⬤ Primary	⬤ 1	⬤ <3 cm
⬤ Recurrent <1 per year	⬤ 2–7	⬤ >3 cm
⬤ Recurrent >1 per year	⬤ 8 or more	

T category	**Grade (WHO 1973)**	**Concomitant CIS**
⬤ Ta	⬤ G1	⬤ No
⬤ T1	⬤ G2	⬤ Yes
	⬤ G3	

Calculate probabilities	**Clear**		**Exit**	
1 Year	2 years	3 years	4 years	5 years

Probability of recurrence

Probability of progression

Source: Sylvester RJ et al. *European Urology* 2006;49:466–477. Reproduced with permission from Elsevier.

destruction of circulating tumour cells and ablating on small overlooked tumours and residual tumour cells at the resection site. It does not influence the rate of tumour progression to a more aggressing type subsequently. Mitomycin treatment may cause an allergic reaction if it gets into contact with the skin and should be omitted if overt or suspected perforation is suspected following extensive transurethral bladder tumour resection.

Based on clinical and pathological factors, patients can be stratified into risk groups – low, intermediate and high – based on their EORTC risk classification score (Table 13.1). When there are recurrences of low-grade superficial tumours (G1–2, Ta-1), the cancer is deemed to have progressed to the intermediate-risk group. Intermediate-risk group bladder cancer is treated with a 6-week course of intravesical mitomycin involving one instillation lasting 2 hours, per week. Patients with high-risk bladder cancer, which includes any grade 3 tumour, CIS and intermediate-risk cancers that recur after a

course of mitomycin, should undergo intravesical instillations of BCG.

BCG immunotherapy

Intravesical immunotherapy with the live attenuated anti-tuberculous vaccine BCG induces a local immune response in the bladder, which reduces the progression of bladder cancer and can cure high-risk disease and CIS. Unlike mitomycin C that reduces just disease recurrence, BCG significantly reduces both recurrence and progression of superficial bladder cancer. The precise immunological mechanism of action is unknown; stimulation of a T-cell-mediated immunologic response occurs. Like mitomycin C, intravesical BCG is conducted over a 6-week period. Maintenance therapy, which involves 3 weeks of treatment every 3 months after the induction course and then 6-monthly, improves efficacy. Intravesical BCG is more toxic than mitomycin C and is usually accompanied by cystitis, a transient fever is also common, and flu-like symptoms may occur and

Table 13.2 Risk group stratification in superficial bladder cancer

Low-risk tumours	Intermediate-risk tumours	High-risk tumours
• Primary • Solitary • Ta, G1 (low grade) • <3 cm • No CIS	All tumours between the low- and high-risk categories	Any of the following: • T1 • G3 • CIS • Multiple and recurrent • Large (>3 cm) • Ta G1 G2

rarely full-blown systemic tuberculosis requiring anti-tuberculous therapy.

Prognosis

Overall 30% of patients with superficial bladder cancer progress to invasive bladder cancer. If there is associated CIS, the figure rises to 60% (Table 13.2).

T2 and T3 bladder cancer

Most of muscle invasive bladder tumours are high grade. The treatment of muscle invasive bladder cancer is by radiation or with surgery. The efficacy of these modalities is similar. Neoadjuvant chemotherapy prior to radiotherapy or surgery has been shown in randomised studies to improve absolute survival by approximately 6%. Patients are given three cycles of chemotherapy over a 3–4-month period prior to proceeding to either radiotherapy or surgery. A combination of chemoradiation with cystectomy reserved for refractory disease has the reported advantage of approximately a third of patients being cured while keeping their bladders.

Radiotherapy

About half of the grade 3 muscle-invading cancers will respond completely to a course of radiotherapy. Doses of 64 Gy to the bladder treated from Monday to Friday over a 6½-week period are used. There is at present no way of predicting which cancer will respond, although the presence of squamous metaplasia staining for beta-human chorionic gonadotropin in the tissue suggest that it will not.

During radiation treatment, the patient commonly complains of cystitis-like symptoms and occasionally of proctitis. These acute symptoms settle over the course of 2–3 months. However patients can be left with long-term late radiation damage due to endarteritis obliterans. Radiation fibrosis that results in a small shrunken bladder is common.

Whether radiotherapy is chosen as the primary treatment or cystectomy, patients are followed up regularly for recurrences. If radiotherapy is chosen, 'salvage' cystectomy can be offered when the cancer fails to respond or recurs. The primary disadvantage of primary radiotherapy is that if cystectomy is needed later on because of persistent or recurrent cancer, complications are greater due to radiation damage to the tissue and impaired healing. For the same reason, it is more difficult to construct a new bladder from bowel, and the patient usually requires an ileal loop diversion. The disadvantage of performing cystectomy as the method of first choice is that it is a far more morbid treatment. The long-term results of the two are much the same and it is usual nowadays to explain the pros and cons of each method to the patient. Local disease recurrence after cystectomy carries a very poor prognosis but can be treated by radiotherapy.

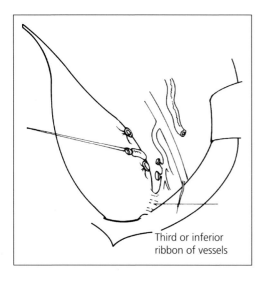

Third or inferior
ribbon of vessels

Figure 13.16 Dividing the main vessels of the bladder.

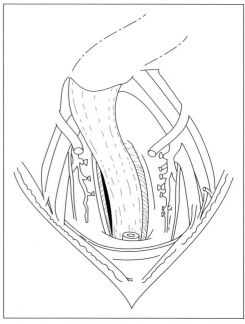

Figure 13.17 The empty pelvis after the bladder has been removed.

Radical cystectomy

The operation removes the whole bladder, the prostate and sometimes the urethra in males and the anterior vaginal wall, cervix and uterus in females. Pelvic lymph node clearance is mandatory as it improves survival. Radical cystectomy is a very morbid operation, which carries approximately a 5% mortality, and the patient needs to understand fully its grave implications. Nearly every male is rendered impotent although it is sometimes possible to protect the nerve supply to the penis and preserve potency. It is essential to discuss all the implications and problems that are associated with various forms of urinary diversion or the reconstruction of a new bladder from small or large bowel.

Operative steps

Bowel preparation is required and the patient optimised medically. All the lymph nodes are dissected from the aorta and common and internal iliac vessels on each side. All the vessels supplying the bladder from the internal iliac artery are divided between ligatures, one after the other (Figure 13.16). The ureters are divided about 5 cm away from the bladder (Figure 13.17). When there are multiple tumours, there is a chance of recurrent cancer in the urethra, so it is removed *en bloc* with the bladder and prostate.

Urinary diversion

(a) Ileal conduit

The ureters are anastomosed to one end of an isolated loop of ileum whose other end is led onto the skin to form a urostomy that is fitted with an adhesive bag (Figure 13.18). Care must be taken in choosing the site for the stoma: it must not rub against the belt or lie in a scar or crease or else the bag will come unstuck.

(b) Continent reservoir

After removing the bladder, a new one is constructed out of intestine. Numerous different methods are in use, but they all share certain principles: the bowel is open and closed in such a way that powerful peristaltic waves do not generate an

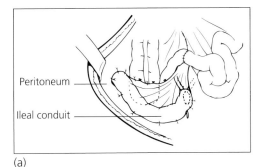

Peritoneum

Ileal conduit

(a)

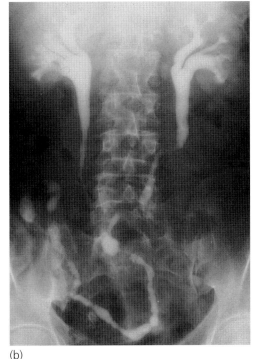

(b)

Figure 13.18 (a) Ileal conduit. (b) Contrast intravenous urography.

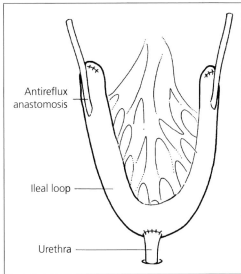

Antireflux anastomosis

Ileal loop

Urethra

Figure 13.19 Neocystoplasty by Camey's method.

increase in pressure, and precautions are taken to prevent reflux of urine from the new bladder up the ureters (Camey's neocystoplasty; Figure 13.19). If the urethra has been removed, a stoma is made onto the skin, which is designed to be continent, so that the patient empties it from time to time with a catheter (Kock's continent pouch; Figure 13.20). If the urethra has not been removed, the reservoir can be sewn onto the stump of the urethra and in many cases normal voiding is established (Kock's pouch; Figure 13.21).

Absorption of urine from the bowel that has been used to make the new bladder still leads to the biochemical complication of hyperchloraemic acidosis, and these patients all need to be carefully followed to make sure that infection and stone formation in the new reservoir are detected and treated. Most of the complications from intestinal neo-bladder reflect the fact that the bowel continues to function as bowel despite acting as urinary bladder.

Carcinoma of the urachus

This is very uncommon. The tumour is found on cystoscopy as a cherry-like swelling at the top of the bladder. Outside it is a much larger mass (Figure 13.22). Biopsy shows adenocarcinoma. It is treated by a wide excision that takes all the

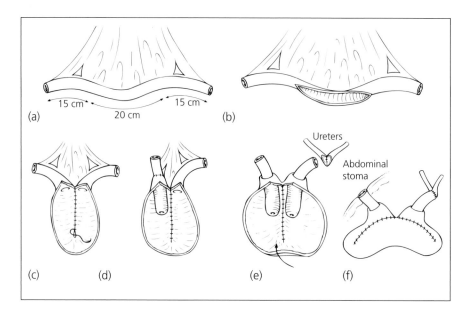

Figure 13.20 Kock's continent pouch: (a) ileal segment chosen measures, (b) window in mesentery, (c) initial step in pouch preparation, (d) one nipple intussuscepted and fixed with staples and (e) second nipple intussuscepted, (f) pouch completed.

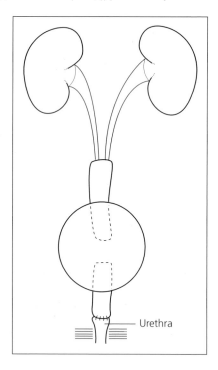

Figure 13.21 A Kock pouch may be anastomosed to the urethra.

triangle of tissue from the umbilicus down to the upper part of the bladder as well as all the regional lymph nodes (Figure 13.23). The small residual bladder is closed but enlarges to its former capacity within a few weeks.

Combination chemotherapy

Combination chemotherapy is used in two settings in patients with bladder cancer: either in the neoadjuvant setting prior to radical treatment with either surgery or radiation or in the palliative setting in patients with metastatic or locally advanced disease. Various combinations of chemotherapeutic agents that are used are similar in both settings. Regimes commonly used are cisplatin and gemcitabine or methotrexate, vinblastine, adriamycin and cisplatin (MVAC). The response rates with both these regimes are in the order of 50%.

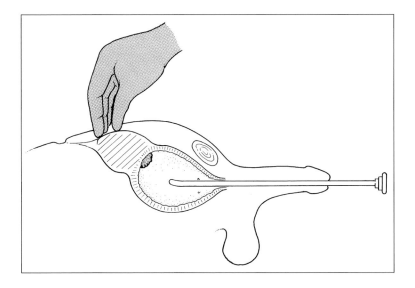

Figure 13.22 Carcinoma of the urachus.

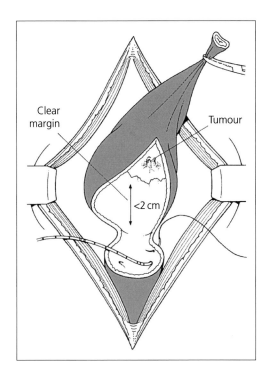

Clear margin

Tumour

<2 cm

Figure 13.23 Subtotal cystectomy for carcinoma of the urachus.

Palliation

When bladder cancer has spread beyond the bladder, it is conventionally treated with chemotherapy, with approximately 50% of patients responding for a median duration of 9 months. For local problems when you are faced with an elderly patient, who has to void bloodstained urine with pain and difficulty every few minutes by day and night, there are a number of options. Palliative radiotherapy given in a few fractions may stop bleeding and control pain without exposing the patient to significant toxicity. A surgical approach such as a palliative urinary diversion with an ileal conduit can be considered to relieve symptoms such as painful frequency.

Pain-relieving medication should be provided at the control of the patient, that is, when needed, not according to the hour, for pain knows no clock. It is important to involve palliative care in the management of these patients as they often require palliation of symptoms.

Part 4

The prostate gland

14

Benign disorders of the prostate gland

Surgical anatomy

The prostate is described as expressing zonal anatomy (McNeal zones), which differ based on their predominant cell type and anatomy. Benign prostatic enlargement mainly arises in the transition zone, and cancer mainly in the peripheral zone. The ejaculatory ducts run through the central zone and empty into the urethra at the verumontanum (Figure 14.1). The peripheral zone is wrapped around the central and transitional zones and is deficient anteriorly where the anterior fibromuscular stroma lies.

Structurally, the prostate is composed of fibromuscular stroma and glandular epithelial cells. In childhood there are very few epithelial glands; they appear and develop in puberty. In old age hypertrophy of one or all three elements in the transition zone around the periurethral area gives rise to the nodules of benign prostatic enlargement.

The prostate is closely related to the three elements of the urethral sphincter in the male; these are as follows:

1. The bladder neck (internal sphincteric mechanism) is a collection of alpha-adrenergic smooth muscle and supplied by sympathetic nerve fibres.
2. The supramembranous external sphincter, partly smooth muscle, partly striated, is just distal to the verumontanum and is also supplied by sympathetic nerve fibres.
3. The levator ani, voluntary striated muscle that forms the pelvic floor looping around the urethra and supplied by the pudendal nerve.

Anatomical relations

Anterior to the prostate is the symphysis pubis. Posteriorly, the prostate is separated from the rectum by the fascia of Denonvilliers. Cephalad to the prostate lie the bladder, seminal vesicles, vasa deferentia and ureters (Figure 14.2).

Physiology

The prostate is an accessory sex gland whose primary function is the support and promotion of male sperm function and fertility. During ejaculation it is thought that the prostate secretes about 0.5–1.0 mL of fluid, which is added to the ejaculate. The acini of these ducts are composed of secretory cells, basal cells and neuroendocrine cells. It is the epithelial secretory cells that produce both prostate-specific antigen (PSA) and prostatic acid phosphatase.

Prostatitis

Prostatitis is overdiagnosed in patients with nonspecific perineal discomfort or lower urinary tract symptoms. In 1998, classification of the prostatitis syndromes addressed the categories of the disease based on the patient history,

Urology Lecture Notes, Seventh Edition. Amir V. Kaisary, Andrew Ballaro and Katharine Pigott.
© 2016 John Wiley & Sons, Ltd. Published 2016 by John Wiley & Sons, Ltd.

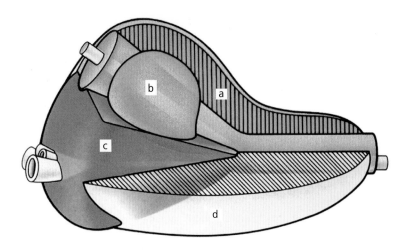

Figure 14.1 Zones of the prostate gland: (a) fibromuscular stroma, (b) transition zone, (c) central zone and (d) peripheral zone.

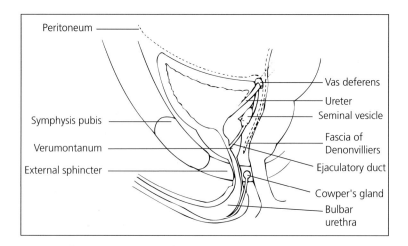

Figure 14.2 Surgical anatomy of the prostate.

physical examination and urine analysis/culture as the cornerstones (Table 14.1).

Acute bacterial prostatitis

Acute bacterial prostatitis is a febrile illness with sudden abrupt onset. There are marked genitourinary symptoms and often a positive bacterial urine culture.

Obstruction downstream to the prostate may force urine up into its ducts, and if the urine is infected, it causes inflammation. Blood-borne infection is equally common.

Whatever the route of the infection, the prostate becomes enlarged and painful on rectal palpation and may cause painful and obstructed micturition. Pathogens may be recovered from the urine. Colour Doppler transrectal ultrasound scanning may show hyperaemia (Figure 14.3). The most common pathogens include *Escherichia coli*, *Klebsiella*, *Proteus mirabilis* and *Enterococcus faecalis*.

Table 14.1 Classification of the prostatitis syndromes

Category	Name	Definition
I	Acute bacterial	Acute infection of the prostate
II	Chronic bacterial	Chronic infection of the prostate
IIIA	Chronic pelvic pain syndrome	Inflammatory Nonbacterial WBC+
IIIB		Non-inflammatory Prostatodynia
WBC: insignificant		
IV	Asymptomatic	Incidental inflammation (prostate biopsy)

Source: National Institutes of Health Summary Statement (1998, November) *First National Institutes of Health International Prostatitis Collaborative Network Workshop on Prostatitis*. NIH, Bethesda, MD.

Treatment

An antibiotic that can reach the alkaline milieu of the prostate is needed, for example, trimethoprim, erythromycin or ciprofloxacin. A good combination is a short course of ciprofloxacin in the acute attack, followed by 4–6 weeks of a low dose of trimethoprim. In most cases acute prostatitis resolves completely. Very rarely there is suppuration, and an abscess forms, which is best drained transurethrally, before it bursts spontaneously into the rectum (Figure 14.4). Acute prostatitis is a disorder that may relapse without warning.

Chronic prostatitis/pelvic pain syndrome

Chronic prostatitis classically presents with persistent discomfort in the perineum with painful ejaculation. Symptoms may vary considerably however and include non-specific pelvic and suprapubic pain and storage lower urinary tract symptoms. To diagnose chronic bacterial prostatitis, bacteria must be isolated. Urine is collected for culture in two parts (VB1 and VB2). Then the prostate is massaged transrectally to express fluid, which is collected (EPS).

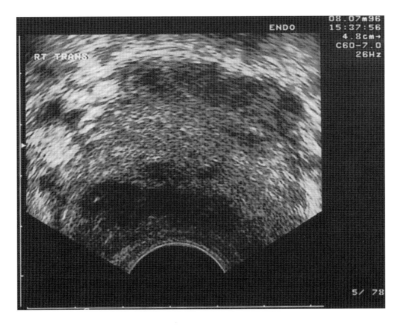

Figure 14.3 Transrectal Doppler scan showing hyperaemia in a case of acute prostatitis.

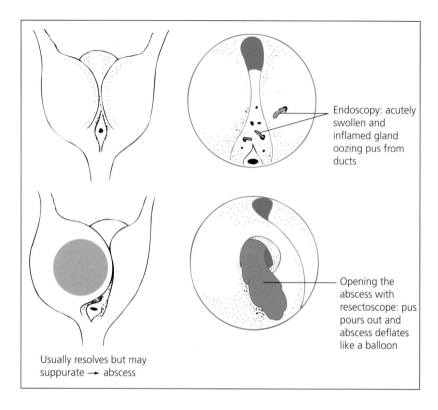

Endoscopy: acutely
swollen and
inflamed gland
oozing pus from
ducts

Opening the
abscess with
resectoscope: pus
pours out and
abscess deflates
like a balloon

Usually resolves but may
suppurate → abscess

Figure 14.4 Acute prostatitis usually resolves but may form an abscess.

Finally a third urine specimen is collected (VB3). A diagnosis of infection in the prostate is made if the colony count of bacteria in EPS and VB3 is more than in VB1 and VB2.

The organisms that are recovered may be the usual *E. coli*, but *Chlamydia trachomatis* and *Trichomonas vaginalis* are found from time to time. Their detection requires special culture techniques. Symptoms of chronic prostatitis in the absence of cultured bacteria is termed chronic pelvic pain syndrome.

Treatment

The principles of the treatment of chronic bacterial prostatitis are the same as for any persistent bacterial infection, with the added difficulty that in the prostate the milieu is alkaline and many of the standard antibiotics do not penetrate the gland. For chlamydia, tetracyclines are usually effective. *Trichomonas* requires a week's course of metronidazole. The addition of an alpha-adrenoreceptor blocking agent and anti-inflammatory drugs improves symptoms.

Localisation of pain in patients with prostatitis-like symptoms

Site	%
Prostate/perineum	46
Scrotum and/or testes	39
Penis	6
Urinary bladder	6
Low back	2

Source: Zermann, D.H., Ishigooka, M., Doggweiler, R. & Schmidt, R. A. (1999) Neurourological insights into the etiology of genitourinary pain in men. *J Urol*, 161 (3), 903–908.

Benign prostatic enlargement

Symptoms resulting from benign prostatic enlargement account for a large proportion of the workload of a general urologist. The prostate is a complex organ consisting of acinar, stromal and muscular tissue. The earliest changes of benign prostatic enlargement occur in the periurethral glands around the verumontanum, where there develops an imbalance between stimulatory and inhibitory prostatic growth factors that results in prostatic hyperplasia and fibromuscular nodule formation. These nodules vary in size and may compress the outer zone of the prostate into a thin shell and deform the prostate so as to give the appearance of having two 'lateral lobes' and one 'middle lobe'. These 'lobes' are not true functional entities, but artefacts caused by the way the prostate is confined by the symphysis and the bladder.

Pathophysiology of symptoms

The development of benign prostatic enlargement occurs over a time period of many years, and the resulting symptoms are generally insidious. The popular term 'prostatism' used broadly in the past to cover benign prostate hypertrophy and lower urinary tract symptoms is now known to be simplistic and inaccurate. A complex interplay exists between symptoms and pathology. The size of the prostate gland is irrelevant: the smallest prostates may cause severe bladder outflow obstruction; huge glands none at all, and patients with bladder outflow obstruction may be asymptomatic and present for the first time in urinary retention.

Compression of the prostatic urethra and the way in which the bladder responds to obstruction are the main factors involved in symptom generation. The storage and voiding lower urinary tract symptoms that may result from bladder outflow obstruction are not specific to either the prostate, benign prostatic enlargement or indeed bladder outflow obstruction (see Chapter 1).

 KEYPOINTS

- **Lower urinary tract symptoms (LUTS):** A progressive group of symptoms that are non-specific, age related and non-organ specific, in both female and male subjects as a combination of storage, voiding and post-micturition symptoms
- **Storage symptoms:** Daytime frequency, nocturia, urgency and urge incontinence
- **Voiding symptoms:** Hesitancy, slow stream, straining, a feeling of incomplete emptying, intermittency and terminal dribbling
- **Post-micturition symptoms:** Sense of incomplete bladder emptying and post-micturition dribble

Patients who are most likely to drive maximal benefit from intervention are those who combine lower urinary tract symptoms and bladder outlet obstruction. Several factors contribute to the generation of lower urinary tract symptoms associated with bladder outflow obstruction.

Bladder neck smooth muscle tone

The alpha-adrenergic smooth muscle fibres in the prostate, especially around the bladder neck, fail to relax as the detrusor contracts. This may be accompanied by hypertrophy of the smooth muscle (Figure 14.5), and endoscopy may show a tight ring at the bladder neck without enlargement of the prostate.

Prostatic enlargement

Enlargement of any or all three 'lobes' of the prostate may physically obstruct the urethral lumen. The middle lobe alone may protrude into the bladder causing a ball-valve type obstruction to the bladder outlet (Figure 14.6). As the inner zone of the prostate enlarges, the outer zone may become compressed and is often, incorrectly, called the 'capsule'. The presence of an enlarged prostate indenting the bladder may stimulate the bladder to initiate a voiding response more frequently than normal.

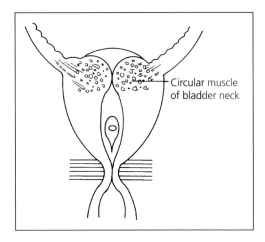

Figure 14.5 Hypertrophy of the smooth muscle of the bladder neck.

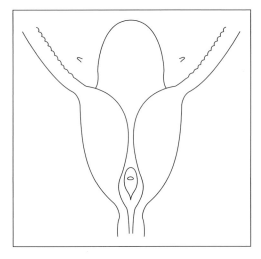

Figure 14.6 The middle 'lobe' may protrude into the bladder.

Bladder neck dysfunction may generate symptoms of urinary hesitancy and difficulty in initiating micturition and a poor and intermittent urinary stream. Hesitancy may also be caused by the longer time it takes for the detrusor to generate a contraction strong enough to overcome the increased outflow obstruction from the compressed prostatic urethra and an intermittent stream by failure to maintain this.

Detrusor dysfunction

The detrusor smooth muscle of the bladder may hypertrophy in response to chronic obstruction and become stronger and more sensitive. These changes are accompanied by complex changes to its structure and physiology characterised by infiltration of the muscle fibres by connective tissue and a poorly characterised complex neuromuscular disorder. This generates symptoms of urinary frequency and urgency and is termed obstructive detrusor overactivity. The hypertrophied fibres cause trabeculation of the bladder, and diverticula form in between them. Bladder diverticula can be large and contribute to incomplete bladder emptying.

The detrusor muscle fibres may also become weaker in response to chronic obstruction and fail to empty the bladder effectively. The residual urine results in shorter periods of time between voids causing frequency and nocturia.

Complications of bladder outflow obstruction

Urinary infections and bladder stones

Incomplete bladder emptying causes stagnant urine, which predisposes to urinary infections as any bacteria that enter the bladder are not washed out. Bladder stones may also form in stagnant urine as the urinary constituents precipitate.

Obstructive uropathy due to high-pressure chronic retention

Hypertrophy of the bladder wall may lead to high bladder pressures as it fills and is unable to empty fully. Disruption of the anti-reflux ureteric valve mechanism results in these high pressures being transmitted to the upper tracts causing dilatation of both the ureter and renal collecting system (hydroureteronephrosis), obstructive uropathy and nephropathy. Detrusor smooth muscle hypertrophy may also cause direct obstruction to the ureter as its terminal part runs through the bladder.

Acute urinary retention

Acute urinary retention is the sudden inability to void urine and is always painful. The condition is not solely the result of benign prostatic enlargement and may be precipitated or spontaneous. Precipitants include any factor that increases bladder outflow resistance or decreases bladder contractility.

It is postulated that large prostates may undergo focal infarction, which increases the outflow resistance due to inflammation and swelling. Kinking of the prostatic urethra due to uneven prostatic enlargement has also been suggested as a mechanism. Detrusor inhibitory factors are better characterised. These include anaesthetic agents, accounting for post-operative retention; alcohol, which may numb the desire to void while acting as a diuretic at the same time; constipation, which generates reflex afferent inhibitory sympathetic nervous activity to the bladder; pelvic pain; and bladder over-distension. Spontaneous urinary retention carries a worse prognosis than precipitated retention as there is no factor that can be reversed. With both precipitated and spontaneous urinary retention, there is usually a degree of underlying clinical or subclinical bladder outflow obstruction.

Chronic urinary retention

Chronic urinary retention is the maintenance of voiding with failure to empty the bladder. If the bladder has responded to insidious outflow obstruction by becoming weaker and distending, it may contain several litres of urine after voiding with no symptoms. In gradual chronic detrusor failure, there is no pain. The big distended bladder is often soft and difficult to feel. A little urine may escapes from time to time – overflow incontinence (Figure 14.7). Patients with chronic urinary retention may develop the sudden inability to pass urine at all; this may or may not be painful and is referred to as acute-on-chronic retention.

If the bladder has responded to the obstruction by becoming hypertrophied and thick walled, high-pressure chronic retention with obstructive uropathy may occur. This is commonly accompanied by the clinical sign of nocturnal enuresis,

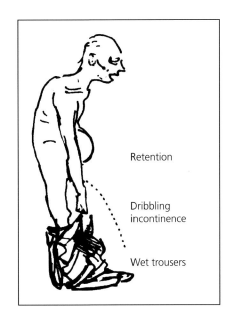

Retention

Dribbling incontinence

Wet trousers

Figure 14.7 Overflow incontinence.

or bed-wetting, which occurs as the bladder overflows and the voluntary inhibitory mechanisms that prevent incontinence during waking hours are overcome.

Diagnosis of prostatic obstruction

History

Men with bladder outflow obstruction seek medical input because of bothersome lower urinary tract symptoms, the complications of obstruction most commonly urinary retention and urinary infections, and because they are concerned that non-bothersome symptoms may be a sign of prostate cancer. Lower urinary tract symptoms and their detrimental impact on the patient known as 'bother' are quantified and documented using the International Prostate Symptom Score (IPSS) (Table 14.2). The IPSS questions cover both obstructive and storage symptoms and enable a numerical score to be attributed both to the severity of the symptoms and the degree of bother they cause. The bother score varies widely between patients with the same symptom scores. Patients are divided into patients with mild score

Table 14.2 International Prostate Symptom Score (IPSS)

	Never	About 1 time in 5	About 1 time in 3	About 1 time in 2	About 2 times in 3	Almost always		
1. Over the past month, how often have you had a sensation of not emptying your bladder completely after you finished urinating?	0	1	2	3	4	5		
2. Over the past month, how often have you had to urinate again less than 2 h after you finished urination?	0	1	2	3	4	5		
3. Over the past month, how often have you found you stopped and started again several times when you urinated?	0	1	2	3	4	5		
4. Over the past month, how often have you found it difficult to hold back urinating after you have felt the need?	0	1	2	3	4	5		
5. Over the past month, how often have you noticed a reduction in the strength and force of your urinary stream?	0	1	2	3	4	5		
6. Over the past month, how often have you had to push or strain to begin urination?	0	1	2	3	4	5		
	None	1 time	2 times	3 times	4 times	5 or more times		
7. Over the past month, how many times did you most typically get up to urinate from the time you went to bed at night until the time you got up in the morning?		1	2	3	4	5		
Total IPSS score S =								
Quality of life due to urinary symptoms								
If you were to spend the rest of your life with your urinary condition just the way it is now, how would you feel about that?	Delighted	Pleased	Mostly satisfied	Mixed. equally satisfied and dissatisfied	Mostly dissatisfied	Unhappy	Terrible	
	0	1	2	3	4	5	6	
Quality of life assessment index L =								

(<7), moderate (8–19) and severe (>20). It should never be a substitute for listening to the patient carefully, especially since these symptom scores do not match objective evidence of obstruction.

Physical signs

Abdominal palpation may reveal a chronically obstructed bladder, but this is a late feature of the disease. Rectal examination cannot distinguish between a tight bladder full of residual urine and a large prostatic adenoma (Figure 14.8), nor can it feel a middle lobe that sticks up into the bladder out of reach of the finger (Figure 14.9).

Investigations

1. *Flow rate*: Flow rates vary from day to day, and a poor flow may not necessarily mean obstruction: it may result from a weak detrusor, while on the other hand if the detrusor has undergone considerable hypertrophy, it can compensate for obstruction and produce a good flow rate. Nevertheless an impaired flow rate of <10 mL/s is a significant part of the clinical pattern (Figure 14.10).
2. *Residual urine*: The volume of urine remaining in the bladder can be measured by abdominal ultrasound. This may vary from day to day and may be caused by bladder outflow obstruction, detrusor failure or both. The abdominal ultrasound may also detect dilatation of the ureters and renal pelves in chronic high-pressure

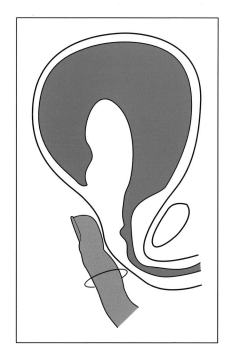

Figure 14.9 The rectal finger cannot feel a large middle lobe.

urinary retention and gross bladder trabeculation and diverticula (Figure 14.11).

3. *Transrectal ultrasound*: The volume of the prostate can be measured from the ultrasound image (width, height and length) and may help in planning treatment (Figure 14.12).
4. *Urodynamic studies*: The only way of making certain that lower urinary tract symptoms are due to bladder outflow obstruction is by means of a cystometrogram (see Chapter 10).

The recommended investigations of lower urinary tract symptoms are urine dipstick to identify inflammatory causes, the frequency volume chart to identify systemic disorders of fluid handling and the IPSS questionnaire to quantify the severity of symptoms and document the baseline to monitor response to treatment. All others are optional.

Management of urinary retention

Treatment of urinary retention involves draining the bladder by passing either a urethral catheter or, if this is not possible, a suprapubic catheter.

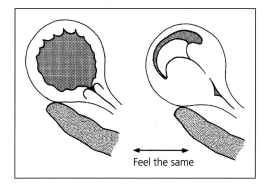

Feel the same

Figure 14.8 The finger in the rectum cannot distinguish urine under pressure in the bladder from a big prostate.

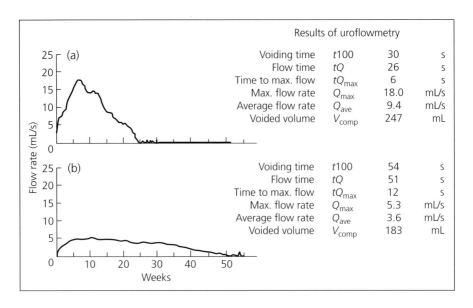

Results of uroflowmetry			
(a)			
Voiding time	$t100$	30	s
Flow time	tQ	26	s
Time to max. flow	tQ_{max}	6	s
Max. flow rate	Q_{max}	18.0	mL/s
Average flow rate	Q_{ave}	9.4	mL/s
Voided volume	V_{comp}	247	mL
(b)			
Voiding time	$t100$	54	s
Flow time	tQ	51	s
Time to max. flow	tQ_{max}	12	s
Max. flow rate	Q_{max}	5.3	mL/s
Average flow rate	Q_{ave}	3.6	mL/s
Voided volume	V_{comp}	183	mL

Figure 14.10 Urine flow rates in (a) normal and (b) benign enlargement of the prostate.

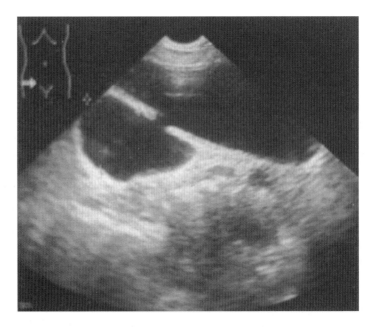

Figure 14.11 Ultrasound after trying to empty the bladder showing large residual as well as a diverticulum.

It is important to record how much urine is drained in the first fifteen minutes after catheterisation, as this gives a valuable clue as to the state of the bladder. A volume of up to approximately 800 mL is consistent with a normal bladder; more than this indicates a degree of prior bladder decompensation and chronic retention.

The patient is assessed to determine whether the retention episode is acute or chronic, precipitated or spontaneous. Any identified reversible

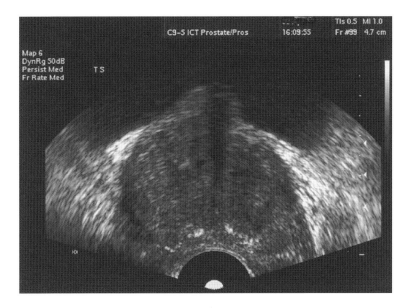

Figure 14.12 Transrectal ultrasound image showing enlargement of the prostate.

precipitants such as drugs or infection should be reversed or treated. A rectal examination is performed to exclude an advanced prostate cancer, other pelvic tumour or impacted stool. The electrolytes should be assessed. If these are normal and the residual urine was less than approximately 1½ L, the patient should be prescribed an alpha-adrenoreceptor blocking drug such as tamsulosin, and a trial without catheter performed after a day. If he is unable to void, then the choice is between permanent and intermittent catheterisation and bladder outflow tract surgery.

In the event of evidence of renal impairment, it is important to determine whether this improves after catheterisation and whether there is evidence of obstructive uropathy. If so high-pressure chronic retention was present prior to catheterisation, a trial without catheter should not be performed. Sometimes, urinary retention associated with obstructive uropathy that is not improved by catheterisation occurs; this is usually caused by locally advanced prostate cancer obstructing both the bladder outlet and the ureters as they enter the bladder trigone adjacent to the prostate.

Treatment

1. *Conservative*

   Many elderly men go through a year or two during which their symptoms irritates them, but not very severely, and then it gets better without any treatment. They may still have to urinate once or twice in the night, but their daytime activities are unaffected. They have a reasonable flow rate and their residual urine is negligible. The patient is advised to come back and report progress in 6 months or so. Some patients are helped by simple management of their fluid intake and manipulation of diuretics to reduce bothersome urinary frequency. Patients with mild symptoms and low levels of bother are most suitable for this.

2. *Pharmacological management*

   (a) *Alpha-blockers*: There are three forms of alpha 1 adrenoreceptors. Alpha 1a is primarily found in the prostate gland. Alpha 1b is found in the walls of blood vessels. Alpha 1d is found in the bladder. There are at least four different subtypes of the alpha 1a adrenoreceptors: alpha 1a 1–4. Selective antagonism of the alpha 1a receptors leads to a reduction of the smooth muscle tone of the bladder neck and prostate and reduces bladder outflow obstruction. Some patients might experience postural hypertension, and absence of ejaculation is common.

(b) *5-Alpha-reductase inhibitor (finasteride and dutasteride):* This class of drug prevents conversion of prostatic testosterone to the more active metabolite dihydrotestosterone causing apoptosis of the glandular part of the prostate. It causes the PSA level to fall and in many patients relieves bothersome symptoms. Response to therapy can take up to 12 months in some cases, and unfortunately only 50% of patients will respond to treatment. Those with larger prostates respond better as they experience greater proportional prostatic size reduction. Those who do respond may continue to receive tablets indefinitely. Finasteride and dutasteride occasionally effect on sexual function with loss of potency (approximately 8%), decreased libido (approximately 5%) and decreased ejaculate volume (approximately 4%) being reported. Dutasteride inhibits two of the three isoforms of 5-alpha-reductase and acts more quickly than finasteride, which inhibits only the type 2 isoform and has a much shorter half-life.

(c) Both alpha-adrenoreceptor blocking agents and 5-alpha-reductase inhibitors may be taken together and result in a greater reduction in symptom scores than the effect of the two individually added.

(d) *Phytotherapy:* These products are not the actual plants but are extracts derived from either the roots, the seeds, the bark or the fruits of the various plants used. Their mechanisms of action vary. Examples include saw palmetto berry (*Serenoa repens*), African plum (*Pygeum africanum*), South African star grass (*Hypoxis rooperi*) and others.

Pharmacological treatment is most suitable for men with moderately symptomatic symptoms refractory to fluid intake modification.

3. *Surgery*

Bladder outflow tract surgery is reserved for patients with bothersome symptoms refractory to pharmacological treatments, for those who do not want to take medication for the rest of their lives and for men who suffer progression of their disease, a term that includes worsening of symptoms and the presence of complications. The more bothered the patient is by his symptoms, the better the result of surgery he is likely to experience.

i. *Open prostatectomy:* Around 1890, it was found almost by accident that the adenoma in the inner zone could be enucleated from the compressed shell of outer zone with a finger. In the early days this was performed via a suprapubic incision into the bladder or through a perineal incision. In 1943, Millin developed the retropubic approach that is still used in some centres for very large glands (Figure 14.13).

ii. *Transurethral resection:* Improved technology made it possible to remove the inner zone adenoma with a telescope passed along the urethra (Figure 14.14). This operation is arguably the 'gold standard' procedure for bladder outflow obstruction. It carries an operative mortality of less than 1%, but there are still complications. Bleeding can be severe during the operation.

Stricture develops in the urethra afterwards in about 3% of men. There is failure to ejaculate commonly; this is due to either disruption of the reflex bladder neck closure mechanism (retrograde ejaculation) or blockage of the ejaculatory ducts (anejaculation). Impotence occurs in 10–15% after prostatectomy and is more likely if there is a pre-existing problem. Incontinence of urine may be the result of a technical mistake whereby the external sphincter is injured or may be due to persistence of overactive bladder contractions that pre-operatively were not expressed as incontinence due to the outflow tract resistance. It is therefore important to warn men with storage symptoms that incontinence may occur; this resolves

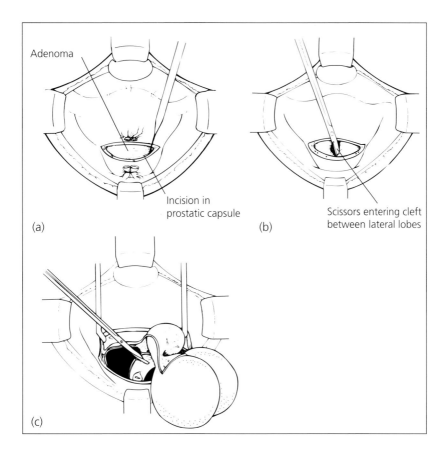

Figure 14.13 Retropubic prostatectomy. (a) Transverse incision in the prostate capsule. (b) Scissors entering the prostatic urethra between the lateral lobes. (c) Enucleation of the prostate exposing the posterior wall of the prostatic urethra being divided.

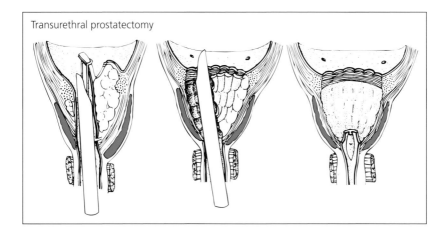

Figure 14.14 Transurethral resection of the prostate.

spontaneously in approximately half of men within 6 months.

Transurethral resection syndrome: It is rare provided that the appropriate precautions are taken and results from systemic absorption of the glycine that is used as an irrigant during the procedure (saline and water cannot be used as they conduct electrical current). The condition is characterised by neurological and cardiovascular dysfunction. The underlying pathophysiology is a dilutional hyponatraemia and the action of glycine metabolites on the central nervous system. The use of a bipolar

resectoscope enables saline irrigant to be used instead of glycine.

iii. *Transurethral incision of the prostate*: Instead of removing the inner zone, an incision is made through the bladder neck and prostate (Figure 14.15). There are less bleeding and a shorter hospital stay. No tissue is removed for histological diagnosis however, and the technique is only useful for small tight prostates and bladder neck obstruction.

iv. *Transurethral ablation of the prostate*: The prostatic tissue can be ablated by a special diathermy current (Figure 14.16). Laser

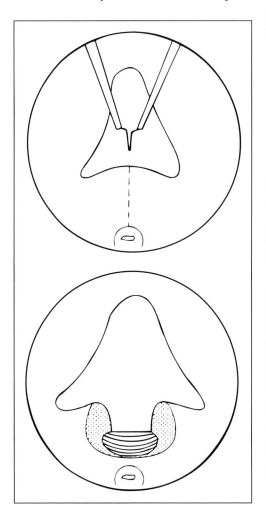

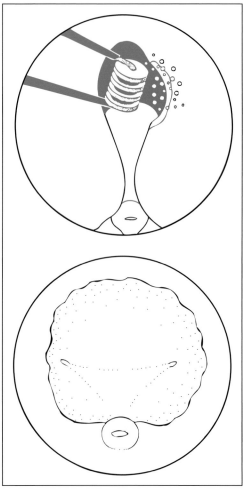

Figure 14.16 Transurethral vaporisation of the prostate using diathermy.

Figure 14.15 Transurethral incision of the prostate.

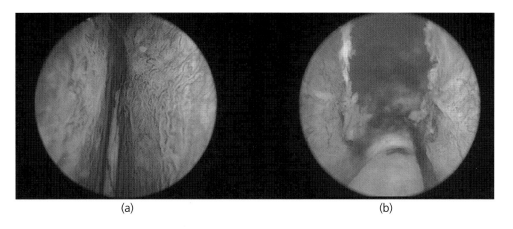

Figure 14.17 Transurethral laser vaporisation of the prostate. (a) Endoscopic view of the prostate. (b) Endoscopic view following completion of vaporisation of the central adenoma.

vaporisation can be performed utilising a non-contact side-firing laser characterised by its green, 532 nm-wavelength emission. The strong absorption of the KTP laser energy by haemoglobin and its minimal absorption by water prevent it from penetrating deep into the tissue; thus the energy gets concentrated into the superficial tissue (depth of 1–2 mm). Its adsorption by haemoglobin renders it very effective at preventing bleeding to the extent that it can be performed on patients taking anticoagulants. The method appears to remove the inner zone tissue in a way that is comparable to transurethral resection (Figure 14.17).

v. *Laser resection of the prostate*: Laser resection is based on the principle of laser vaporisation. Holmium: YAG is the most widely used laser for this technique. The procedure is often referred to by the acronym HoLEP (holmium laser enucleation of the prostate). The energy is delivered to the prostate through an end-firing 0.55 mm laser fibre. The procedure does not completely vaporise the tissue. Instead, the energy is directed such that prostatic adenoma is enucleated (Figure 14.18). The challenge then is to remove the intact prostatic lobes from inside the bladder. This is done with a mechanical tissue morcellator.

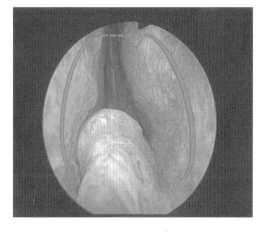

Figure 14.18 Transurethral laser enucleation of the prostate

Post-operative care

After all forms of prostatectomy, a catheter is left in the bladder, usually a three-way catheter, which allows saline to run in and out of the bladder to dilute blood and prevent clots from blocking the catheter (Figure 14.19). Some surgeons rely on natural formation of urine to irrigate the bladder and encourage this with a diuretic. If a chip of prostate or a blood clot does block the catheter, an attempt is made to wash it out with a bladder syringe using strict aseptic precautions. If this fails, the catheter is removed and a new

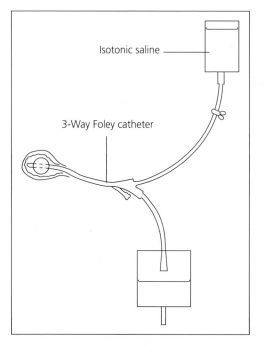

Isotonic saline

3-Way Foley catheter

Figure 14.19 Irrigation of the prostatic fossa with a three-way catheter.

one is passed. The bleeding has usually stopped within 24–48 h, and the catheter is then removed. After HoLEP there is usually minimal bleeding, and the procedure may be performed as a day case.

Patients usually go home after 2 days, but the empty cavity from which the inner zone tissue has been removed is still raw and unhealed, and secondary haemorrhage may occur at any moment. It makes sense to advise him to avoid strain; at around the 10th post-operative day, there is often a little haematuria. Patients understand this if it is explained beforehand that it may bleed a little when the 'scab' comes away. Very rarely the patient must be readmitted to have clot irrigated out of the bladder.

Recovery is not complete until the prostatic fossa has been completely relined with the urothelium. This takes about 6 weeks. Until then the patient may notice some frequency and urgency, and the urine will continue to be a little cloudy, raising the suggestion of infection. Antibiotics are not needed, however, unless there is a significant growth of bacteria.

15

Prostate cancer

There are unexplained differences in the incidence of prostate cancer in different parts of the world: it is relatively uncommon in men of Japanese and Indian ancestry and more common in those of African ancestry. It is twice as common in men of African-American descent and is more likely to present at an advanced stage (Figure 15.1). The number of reported cases seems to be increasing, but this may be due to an increased awareness, the growing number of elderly men who are surviving and better ways of making the diagnosis. Prostate cancer in males in the United Kingdom in 2011 was the most common in new cancers (Figure 15.2). The rate of men dying from prostate cancer varies depending on race and ethnicity. In the United Kingdom, prostate cancer was the fourth most common cause of cancer death in 2012. The crude mortality rate shows that there are 35 prostate cancer deaths for every 100 000 males in the United Kingdom. In 2011 black men were more likely to die of prostate cancer than any other group of the population in the United States (Figure 15.3).

Introduction of the prostate-specific antigen (PSA) blood test in the late 1980s enhanced prostate cancer detection. A dramatic increase in the detection rate in the early 1990s was followed by a subsequent decline and was thought to be due to detection of early small tumours. Cancer that is found by an elevated PSA or a prostate nodule on digital rectal examination is referred to as a clinical cancer. Cancer found only at autopsy is called a latent tumour. Today carcinoma of the prostate is most often detected by screening with PSA.

Knowing that little islands of cancer are present in most elderly men, it is surprising that cancer is not detected more often. However, the total annual number of new cases shows an increase, and this is frequently interpreted in an alarmist way to justify programmed screening.

There is currently no role for general population screening for prostate cancer in the United Kingdom mainly because there are no accurate enough tools. Groups with higher-risk status, for example, those with two first-degree relatives with the disease, may undergo PSA screening with the appropriate counselling.

There are no tools to achieve primary prevention of prostate cancer evolution, and various nutrients and pharmacological agents are debated. No single dietary or lifestyle modification provided a strong evidence of efficacy. Advice to usually adopt a physically active lifestyle and eating a healthy balanced diet high in vegetable intake is recommended.

 KEYPOINTS

Putative protective dietary and pharmacological agents

- Nutrients:
  Possibly: selenium, vitamin D, vitamin E, green tea and lycopene
- Pharmaceuticals:
  Possibly: statins, 5-alpha-reductase inhibitors and non-steroidal anti-inflammatory agents

---

Urology Lecture Notes, Seventh Edition. Amir V. Kaisary, Andrew Ballaro and Katharine Pigott.
© 2016 John Wiley & Sons, Ltd. Published 2016 by John Wiley & Sons, Ltd.

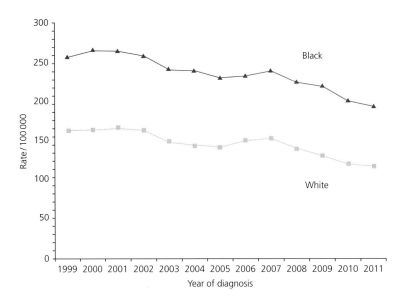

Figure 15.1 The US prostate cancer incidence rates by ethnicity, 1999–2011. Modified from the National Program of Cancer Registries.

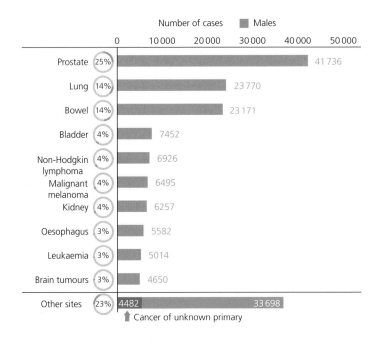

Figure 15.2 The 10 most common new cancer numbers in males in the United Kingdom in 2011.

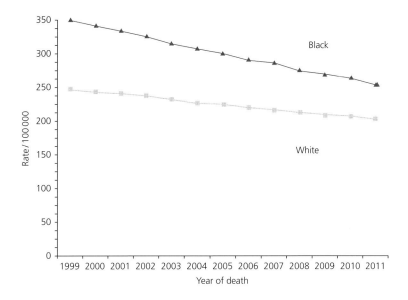

Figure 15.3 The United States prostate cancer death rates by ethnicity, 1999–2011. Modified from the National Program of Cancer Registries.

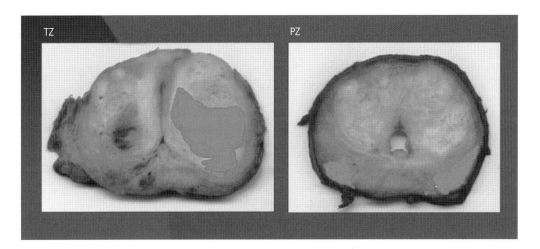

Figure 15.4 Cancer arises mostly in the outer zone of the prostate.

Pathology

Prostate cancer usually arises in the peripheral zone, which may be compressed into a shell by benign enlargement of the central zone (Figure 15.4). It is not uncommon that cancer does also arise in the inner zone.

Most prostate adenocarcinomas are composed of acini arranged in patterns variable in space, size and shape. Mucin and crystalloids are often present in the acinar lumens. The stroma frequently contains collagen. Perineural and microvascular invasion is a strong indicator of poor prognosis.

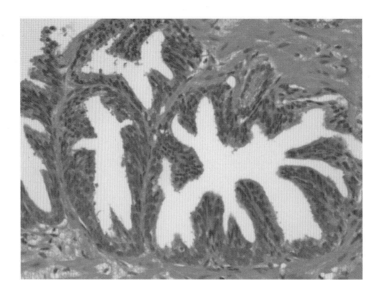

Figure 15.5 Prostatic intra-epithelial neoplasia.

Prostatic intra-epithelial neoplasia

This pathological change is characterised by cellular proliferation within pre-existing ducts and acini with cytological changes mimicking cancer, including nuclear and nucleolar enlargement. Despite these changes, an intact or fragmented basal cell layer is retained unlike cancer where a basal cell layer is lacking or breached. There are two grades: low-grade prostatic intra-epithelial neoplasia (PIN) and high-grade intra-epithelial neoplasia (HGPIN) (Figure 15.5). A high level of inter-observer variability with low-grade PIN limits its clinical value, and indeed many pathologists do not report it. HGPIN is now generally accepted as a potential likely preinvasive stage of adenocarcinoma, and its presence in prostate biopsies warrants repeat biopsy for concurrent or subsequent invasive adenocarcinoma.

Histological grade

The Gleason system is based on the assessment of the pattern of differentiation seen in two low-power fields (Figures 15.6 and 15.7), each assigned a number from 1 to 5. The two numbers are added together to provide a Gleason sum score between 2 and 10. The Gleason system

provides important prognostic information. It correlates very well with the clinical behaviour of the tumour and its response to treatment.

Tumour markers

Biomarkers that help clinicians determine whom to biopsy

- **PSA**

  This is an androgen-regulated protease in the kallikrein family (hk3) that originates as a 17-amino-acid chain. It is secreted only by prostate cells whether benign or malignant. It is normally secreted into semen or lost in urine. It liquefies semen through its action on gel-forming proteins within the semen following ejaculation. It spills over into the bloodstream where it can be measured. It can also be detected by immunofluorescent methods in histological sections. Production of PSA by both normal and malignant prostate glands is dependent on male hormones (androgens) being present in the body at normal levels. The presence of an elevated PSA suggests that either the prostate is enlarged or an abnormal condition exists within it (inflammation, infection, trauma or

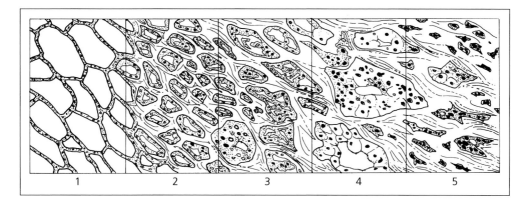

Figure 15.6 The Gleason system: for each tumour, two low-power fields are assigned a score from 1 to 5; the Gleason score is the sum.

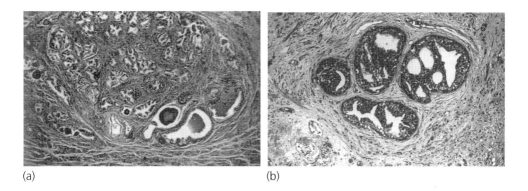

(a)   (b)

Figure 15.7 (a) Benign hyperplasia and (b) cancer – an area of Gleason 2 is surrounded by anaplastic Gleason 5.

cancer). An elevated PSA is not therefore cancer specific. Even at low serum PSA can occur (Table 15.1).

- *Free and total PSA*
  PSA in the plasma may exist in either a free form or one bound to proteins in the blood (alpha 2-macroglobulin or alpha 1-antichymotrypsin). Men with prostate cancer have a greater fraction of complexed bound PSA fraction and lower unbound free PSA in the serum.

  For any given total PSA value with levels between 4 and 10 ng/mL, the percentage of free PSA significantly improves the ability to distinguish between men with or without cancer compared with level of total PSA alone. This aids in optimising sensitivity and specificity for prostate cancer detection depending on

Table 15.1 Risk of prostate cancer in relation to low PSA values

PSA level (ng/mL)	Risk of prostate cancer	Risk of Gleason ≥7%
0.0–0.5	6.6	0.8
0.6–1.0	10.1	1.0
1.1–2.0	17.0	2.0
2.1–3.0	23.9	4.6
3.1–4.0	26.9	6.7

prostate size. The value of free/total PSA ratio when total PSA levels are less than 4.0 ng/mL is unclear regarding prostate cancer being present.

Table 15.2 Total PSA age reference ranges

Age range (years)	Reference range (ng/mL)
40–49	0–2.5
50–59	0–3.5
60–69	0–4.5
70–79	0–6.5

 KEYPOINTS

- PSA is prostate gland specific but not prostate cancer specific.
- To have a routine PSA measurement in asymptomatic non-high-risk man should be clearly counselled in advance and implications understood.
- False negative results do occur.
- A PSA test may detect a slow-growing tumour that could never give any problems and may not warrant treatment.

For men with a slightly elevated total PSA of between 6 and 10 ng/L and a percentage of free PSA more than 25, the risk of prostate cancer being present may be so low that prostate biopsy may be avoided or delayed. This characteristic should not be used as a sole indicator, and other factors such as the digital rectal examination should be taken into account.

- **Age-specific PSA levels**
There is a consistent rise in the size of the prostate in the ageing male (range 0.4–1.2 g/year). So, PSA increases with age (Table 15.2). The use of age-specific PSA levels enhances the specificity and sensitivity of the test and may avoid unnecessary biopsies. One should be suspicious of prostate cancer if the patient's age-specific PSA level is abnormal. The PSA cut-off levels are continuously being challenged in an attempt to improve prostate cancer detection at an earlier age and stage.

- **PSA density**
An enlarged prostate gland of benign nature might produce an elevated PSA. In order to allow for the contribution of benign hyperplasia, a calculation to enhance PSA specificity was proposed by dividing the serum PSA by prostate volume (cc). PSA density values of 0.15 or more might indicate a risk of prostate cancer and prostate biopsy is recommended. There is no complete agreement in the literature about the accuracy of this tool, which many urologists consider useful. It can be an additional tool of value in risk assessment for counselling patients with PSA levels of 4–10 ng/mL regarding the need for prostate biopsy or repeat biopsy if PSA is persistently elevated.

- **PSA velocity**
This is a measurement of change in PSA serum levels in nanograms per millilitre per year (ng/mL/year). A series of at least three PSA blood tests must be obtained. If the PSA increase is more than 0.75 ng/mL/year, one ought to suspect that prostate cancer might be causing the rise.

- **Doubling time**
Evaluation of the rate of PSA change in men with prostate disease may provide a means to improve management. In patients with prostate cancer, PSA changes seem to have both a linear and an exponential phase. During the exponential phase, PSA doubling time for patients with local/regional carcinoma seems to range from 1.5 to 6.6 years (median 3 years). In those with advanced/metastatic disease, the range is 0.9–8.5 years (median 2 years). The PSA doubling time may be helpful in guiding the diagnosis and treatment of prostate cancer patients.

- **PCA3**
PCA3 gene is a non-coding messenger RNA specific to the prostate cells and is overexpressed only by malignant tissue. It is significantly up-regulated 60- to 100-fold in prostate cancer. Massaging the prostate gland releases prostate cells into the urinary tract where they can be collected in the first urine that is passed. The prostate cells are harvested and the expression of mRNA from the PCA3 gene assessed. PCA3 mRNA along with the mRNA of PSA is measured quantitatively and examined

as a ratio. High ratios have been shown to be indicative of prostate cancer. It is of particular value in the follow-up treatment of patients with an elevated serum PSA and negative biopsy results. PCA3 is also considered to be helpful in deciding when to re-biopsy and in the follow-up of patients under active surveillance.

The test has shown a sensitivity of 67% and a specificity of 89% claiming an overall accuracy of 81% for the detection of prostate cancer in comparison to PSA of approximately 40%. PCA3 has been shown to be elevated in >90% of men with prostate cancer but not significantly elevated in normal prostatic glands or in benign prostatic hypertrophy.

Biomarkers that help clinicians determine when to re-biopsy

- **Prostate Health Index (phi)**
  The phi has been developed as an additional diagnostic biomarker in men with a serum PSA level of 2–10 ng/mL: phi = [−2] proPSA/fPSA × PSA1/2. (ProPSA is a PSA subtype and fPSA is a free PSA.)

  Elevated proPSA/fPSA ratios are associated with prostate cancer. In a recent prospective cohort of men enrolled into active surveillance for prostate cancer, higher serum and tissue levels of proPSA at diagnosis were associated with the need for subsequent treatment.

- **PTEN gene**
  PTEN is a tumour suppressor gene involved in cell cycle regulation. Dysregulation is consistently associated with poor prognosis in prostate cancer. Deletion of *PTEN* is associated with higher Gleason grade, risk of progression and recurrence after therapy. Additionally, it is associated with advanced localised or metastatic disease and death. The PTEN assay is a prognostic fluorescence *in situ* hybridisation (FISH) test. Typically it is ordered in conjunction with prostate biopsy tests to indicate partial (hemizygous) or complete (homozygous) deletions in the gene. For patients with a cancer diagnosis (e.g. low-intermediate Gleason scores of 6/7), the PTEN assay may help determine the rate of progression and subsequent appropriate therapy. For patients with HGPIN or an atypical diagnosis, it is an effective screening tool that allows clinicians to distinguish nonaggressive HGPIN or an atypical diagnosis from men at higher risk of prostate cancer.

- **Prostate Core Mitomic Test (PCMT)**
  Mitochondrial and nuclear genomics allows detection of depletion in mitochondrial DNA indicating cellular change associated with undiagnosed prostate cancer in a tumour field effect. The test detects the presence of malignant cells in normal-appearing prostate tissue across an extended area using existing prostate biopsy tissue.

- **ConfirmMDx**
  This is an epigenetic assay to help distinguish patients who have a true negative biopsy from those who may have occult cancer. It detects an epigenetic field effect with the 'cancerisation' process at the DNA level. This field effect around the cancer lesion can be present despite the normal appearance of cells. Detection of field effects extends the coverage of the biopsy, helping to rule in, or rule out, occult cancers. It provides actionable information to help men without prostate cancer avoid unnecessary repeat biopsies, with their inherent risk, and to identify men who require repeat biopsies and potential treatment.

- **ProMark**
  This is an automated quantitative multiplex immunofluorescence *in situ* imaging that identifies as predictive protein biomarkers (phospho-S6 and phospho-PRAS40) for prostate cancer. It is thought to/can differentiate indolent from aggressive disease, based on standard formalin-fixed, paraffin-embedded tissue.

Presentation

- *Chance finding at transurethral prostate resection*
  Carcinoma is found by chance in about 10% of patients undergoing transurethral resection of the prostate (TURP) for what was until then thought to be a benign enlargement of

the prostate. Knowing the true incidence of cancer in the prostate, one would expect the figure to be higher, but of course TURP takes out mostly the inner zone tissue and spares the compressed outer zone where most of the cancers arise.

- **Local symptoms**
  - *Obstructive uropathy*: Compression of the urethra may cause symptoms identical with those due to benign enlargement.
  - *Rectal obstruction*: If the cancer is encircling the rectum, the patient may complain of pencil-thin stools and progressive constipation.
  - *Uraemia*: Ureteric obstruction may lead to hydroureter and hydronephrosis and, if bilateral, to uraemia.
- **Distant metastases effects**

  Metastases may occur anywhere but usually affect the lumbar vertebrae, pelvis and femora. These may cause bone pains characteristically waking the patient at night, pathological fractures or spinal cord compression. In an X-ray these metastases are typically denser than the normal bone (osteosclerotic) (Figure 15.8). Osteolytic bone lesions are also found but much less often. Occasionally fibrinolysins produced by metastases can cause bruising and haemorrhages; anaemia is not uncommon. Soft tissue metastases lead to symptoms according to the affected site, for example, chronic cough in lung metastatic disease.

Investigations

- **Trans-rectal ultrasound**
- The glandular tissue element of the prostate shows a stippled grey appearance that is isoechoic. Less echogenic tissue, for example, cancer, will be designed hypoechoic, and calcification would be hypoechoic (Figure 15.9). Any suspicious area is biopsied using a biopsy needle placed under ultrasonic control. Often a prostate harbouring cancerous changes shows normal echogenic features where the examination is driven by an elevated PSA value in the presence of a normal digital rectal examination. Antibiotic prophylaxis therapy is routinely given, and the complications of bleeding or infection are rare. Local anaesthesia may be given. The biopsies are obtained in a predetermined pattern to sample the peripheral zone. Transition zone biopsies are added when necessary.

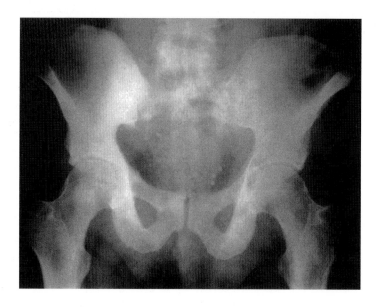

Figure 15.8 X-ray of pelvis showing areas of increased density caused by metastases.

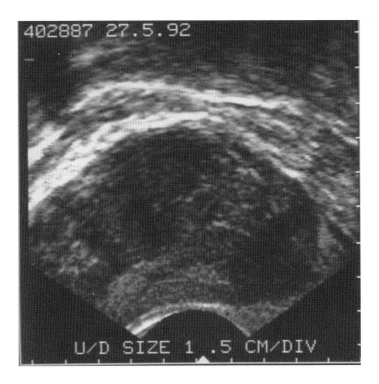

Figure 15.9 Trans-rectal ultrasound showing cancer breaching the capsule on the left side.

The ultrasound image may show that cancer has invaded the seminal vesicles or the periprostatic fat and so help to stage the case. At the time of biopsy, determination of the prostate size and shape is obtained, and any anatomical abnormalities are detected. Trans-perineal prostate biopsy is also performed and reduces the risk of sepsis. Using the trans-perineal route also enables biopsies to be taken in a more systematic manner with the aid of a template.

- *Magnetic resonance imaging*
  An MRI scanner uses a magnetic field and radio waves to build up detailed pictures of various parts of the body by picking up signals sent out by water molecules. This relies on the characteristics of tissues to provide two-dimensional pictures with different orientations as outlined in Chapter 2. These images may be even more precise in staging the cancer (Figure 15.10) and are often performed before biopsy in order to aid targeted biopsies and to allow accurate radiological staging. MRI following biopsy

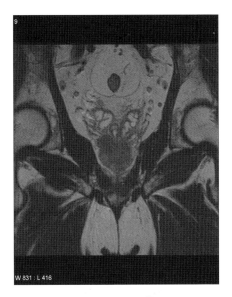

Figure 15.10 Magnetic resonance imaging (MRI) T2-weighted image showing invasion of the seminal vesicle on the right side.

can be difficult to interpret due to haemorrhage in the first 3–6 months. Multiparametric 3T modality demonstrates the best evaluation of the prostate gland. Fusing the prostate views and live trans-rectal ultrasound prostate scan can facilitate and identify target areas that improves the precise outcome of biopsies

- *Computerised tomography of the abdomen and pelvis*

  Computerised tomography (CT) might reveal enlarged pelvic lymph nodes and invasion of the seminal vesicles (Figure 15.11) as well as spread of cancer to the liver and other organs. Although magnetic resonance imaging is increasingly more utilised than CT, there are patients who are not suitable to be in a magnetic field and CT can be performed instead.

- *Positron emission tomography*

  This is a medical imaging technique in which a small amount of a radioactive tracer is given to the patient, normally by injecting it into a vein. The most commonly used tracer in staging prostate cancer is choline C-11. This is a radioactive form of the vitamin choline, which prostate

cancer cells readily absorb. Choline C-11 positron emission tomography (PET) scans may be used when other imaging is not helpful. PET and CT can be combined to provide important information about many conditions affecting the different organs of the body (Figure 15.12).

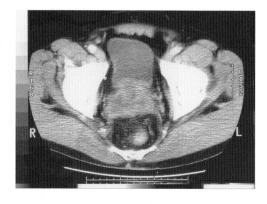

Figure 15.11 CT scan showing carcinoma of the prostate with impending ureteric obstruction due to extra prostatic invasion of the bladder base.

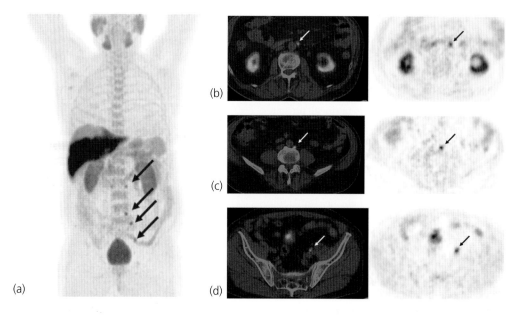

Figure 15.12 18-Fluorocholine PET/CT study. A 77-year-old postradical radiotherapy for prostate carcinoma. Biochemical relapse PSA 7 ng/mL. Maximum intensity projection (MIP) image (a) shows focal activity in several nodes. On the axial fused and PET slices, these correspond to small retroperitoneal and pelvic nodes (b–d, arrowed) not enlarged by CT size criteria. Reproduced with permission from Tara Barwick.

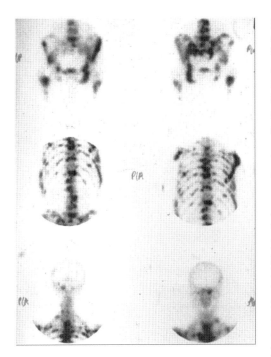

Figure 15.13 Bone scan showing multiple 'hot spots' from metastases.

- **Bone scan**
  The radionuclide ^{99m}Tc-MDP (methylene diphosphonate) is taken up by the bone in proportion to the blood flow, so the increased vascularity of a metastasis shows a 'hot spot' (Figure 15.13). False positives are common from osteoarthritis and old fractures of the ribs. When the bones are so very widely invaded as to be almost uniform, there may be a 'superscan'.

Staging of prostate cancer

Staging of prostate cancer takes into account its method of spread, which is directly up into the bladder and seminal vesicles. It seldom goes through Denonvilliers' fascia into the rectum but instead can grow around it to cause rectal and ureteric obstruction. It quickly invades the pelvic lymph nodes and spreads by the veins and lymphatics into the marrow of the lumbar spine, pelvis and femora. The T staging in the TNM classification system (Sobin LH, Gospodarowicz M, Wittekind C. *HYPERLINK "/australia/Citation: Sobin_LH,_Gospodarowicz_M,_Wittekind_C_2009"TNM classification of Malignant Tumours.* Seventh Edition. UICC International Union Against Cancer. New York: Wiley-Blackwell 2009 Jan 1.) is set out in Figure 15.14.

Treatment

A number of factors need to be taken into account when considering the treatment options for patients. These include familial history, ethnic origin, life expectancy and the disease stage whether localised or metastatic and patient choice. Given the considerable debate that exists as to the preferred choice of treatment, the pros and cons of each different method of treatment should be explained to the patient by the different disciplines involved in the management of prostate cancer so that an informed choice can be made. To advise patients one must be able to predict the outcome of each method of treatment. Here nomograms may be helpful. A nomogram is a graphic representation of a statistical model that incorporates several variables to predict a particular end point. Predictive pretreatment nomograms make outcome predictions based on the characteristics of individual patient: clinical stage, biopsy Gleason sum, pretreatment PSA level, receipt of neoadjuvant hormonal deprivation therapy and total radiation dose as predictor variables. An example is shown in Table 15.3. Some men find it repugnant to think that they might be walking around with cancer. Others find the prospect of the potential side effects associated with treatment such as incontinence and impotence no less undesirable and prefer to take their chance.

Localised disease

Taking into account the prognostic parameters that have been identified, patients are divided into risk groups: low, intermediate and high (Table 15.4).

The options in localised prostate cancer include watchful waiting/active surveillance, surgery, irradiation and methods of ablation

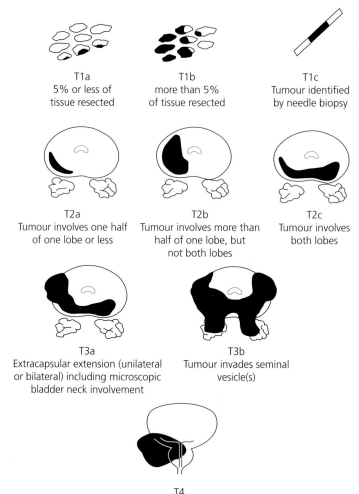

T1a
5% or less of
tissue resected

T1b
more than 5%
of tissue resected

T1c
Tumour identified
by needle biopsy

T2a
Tumour involves one half
of one lobe or less

T2b
Tumour involves more than
half of one lobe, but
not both lobes

T2c
Tumour involves
both lobes

T3a
Extracapsular extension (unilateral
or bilateral) including microscopic
bladder neck involvement

T3b
Tumour invades seminal
vesicle(s)

T4
Tumour is fixed or invades adjacent structures other than seminal vesicles:
external sphincter, rectum, levator muscles, and/or pelvic wall.

Figure 15.14 The T staging in the TNM classification of prostate cancer.

including cryosurgery and high-intensity focused ultrasound.

- **Active surveillance**

  In certain patients a policy of observation and monitoring might be a preferred management option. In an incidental prostate cancer found at transurethral prostate resection (T1a), the probability of disease progression may be very low. Patients who have reduced life expectancy might be monitored with regular PSA measurements, proceeding to therapy only if there was

clear evidence of disease progression. Gleason histological grading is believed to be the best indicator of the probability of significant disease progression. NICE proposed a guide protocol to be acknowledged by clinicians and patients. The purpose of active surveillance is to identify the small number of prostate tumours that are likely to progress and cause morbidity within the patient's natural lifespan, so they can be treated, while sparing the majority of patients with clinically insignificant disease from the

Table 15.3 Prostate nomogram

Prostate nomogram results: pretreatment

Pretreatment PSA	9.1	Organ-confined disease	49%
Biopsy primary Gleason	3	Extra-capsular penetration	40%
Biopsy secondary Gleason	4	Seminal vesicle involvement	8%
Biopsy Gleason score	7	Lymph node involvement	3%
Clinical tumour stage	T1c	5-Year progression-free probability Postradical prostatectomy	77%
Prescribed external radiation dose (64.8–86.4 Gy)	86.4	5-Year progression-free probability Post-external beam radiotherapy	87%
Neoadjuvant hormones	No	5-Year progression-free probability Post-brachytherapy	72%
Neoadjuvant radiation	No		

Table 15.4 Predictive risk groups' criteria in prostate cancer

Low	Intermediate	High
Clinical T1a or T1c	Clinical T1b or T2a	Clinical T2b–T3
PSA <10	PSA <10	PSA 10–20
Gleason score <6	Gleason score 6 or 7 (3 + 4)	Gleason score ≥7
Biopsy: unilateral or <50% core +ve	Biopsy: bilateral	Biopsy: >50% core +ve or perineural invasion or ductal/neuroendocrine differentiation

harms of over treatment. A guide for active surveillance is recommended by NICE (Table 15.5).

- **Radical prostatectomy**

  There is a heated debate between those who favour radical prostatectomy for cancers that appear to be confined to the prostate and those who are against it.

  The arguments in favour of radical surgery are as follows:

  - More of those who survive for 10–15 years after radical surgery do so without residual cancer.
  - Improved surgical techniques can achieve potency preservation and continence.

The arguments against radical prostatectomy are the following:

- Almost every elderly man has a small cancer in his prostate, but less than 0.5% die of it; that is, 99.5% do not.

Table 15.5 Prostate cancer protocol for active surveillance guide

Timing	Tests
Year 1	• PSA/3 months. Kinetics • DRE/6–12 months • At 12 months: prostate re-biopsy
Years 2–4	• PSA/3–6 months. Kinetics • DRE/6–12 months
Year 5 and yearly thereafter	• PSA/6 months. Kinetics • DRE/12 months

Source: NICE (Prostate cancer: protocol for *active surveillance*. Implementing the *NICE* guideline on prostate cancer (CG175). Published: January 2014).

- The only prospective controlled studies to have been carried out showed no differences in survival after 20 years between men treated by radical surgery or surveillance.
- Larger retrospective studies show no difference in survival between those undergoing radical surgery and surveillance.
- The morbidity of radical prostatectomy includes incontinence, stricture and impotence in a (debated but large) proportion of patients.

Open retropubic surgical excision was initially introduced more than 25 years ago and gradually became the popular surgical modality offered. Trans-perineal prostatectomy, a different surgical approach, was offered to selected patients where no lymphadenectomy is contemplated. Laparoscopic approach gained wide appeal. Gradually open surgery has been challenged and robotic techniques are becoming more popular. All techniques rely on the expertise of the urological surgeon and meticulous patient selection. The anatomical steps are more or less the same.

The prostate is approached retropubically, the dorsal veins of the penis are doubly ligated and divided behind the symphysis, and the neurovascular bundles going to the penis are pushed aside out of harm's way (Figure 15.15). The urethra is transected, and the prostate lifted up, to reveal the seminal vesicles, whose vessels are ligated. The bladder is then cut across at the level of the bladder neck, which is then narrowed, and sutured to the stump of the urethra over a catheter (Figure 15.16). The lymph nodes along the internal iliac and obturator vessels are dissected and removed unless no lymphadenectomy is contemplated.

Staging lymph node dissection

Most surgeons consider that radical prostatectomy is futile if the lymph nodes are involved and usually sample the lymph nodes around the obturator nerve and vessels before going ahead with radical surgery. This can be performed laparoscopically a few days before surgery is planned or as the first stage of the operation.

- Radiotherapy

There are numerous ways to deliver therapeutic radiation including external beam radiotherapy with the linear accelerator and brachytherapy (inserting radioactive sources into the prostate under trans-rectal ultrasound control (Figure 15.17). There is no clear consensus as to which method of radiotherapy is best. What is clear is that certain patients may be better suited for one or another or, in fact, a combination of these modalities. Pre-treatment PSA levels and Gleason histological score are very important tools for prediction of response. It is important to define the patient's risk status (high, intermediate or low) to determine the method of choice offered to the individual patient. No randomised prospective controlled study has ever shown that any type of radiation is better or worse than surveillance or radical prostatectomy. Survival is much the same, but residual cancer is found more often after radiation in the survivors than in those treated by surgery, even though it does not necessarily cause symptoms. Neoadjuvant and adjuvant hormone suppression combined with radiotherapy improves local control, may prolong disease-free survival and may delay

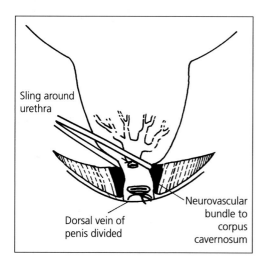

Sling around urethra

Dorsal vein of penis divided

Neurovascular bundle to corpus cavernosum

Figure 15.15 Radical retropubic prostatectomy: the neurovascular bundles to the penis can be preserved.

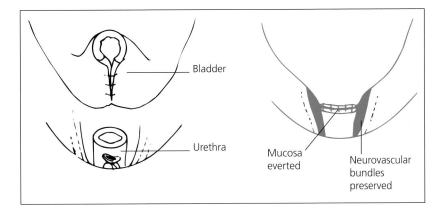

Figure 15.16 After the prostate has been removed, the bladder is sutured to the stump of the urethra.

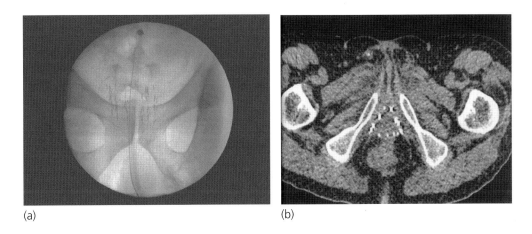

(a)

(b)

Figure 15.17 Brachytherapy: (a) iodine seeds and (b) gold grains.

the time to the development of metastatic disease and extend overall survival in some subsets of patients.

Painful proctitis is a common early sequel of radiation, and impotence occurs in a proportion, probably as a result of radiation arteritis.

- Cryosurgery

Complete cell destruction occurs in response to freezing down to temperatures reaching −40°C. The direct effects of cryosurgery on cells include the following:

- Crystallisation of extracellular fluid leading to cellular dehydration.

- Cellular pH changes leading to electrolyte abnormalities resulting in denaturation of cellular proteins.
- Lipoproteins are damaged in response to the thermal shock.
- Cellular membrane disruption occurs as a result of intracellular crystallisation.
- Membrane disruption occurs due to fluid influx during thawing following freezing.
- Thrombosis and vascular stasis occurs after freezing.

Cryosurgery clinical experience continues to advance. Improvements and refinement of the

> **🔑 KEYPOINTS**
>
> **Localised disease management modalities**
>
> | | Low risk | Intermediate risk | High risk |
> |---|---|---|---|
> | Watchful waiting | Yes[a] | Yes[a] | Yes[a] |
> | Active surveillance | Yes[b] | No | No |
> | Radical prostatectomy | Yes[b,c] | Yes[b] | Yes[b] |
> | Radiotherapy | Yes | Yes | Yes (MDT) |
> | | EBR or brachytherapy | Androgen deprivation 4–6 months | Androgen deprivation 2–3 years |
>
> [a] <10 years life expectancy.
> [b] >10 years life expectancy.
> [c] Biopsy minimal core involvement <50% cancer.

delivery systems are promising and may lead to increase in its use.

- High-intensity focused ultrasound therapy (HIFU)

  A recent method of treatment carried out under a spinal or general anaesthetic is thought to be offering an advance in prostate cancer management. A beam of ultrasound emission from a rectal probe targets the prostate gland. It is focused to reach a high intensity in the target tissue where absorption of the ultrasound energy creates an increase in the temperature, which destroys tissue. A cooling balloon surrounds the probe to protect the rectal mucosa from the high temperature. A urethral or a suprapubic catheter is inserted after the procedure to aid urinary drainage during the time the necrotic debris is expelled. The long-term clinical outcome and impact on quality of life are currently being studied.

Advanced/metastatic disease

Hormonal manipulation

Malignant prostate cells start off by requiring a daily supply of testosterone – without which they die. Largely as a result of these and other anecdotal experiences, there was a feeling that no harm arose from deferring the treatment until metastases began to cause symptoms. This was the subject of a recent Medical Research Council controlled prospective trial, but this showed an unacceptably high incidence of serious metastatic complications in patients for whom hormone therapy had been deferred.

The different ways of hormonal manipulation and the adverse effects encountered are illustrated in Figure 15.18. The testosterone metabolic pathway in Figure 15.19 demonstrates the effects of the withdrawal of testosterone and its metabolites or antagonism for the metabolites only on target tissue. The supply of testosterone can be cut off or interfered within a number of ways:

1. *Orchidectomy*: The testicles may be removed, or a subcapsular orchidectomy may be performed, which leaves something behind that feels like a normal testicle.

2. *Diethylstilboestrol*: This is a synthetic oestrogen that blocks the products of metabolism of testosterone. It is not commonly used to treat prostate cancer now because the synthetic version – diethylstilbestrol – has been shown to cause serious cardiovascular problems and is no longer used.

3. *Luteinising hormone-releasing hormone* (LHRH) *agonist*: LHRH overstimulates the anterior pituitary gland and initially more

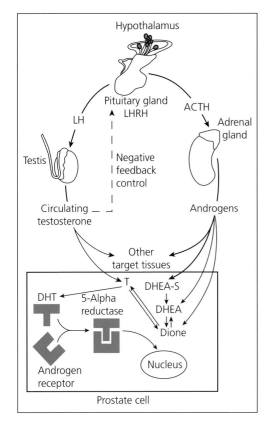

Figure 15.18 Androgen hormonal pathway and metabolic changes demonstrating sites of various treatment approaches.

luteinising hormone is released during the first 2 weeks of treatment and thus an increased testosterone secretion. This may cause a 'flare-up' with pain and other complications from metastases; thus, LHRH agonists are given in combination with drugs that block the action of testosterone in the cells – anti-androgens (see later). However, downregulation of the prostate cell receptors leads to a decreased luteinising hormone production, which in turn results in the testes no longer secreting testosterone with maintenance therapy.

4. *Gonadotrophin-releasing hormone antagonist*: Recent interest in novel gonadotrophin-releasing hormone antagonist formulation degarelix is appealing as it can provide a faster onset of castration than with agonists and no testosterone surge without concomitant anti-androgen treatment. Furthermore, data suggest that it improves disease control and might delay the onset of castrate-resistant disease.

5. *Anti-androgens*: Dihydrotestosterone acts on receptors in the cytosol of the prostate cell. These receptors are blocked by two types of anti-androgen:
   i. Steroids such as megestrol and cyproterone
   ii. Non-steroids such as flutamide, nilutamide and bicalutamide

6. *Aromatase inhibitors*: These prevent the action of *aromatase*, an enzyme in the prostate cell that converts adrenal steroids into testosterone.

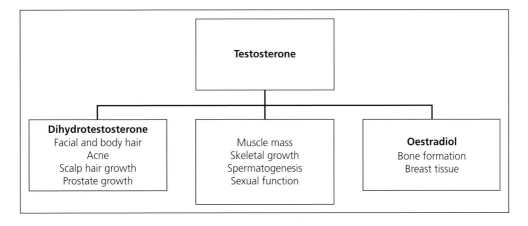

Figure 15.19 The testosterone metabolic pathway.

Maximal androgen blockade

A combination of LHRH agonists given together with anti-androgens is claimed to give a small improvement (a matter of weeks) in survival, but not everyone is convinced that this is justified by the side effects, let alone the expense of this additional therapy.

Side effects of hormonal therapy

We have become more aware of the side effects of hormonal treatment. Orchidectomy, LHRH analogues and LHRH antagonists can all cause similar effects due to changes in the level of hormones such as testosterone and oestrogen. These side effects include:

- Reduced or absent libido (sexual desire)
- Impotence (erectile dysfunction)
- Shrinking of testicles and penis
- Hot flashes, which may get better or even go away with time
- Breast tenderness and growth of breast tissue
- Osteoporosis (bone thinning), which can lead to broken bones
- Anaemia (low red blood cell counts)
- Decreased mental sharpness
- Loss of muscle mass
- Weight gain
- Fatigue
- Increased cholesterol
- Depression

Some research has suggested that the risk of high blood pressure, diabetes, strokes, heart attacks and even death from heart disease is higher in men treated with hormone therapy, although not all studies have found this.

Castrate-resistant prostate cancer (CRPC)

Cancer of the prostate is a heterogeneous disease, and our knowledge of the mechanisms involved in androgen independence remains incomplete. After the initiation of androgen deprivation therapy (ADT), the vast majority of prostate cancer patients will show some evidence of clinical response. The magnitude and rapidity of that response remain the best predictors of its durability. Assuming ADT effectively targets the androgen-sensitive population of prostate cancer cells, an incomplete or sluggish response raises the possible evolution of an androgen-refractory population. Early in the clinical use of PSA as a biomarker of prostate cancer response, it was recognised that declines in PSA could predict response. For example, patients who had more than an 80% drop of PSA within 1 month of initiating ADT had a significantly longer disease-free progression. Likewise, the nadir PSA predicted the progression-free interval, as did pretreatment testosterone levels. In cancer, mutant clones eventually emerge, which no longer depend on testosterone, and this (on average) occurs in about 80% of men within 2 years of the diagnosis of metastases; however, among the 20% who do not develop metastases within 2 years, there are many who survive for decades without any other treatment. A rise in PSA level, which is evidence of the emergence of castrate-resistant disease, preceded bone metastatic progression by several months, with a mean lead time of 7.3 months.

The androgen receptor (AR) is a modular cytoplasmic protein that binds to the DHT component forming an androgen complex component, which is thought to undergo a conformational change allowing nuclear translocation and driving gene transcription. The adrenal cortical androgen contribution, 5%, is recognised. In addition, it is acknowledged that testosterone is synthesised directly from cholesterol by the CYP11A and CYP17 enzymes. An alteration in normal androgen signalling is thought to be central in the pathogenesis of androgen-independent prostate cancer.

AR-independent mechanisms may be associated with the deregulation of apoptosis through the deregulation of oncogenes. High levels of *bcl-2* expression are seen with greater frequency as prostate cancer progress, and the regulation of microtubule integrity may be a mechanism through which *bcl-2* induces its anti-apoptotic effect. Indeed, most active chemotherapeutics in hormone-resistant prostate cancer work by inhibiting microtubule formation. The tumour suppressor gene *p53* is more frequently mutated in androgen-independent prostate cancer. Overexpression of *bcl-2* and *p53* in prostatectomy specimens has been shown to predict an aggressive clinical course.

AR possible changes contributing to castrate evolution are demonstrated in Figure 15.20a–c. AR amplification may lead to AR hypersensitivity. AR mutations may lead to a functional change in AR function. Because AR mutations are found in only a subpopulation of tumour cells, they are unlikely to be responsible for the entire spectrum of the AR-independent state. The AR mutations might be related to the selective pressure of anti-androgens. The recent discovery of gene fusion between the androgen-driven TMPRSS2 and the EGR–ETS oncogene family raises the question of oncogene regulation through androgen regulation pathways. The mechanism of gene fusion is based on the association of an androgen-responsive element from an androgen-regulated gene with genes that are usually not androgen regulated leading to their androgen regulation.

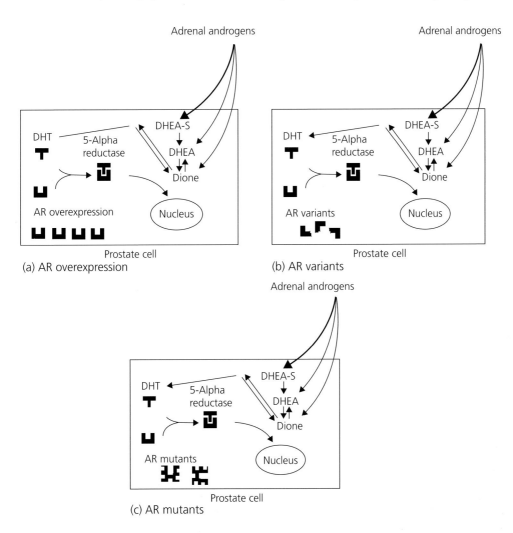

Figure 15.20 (a–c) Androgen receptor possible changes contributing to castrate resistance evolution.

Even in castrated patients, metastatic tissues have repeatedly shown high levels of androgens, suggesting a high level of intracrine synthesis. It is possible that a high intraprostatic cholesterol level can activate specific androgen pathways.

Definition of HRPC

- Castrate serum testosterone <50 ng/dL or 1.7 nmol/L plus metastases progression
- Biochemical progression: three consecutive rises of PSA – 1 week apart resulting in two 50% increases over the nadir with PSA >2 ng/mL
- Radiological progression: 2 or more bone lesions (bone scan) or progression of soft tissue lesions using response evaluation criteria in solid tumours (RECIST)

EAU Guidelines on Prostate Cancer 2015

Management

(A) Secondary hormonal therapy
- **Ketoconazole**: Non-specific CYP17 inhibitory properties are used to achieve adrenal androgen androstenedione suppression and are usually given with hydrocortisone 20 mg twice daily. Ketoconazole seems to be less effective in patients with low levels of androgen at baseline.
- **Abiraterone acetate** is a selective inhibitor of androgen biosynthesis that potently and irreversibly blocks CYP17, a crucial enzyme in testosterone and oestrogen synthesis resulting in virtually undetectable serum and intratumoural androgens. In castrate-resistant prostate cells, the intracellular androgen level is increased compared to androgen-sensitive cells, suggesting an adaptive mechanism, through an increase of androgen biosynthesis enzymes. Mineralocorticoid-related adverse events, hypokalaemia, hypertension and fluid retention reported in trials were mitigated by administration of prednisone as concomitant treatment. It has shown a significant overall improvement in survival.

- **Enzalutamide** (MDV3100): A novel anti-androgen that blocks the androgen AR transfer to the nucleus with a higher affinity compared to bicalutamide. It blocks the transfer of ARs to the nucleus so that no agonist-like activity should ever occur. In contrast, currently available drugs still permit the transfer of ARs to the nucleus. The ability of enzalutamide to block AR transfer is important because overexpression of the AR has been observed in CRPC. It has shown a significant overall improvement in survival.

(B) Cytotoxic agents (taxanes)
- Docetaxel is considered the standard first-line therapy in castrate-resistant prostate cancer patients. It is given at a dose of 75 mg/m^2 at 3-week intervals in combination with prednisone. It has demonstrated both a survival benefit and a palliative benefit in symptomatic disease.
- Cabazitaxel: A tubulin-binding taxane cabazitaxel in combination with prednisone significantly extends overall survival in men with hormone-refractory prostate cancer previously treated with a docetaxel-containing regimen overcoming taxane resistance.

(C) Bone-targeted agents
- Radium-223 is a calcium-mimicking radionuclide that is incorporated into areas of new bone formation, accumulating preferentially at sites of osteoblastic metastases. Radium-223 emits high-energy alpha particles, leading to highly localised tumour cell death while minimising damage to surrounding healthy tissue. It was well tolerated in initial trials and showed no evidence of myelodepression and significant improved overall survival treatment benefit.
- Zoledronic acid: Bisphosphonates are potent inhibitors of bone resorption. Zoledronic acid is the only bisphosphonate to demonstrate a beneficial effect in patients with castrate-resistant prostate cancer. Longer therapy seems to confer continued prolonged benefit. Toxicity includes osteonecrosis of the jaw, hypocalcaemia and nephrotoxicity.

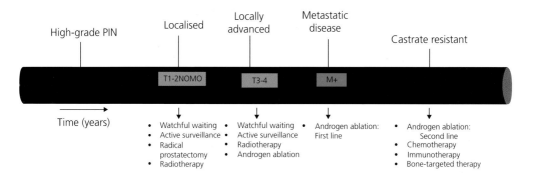

Figure 15.21 Prostate continuum and management strategies.

- Denosumab: Although prostate bone metastases are predominantly osteoblastic, analysis of bone turnover markers support the view that excess osteoclastic activity induces bone destruction in these metastases. Receptor activator of nuclear factor kappa B ligand (RANKL) is the main driver of osteoclast formation, function and survival. Denosumab is a human monoclonal antibody against RANKL, which has an inhibitory effect on osteoclast-mediated bone destruction.

(D) Targeted immunotherapy
- Sipuleucel-T: This is classified as an autologous cellular immunotherapeutic preparation designed to induce an immune response targeted against prostatic acid phosphatase (PAP). The patient's peripheral blood mononuclear cells are obtained and activated during a defined culture period with a recombinant human protein linked to a granulocyte-stimulating factor, an immune cell activator. The patient's peripheral blood mononuclear cells are obtained approximately 3 days prior to the infusion date. The cellular composition of sipuleucel-T is dependent on the composition of

cells obtained from the patient's leukopheresis. It contains T cells, B cells, natural killer cells and other cells. Each dose contains a minimum of 50 million autologous activated cells suspended in 250 mL of lactated Ringer's solution. The recommended course is three complete doses given approximately 2 weeks interval. The precise mechanism of action is unknown.

Key message

The prostate continuum and management strategies are demonstrated in Figure 15.21. Urologists are well trained in the management of patients on androgen ablation. It is recognised that eventually prostate cancer cells either adapt to low testosterone status, use adrenal androgens or probably synthesise androgens directly. An explosion of new treatments for castrate escape prostate cancer appeared over the last few years searching for effective second-line androgen deprivation and chemotherapy. Extensive clinical study programmes are ongoing to identify the best regimen protocols to offer patients. The golden goal should always be to achieve the best possible quality of life preservation issues.

Part 5

Male genitalia

16

The urethra

Anatomy

The male urethra is usually 16–18 cm in length and comprises prostatic, membranous, bulbar and penile sections; the later includes a short dilatation just proximal to the meatus called the fossa navicularis. The prostatic urethra is lined with transitional cell urothelium, and the remainder is pseudostratified columnar changing to stratified squamous epithelium close to the external urethral meatus. The female urethra is 3 cm in length and lined by pseudostratified columnar and squamous epithelium only. Paraurethral glands known as Cowper's and Littre's glands secrete mucous into the bulbar and penile urethra, respectively (Figure 16.1).

The urethra of both sexes is surrounded by the corpus spongiosum and in males expands to form the glans penis and in females the glans clitoris. Each corpus spongiosum is supported by a pair of corpora cavernosa, which are attached to the medial aspect of the ischiopubic rami (Figures 16.2 and 16.3).

Congenital disorders of the urethra

Errors in the genital folds

Hypospadias

As the embryonic *genital folds* roll in to form the male urethra and corpus spongiosum, they may fail to fuse, resulting in a urethra that opens on the ventral aspect of the penis – hypospadias (Figure 16.4). There are different degrees of hypospadias according to how far down the urethra the defect opens (Figure 16.5). Hypospadias also involves the additional deformities of a 'hooded' foreskin that is deficient ventrally and fibrous bands called cordee that may deform the penis so that it curves ventrally:

Glandular hypospadias: Here the urethra opens on the underside of the glans, but there is no other deformity. It causes no trouble in later life and it is questionable whether anything needs to be done about it at all. It can be

Urology Lecture Notes, Seventh Edition. Amir V. Kaisary, Andrew Ballaro and Katharine Pigott.
© 2016 John Wiley & Sons, Ltd. Published 2016 by John Wiley & Sons, Ltd.

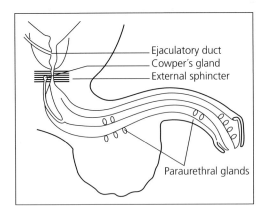

Figure 16.1 Anatomy of the male urethra.

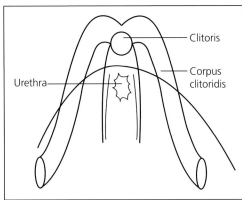

Figure 16.3 Anatomy of the female urethra and clitoris.

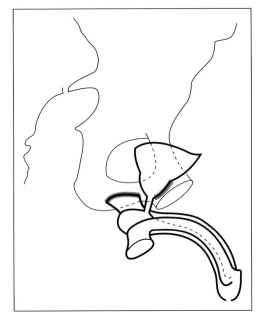

Figure 16.2 The fixed attachments of the corpora cavernosa to the ischiopubic rami below and the prostate to the symphysis pubis above: the membranous urethra is the weak link.

corrected by an operation, but it is doubtful whether this is justified merely on the basis of cosmetic advantage.

Penile hypospadias: Here the urethra opens onto the penile shaft. Correction is necessary and performed in early life, and the important thing is to refer the baby to a paediatric urological centre where these operations are done often enough to give the team experience. In specialised centres a one-stage operation is often successful (Figure 16.6).

Complete hypospadias: Here the meatus opens at the base of the penis, and a complex penile reconstruction is required. Correction of hypospadias is most effectively performed between 12 and 24 months of age; urethral scarring can necessitate multiple revision operations.

Errors in the development of the cloacal membrane

Bladder exstrophy and epispadias complex is a complex congenital abnormality of the genital tubercle and urethra. The condition affects both sexes with male predominance and is characterised by exposure of the urethral mucosa for a variable extent on its dorsal aspect. This may be confined to the penis, although underlying bladder neck abnormalities coexist, or may extend proximally resulting in splitting of the symphysis pubis, and the entire bladder may open to the anterior abdominal wall. In females the urethral plate is exposed dorsally and the clitoris is bifid. Complex reconstruction is required and normally takes place before 2 years of age.

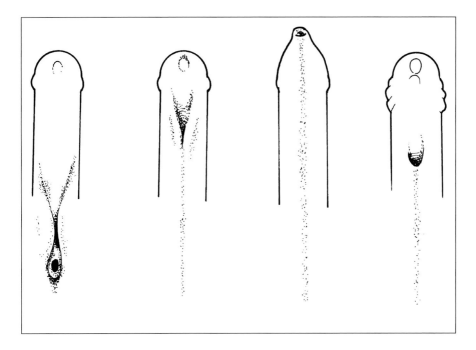

Figure 16.4 Incomplete inrolling of the genital folds results in different degrees of hypospadias.

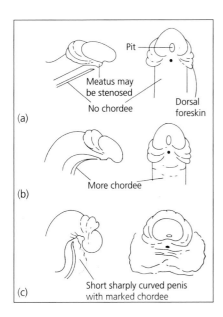

Figure 16.5 Varying degrees of hypospadias: (a) glandular, (b) coronal and (c) penoscrotal and perineal.

Congenital posterior urethral valves

Posterior urethral valves are thought to arise either from anomalous insertion of the mesonephric duct into the urogenital sinus or an abnormality of the cloacal membrane. There is a thin tough urethral membrane with a small aperture, which originates just distal to the verumontanum and extends anteriorly and distally beyond the sphincter (Figure 16.7) causing bladder outflow obstruction. The bladder responds to the obstruction by undergoing hypertrophy and trabeculation, and a range of associated renal and bladder dysfunction with vesicoureteric reflux and obstructive nephropathy may result. The condition accounts for a quarter of paediatric renal transplants. Posterior urethral valves are usually detected antenatally when vesicoamniotic shunting can be performed. Once the child has been delivered, the membrane is ablated endoscopically with a hook equipped with diathermy (Figure 16.8).

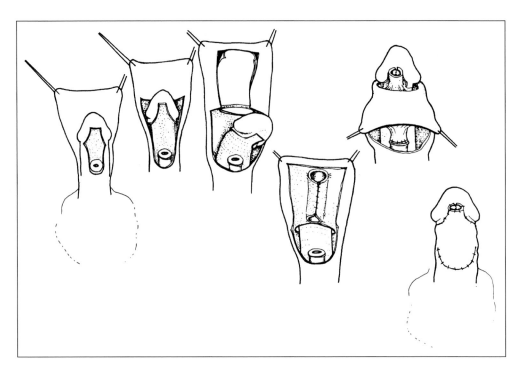

Figure 16.6 One-stage operation for hypospadias.

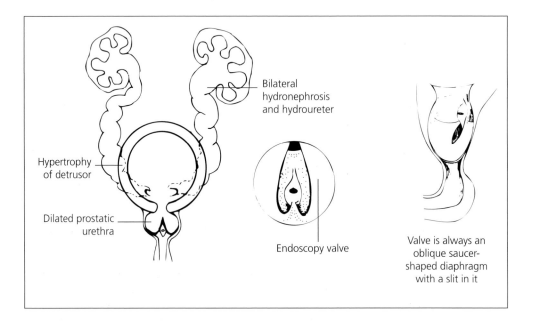

Bilateral
hydronephrosis
and hydroureter

Hypertrophy
of detrusor

Dilated prostatic
urethra

Endoscopy valve

Valve is always an
oblique saucer-
shaped diaphragm
with a slit in it

Figure 16.7 Congenital posterior urethral valves.

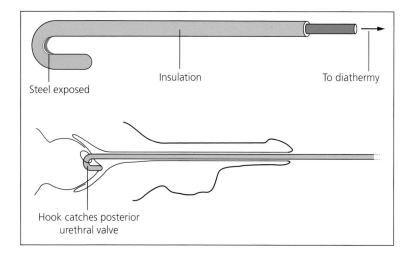

Steel exposed

Insulation

To diathermy

Hook catches posterior
urethral valve

Figure 16.8 Insulated diathermy hook for destroying posterior urethral valve.

Inflammation of the urethra

Gonorrhoea has been with mankind from time immemorial. Pharaohs took catheters with them to the afterlife, and Socrates made jokes about it. Infection with *Neisseria gonorrhoeae* causes acute inflammation in the periurethral glands. There is a profuse discharge of yellow pus in which a Gram stain will show the typical Gram-negative intracellular diplococci. The patient suffers painful urination, and the oedema and inflammation may cause the penis to bend when erect. There may be a urethral discharge. Eventually the inflammation subsides, but, if not treated promptly with antibiotics, leads to scarring in the periurethral tissues, which contracts and causes a stricture (Figure 16.9).

There are other bacterial causes of urethritis, notably *Chlamydia trachomatis, Ureaplasma and Mycoplasma* in which the organism is more difficult to identify, but which can also progress to a stricture. In the absence of gonococcal infection, urethritis is termed non-gonococcal or non-specific urethritis and is most appropriately treated with doxycycline or azithromycin.

Urethral trauma

Iatrogenic trauma

Instrumental injury to the urethra is common. A clean cut may heal with an inconspicuous scar and no stricture. However, when the injury is caused by the chronic pressure of a catheter leading to ischaemic necrosis or urethral rupture due to the blowing up of a catheter balloon in the urethra, healing may lead to a stricture. Iatrogenic strictures most commonly occur near the meatus due to introduction of a cystoscope through a tight meatus without first dilating it, at the penoscrotal junction where the urethra deviates and is prone to false passage formation during catheter insertion and endoscopic manipulation or at the level of the external sphincter (Figure 16.10).

There is one important variation on this theme. After open heart or aortic surgery, multiple strictures may occur along the length of the urethra. At first these were thought to be caused by some toxic chemical in latex catheters. It is now thought that the strictures are contributed to by urethral ischaemia due to haemodynamic effects of cardiopulmonary bypass (Figure 16.11).

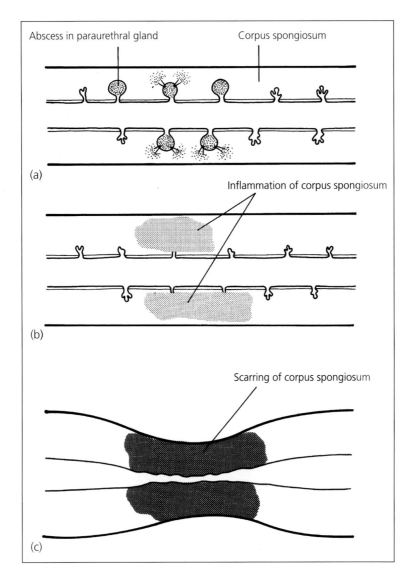

Figure 16.9 Sequential progress of acute gonorrhoea followed by scarring: (a) abscess in paraurethral gland, (b) inflammation of corpus spongiosum and (c) scarring of corpus spongiosum.

Blunt force injury

The blunt force of a fall astride injury, onto the crossbar of a bicycle, for example, leads to compression of the bulbar urethra against the inferior edge of the symphysis and tearing of the corpus spongiosum and urethra (Figure 16.12). Because the corpus spongiosum is firmly attached to the corpora cavernosa, its ends do not retract (Figure 16.13). Urine and blood escape into the scrotum, in a space that is limited by the fasciae of Scarpa and Colles. In the presence of infection, and particularly if there is faecal contamination of the extravasated urine due to concomitant bowel injury, necrotising fasciitis of the fat and overlying skin (Figure 16.14) may occur.

Management

The first priority is to treat the patient according to trauma protocols as associated injuries may be life threatening. The next step is to divert the urine. It is reasonable to gently attempt to pass a urethral catheter under antibiotic cover; if the urethral injury is incomplete, it may pass. If this fails, a suprapubic catheter is inserted under imaging control.

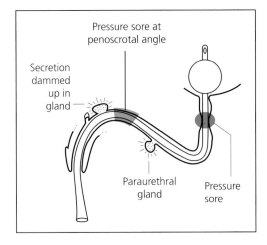

Figure 16.10 Dangers of a snugly fitting catheter.

About 10 days later the urethra is examined with the flexible cystoscope: in some cases it will be found to have healed completely. Alternatively the scar contracts and causes a stricture.

Fractured pelvis with rupture of the membranous urethra

The membranous urethra is thin and connects two fixed points, the prostate above, which is firmly attached to the symphysis, and the bulbar urethra below, which is bound to the corpora cavernosa on either side: these are in turn fixed to the ischiopubic ramus. If a fracture separates these two fixed points, the membranous urethra is first stretched and may be torn across completely. There are three types of injury: (i) minimal displacement of the pelvis, (ii) gross displacement of the pelvis and (iii) combined urethral and rectal injuries.

Minimal displacement of the pelvis

When the pelvic ring is compressed from front to back, for example, by a car backing into a man leaning over a wall, it gives way where it is thinnest – at the pubic and ischial rami on

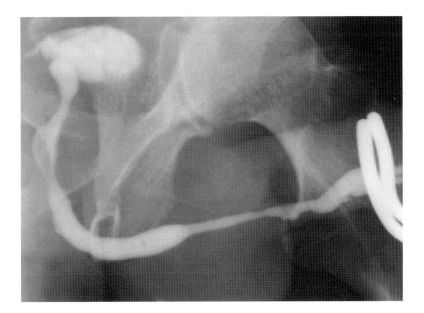

Figure 16.11 Long urethral stricture following cardiac surgery.

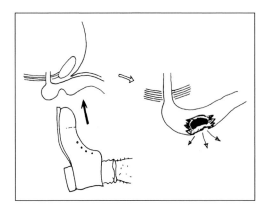

Figure 16.12 Perineal injury to the urethra.

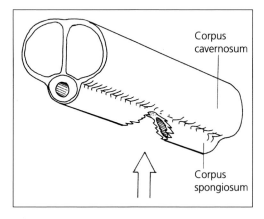

Figure 16.13 The attachments to the corpora cavernosa prevent the ends of the injured urethra from retracting.

either side of the symphysis (Figure 16.15). The symphysis carries the prostate back with it, while the bulbar urethra remains attached to the ischiopubic rami. The membranous urethra is first stretched and may be torn completely or incompletely. The car backs off and the pelvic ring springs back almost to its original position, but in practice the symphysis ends up being displaced a little posteriorly to its original position. If the lumen of the urethra is intact, it will now have an S-shaped bend. If torn completely, the prostatic urethra will come to lie behind the bulb (Figure 16.16).

Management

In the accident and emergency department, X-rays show the typical fracture. Blood escaping from the urethra shows that there has been some damage. Using sterile precautions, about 20 mL of soluble contrast medium is gently injected into the urethra: extravasation confirms that the urethra has been damaged. *At this stage, do not try to pass a catheter: put in a suprapubic tube.*

The next step depends on the general state of the patient. Usually there are other more important injuries to be taken care of, and it takes several days for the patient to recover sufficiently for the urethral injury to be investigated. A flexible cystoscope is passed. In an *incomplete injury* the way can be seen into the bladder, and nothing more need be done at this stage. About 2 weeks later the cystoscopy is repeated and at worst may show the S-shaped bend whose thin septa can easily be incised (Figure 16.17).

If the urethra has been *completely* torn and the flexible cystoscope does not show any way into the bladder, the bulbar urethra is exposed through a perineal incision, the haematoma is evacuated, and the separated ends are anastomosed together over a silicone catheter (Figure 16.18). The sooner this can be done the easier it is, but the timing of this operation is nearly always determined by the patient's other injuries.

Gross displacement of the pelvis

Here the anatomy of the injury is different. The patient has usually been driving a car with an outstretched lower limb, and the force of the impact is transmitted along the limb, forcing the head of the femur through the acetabulum, dislocating one half of the pelvis upwards, fracturing the pubic and ischial rami and dislocating the sacroiliac joint (Figure 16.19). The half-pelvis carries up the bladder and prostate. If the bulbar urethra rides up as well, then the urethra may escape damage, but more often the bulbar urethra remains attached to the opposite half of the pelvis and the membranous urethra is torn across. The gap between the severed ends of the

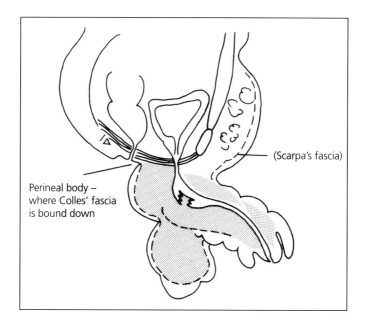

(Scarpa's fascia)

Perineal body –
where Colles' fascia
is bound down

Figure 16.14 Urine and blood escape into the scrotum and perineum.

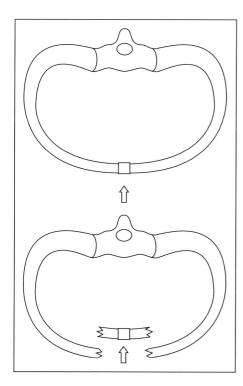

Figure 16.15 Anteroposterior injury: the pelvic ring gives way at its thinnest part.

urethra is now equal to the distance between the dislocated halves of the pelvis.

Management

In this type of injury the two halves of the pelvis do not spring back together: on the contrary, reduction can be very difficult. There is always severe internal haemorrhage from torn pelvic vessels as well as other major injuries, for example, to the head, liver and chest. For the first 48 h the priority is *resuscitation* and saving life. One of the best ways to limit the internal bleeding is to reduce the dislocated pelvis and maintain the correct position with an external fixator (Figure 16.20).

An urethrogram performed (as mentioned Chapter 2) in the accident and emergency department will show whether or not the urethra is damaged. If there is no extravasation, it is safe to pass a urethral catheter. But if there is extravasation or if there is any doubt, it is better to put in a suprapubic tube. This can be difficult in the presence of the pelvic haematoma but is greatly helped by using ultrasound to locate the bladder and make sure the suprapubic tube is in the right position.

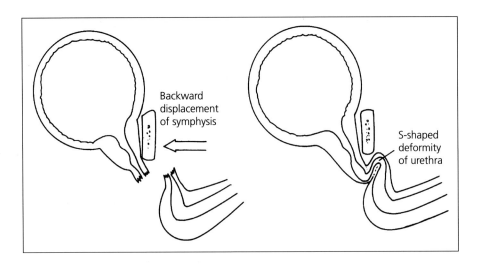

Figure 16.16 The displaced segment of pelvic ring returns almost to its original position, but the prostatic end now lies posterior to the bulbar end of the ruptured urethra.

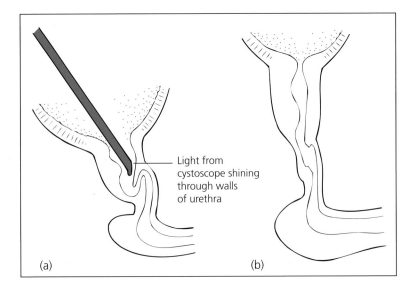

Figure 16.17 Urethroscopy may show an S-shaped bend (a), whose walls can be incised (b).

Correct reduction of the dislocated pelvis will bring the separated ends of the urethra nearly together. When the general condition of the patient permits, a combination of cystogram and urethrogram (*an 'up-and-down-a-gram'*) shows where the separated ends of the urethra are lying and an operation is performed to anastomose them together. The timing of this operation is determined by the general condition of the patient, and it is seldom possible for several weeks.

The bulbar urethra is mobilised through a perineal incision, and the prostatic urethra exposed through a retropubic incision. In practice the prostate may have to be mobilised so that the torn ends can be brought together without tension (Figure 16.21).

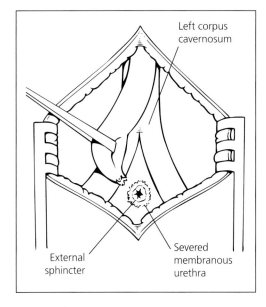

Figure 16.18 End-to-end anastomosis of the ruptured urethra through a perineal approach.

Unreduced dislocation

Sometimes it proves to be impossible to effect an accurate reduction of the dislocated half-pelvis, and by the time the patient is ready to undergo any urological reconstruction, the pelvis is fixed and the severed ends of the urethra are separated by a long gap. To reconstruct this is exceedingly difficult. Essentially part of the malunited callus has to be removed to allow the mobilised bulbar urethra to be brought up to the lower end of the prostate. There are a number of different methods for doing this, which indicates that none of them is always successful (Figure 16.22).

Combined urethral and rectal injuries

Combined urethral and rectal injuries may be caused by gunshot wounds that are rare and very dangerous. In civilian cases the cause is usually a rolling–crushing injury (Figure 16.23). If the rectum is torn, it is essential that faeces are diverted as soon as possible as necrotising fasciitis may occur. A colostomy is performed and the distal colon and rectum

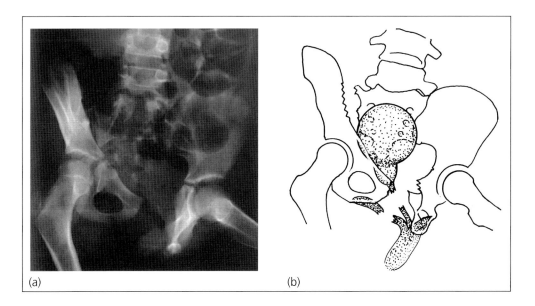

(a) (b)

Figure 16.19 Pelvic fracture X-ray showing gross displacement of one half-pelvis (a). Diagram clarification (b).

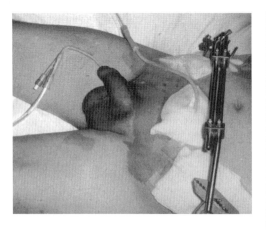

Figure 16.20 External fixation after reduction of a displaced fracture of the pelvis.

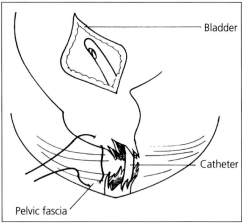

Figure 16.21 It may be necessary to mobilise the prostate through a retropubic approach.

thoroughly washed out. A careful débridement of the wound is performed, bleeding controlled, and a suprapubic tube inserted. The wound is packed. No attempt is made to repair the urethra primarily. When the patient has been stabilised, plans can be made for delayed reconstruction.

Complications of urethral injuries

- *Stricture:* Stricture is a common result of any type of urethral injury.
- *Impotence:* Impotence can occur after pelvic fractures without urethral injury and is caused by damage to the neurovascular bundle of the penis or the pelvic autonomic nerves by the fracture and dislocation of the pelvic bones.
- *Impaired ejaculation:* Damage to the sympathetic nerves may cause paralysis of the bladder neck and seminal vesicles resulting in retrograde or dry ejaculation.
- *Incontinence:* If the bladder neck has been denervated or destroyed or if the supramembranous intramural sphincter is damaged by the injury, then the patient may be incontinent.

Urethral stricture

A urethral stricture is a circumferential scar of the urethra. Scarring can results from a wide variety of insults; the most common affecting the urethra other than trauma is infection. Urethral strictures occur most commonly in the bulbar urethra, as this is where the urethral glands from which infection commonly originates are predominant and also where the urethra is most susceptible to iatrogenic trauma due to its tortuous path. The urethral meatus and penile urethra may also be involved with *balanitis xerotica obliterans*, which is a chronic, progressive, sclerosing inflammatory dermatosis of unclear aetiology, similar to lichen sclerosus.

Clinical features of a stricture

The symptoms of a urethral stricture are those of bladder outflow obstruction, predominantly voiding lower urinary tract symptoms. Bladder dysfunction may occur in chronic cases causing storage symptoms in addition, that is, symptoms may indistinguishable from those caused by an enlarged prostate. There may be a history of pelvic injury, traumatic catheterisation or urological instrumentation; there may also be a history of urethritis, that is, dysuria and urethral discharge.

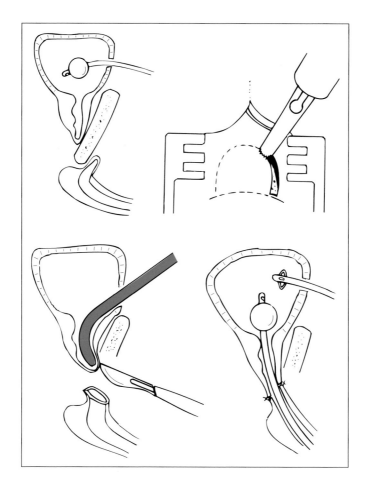

Figure 16.22 Unreduced displaced fracture of pelvis: end-to-end anastomosis after removing a window of symphysis.

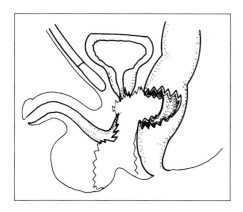

Figure 16.23 Massive crush injury with laceration of rectum.

Physical signs

There are usually no physical signs, but in long-standing strictures palpation of the urethra will reveal thickening and induration in the corpus spongiosum. *Balanitis xerotica obliterans* may be evident as a pale fibrous plaque on the glans penis.

Complications of a stricture

Urinary infection: Infected urine upstream of the stricture, whatever the cause, may be forced into the paraurethral ducts proximal to the stricture and cause further urethritis, with a progression of the stricture along the urethra (Figure 16.24).

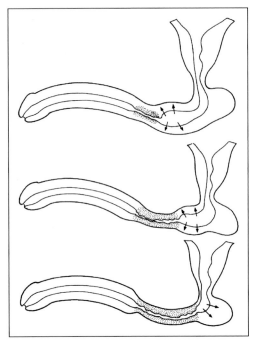

Figure 16.24 Progression of a stricture.

Paraurethral abscess: An infected paraurethral gland may suppurate, and pus may point in the scrotum, and after it has been incised or has discharged, urine may leak through a fistula. When these are multiple, the result is a *watering-can perineum*. Stones may form in these fistulae (Figure 16.25).

Sterility: Even though urine may flow, the thicker semen may be obstructed by the stricture and lead to sterility.

Cancer: In complex strictures complicated by chronic inflammation, squamous cell cancer may arise.

Investigations

A flow rate will document the progress of a stricture but may give a false reassurance that all is well since flow is a factor of both bladder contractility and outflow tract resistance, which itself is inversely proportional to the forth power of the lumen radius.

Urethrography using a water-soluble contrast medium shows the stricture (Figure 16.26); the

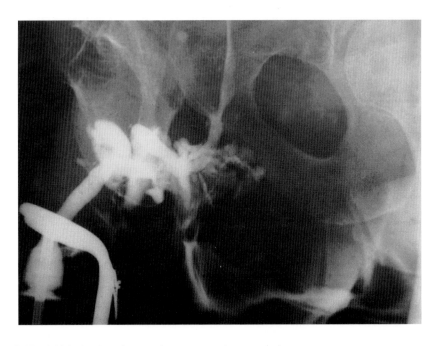

Figure 16.25 Multiple fistulae after a stricture – watering-can perineum.

fibrous changes in the corpus spongiosum are better imaged with ultrasound scan (Figure 16.27) or MRI.

The flexible cystoscope is an easy way to examine the stricture directly.

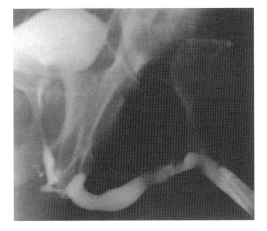

Figure 16.26 Urethrogram showing typical post-traumatic stricture with backward displacement of upper prostatic part.

Treatment

Regular intermittent dilatation: This is the traditional method of managing a stricture. Ancient instruments were adapted from wax tapers, and the best wax came from the Algerian port of Bujiyah, so flexible dilators are still called *bougies* even though they are nowadays made of plastic, not wax. Curved polished steel dilators are usually called *sounds* because they resemble the ancient instrument used before the days of X-rays to 'sound' for stone in the bladder (Figure 16.28). Whether flexible or rigid, dilators come in sets of gradually increasing size. They are used to stretch the stricture. Today, patients are given a self-lubricating catheter that they pass themselves to keep the stricture dilated just as they used to do in ancient Greece. Repeated dilatation of a stricture is rarely curative and may perpetuate and exacerbate scarring and underlying fibrosis of the corpus spongiosum.

Internal visual urethrotomy: When a stricture is too tight to allow a dilator to be passed, the scar tissue is incised under direct vision with the Sachse optical urethrotome (Figure 16.29).

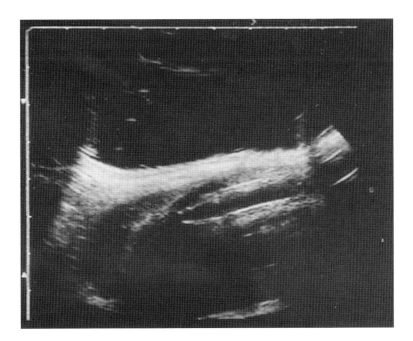

Figure 16.27 Ultrasound image of urethra showing periurethral fibrosis.

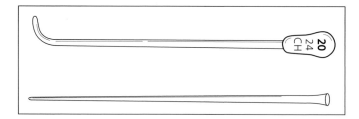

Figure 16.28 Urethral sound and bougie.

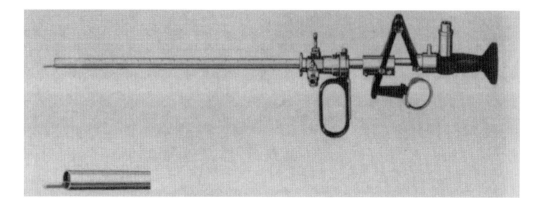

Figure 16.29 Sachse optical urethrotome.

The long-term results of dilatation and incision of urethral strictures are similar and poor. For short bulbar strictures, a single dilatation or incision may be curative. For longer bulbar strictures and those with significant underlying spongiofibrosis and penile strictures, there is a high chance of recurrence and worsening of the stricture, which may compromise the results of subsequent urethroplasty.

Urethroplasty: To prevent scar tissue from contracting after burns in the skin, plastic surgeons apply a skin graft, and there are many ways of adapting this principle to the urethra. The graft can be made of buccal mucosa, split skin or whole thickness skin used as a free graft or on a pedicle of Dartos (Figure 16.30). There are many variations of this principle and all have a failure rate. Sometimes in short traumatic strictures the stricture can be excised the urethra spatulated and rejoined without the need for a substitution graft. Urethroplasty is used when urethrotomy and regular dilatation fail to keep the stricture well controlled and in patients requiring the best chance of a cure of their stricture and willing to suffer the significantly short-term morbidity of the reconstruction.

Urethral carcinoma

Primary urethral carcinoma

The first carcinoma in the urinary tract is detected in the urethra. Primary urethral cancer is very rare and accounts for less than 1% of cancers. The tumour may be transitional cell, squamous or adenocarcinoma and deeply invades locally and metastasises to adjacent organs. Urethral tumours often presents late, as their symptoms are non-specific; they are usually picked up by vaginal examination in women or flexible cystoscopy in males.

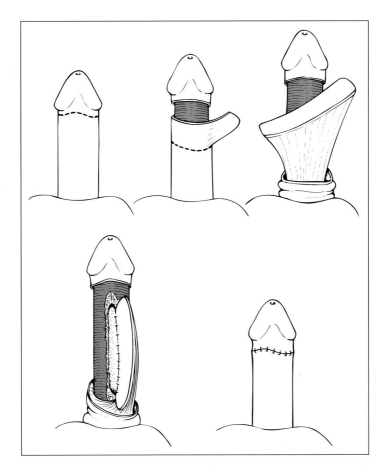

Figure 16.30 Pedicled skin graft urethroplasty.

Secondary urethral carcinoma

Recurrent carcinoma after prior diagnosis and treatment of carcinoma elsewhere in the urinary tract, mostly after radical cystectomy for bladder cancer.

Predisposing risk factors and aetiology

Various predisposing factors have been reported:

- *Males:* Urethral strictures
  - Chronic irritation after intermittent catheterisation/urethroplasty
  - Chronic urethral inflammation/urethritis following urethral transmitted diseases

- External beam radiotherapy and radioactive implantation
- *Females:* Urethral diverticula and recurrent urinary tract infections

Diagnosis and staging

Most patients present with symptoms associated with locally advanced disease including macroscopic haematuria and urethral discharge, extra-urethral mass, bladder outlet obstruction, dyspareunia, pelvic pain and abscess formation. Investigations include diagnostic urethroscopy and biopsy. Radiological imaging, such as MRI and CT, aims at assessing the local tumour extent and detect metastases.

TNM classification (Table 16.1)

Table 16.1 TNM classification

T – primary tumour (men and women)

TX	Primary tumour cannot be assessed
Tis	Carcinoma *in situ*
T0	No evidence of primary tumour
Ta	Non-invasive papillary carcinoma
T1	Tumour invades subepithelial connective tissue
T2	Tumour invades any of the corpus spongiosum, prostate and periurethral muscle
T3	Tumour invades any of the corpus cavernosum, beyond prostate capsule, anterior vaginal wall and bladder neck
T4	Tumour invades neighbouring organs

T – transitional cell carcinoma of the prostate

Tis	Carcinoma *in situ* in the prostatic urethra or ducts
T1	Tumour invades subepithelial connective tissue
T2	Tumour invades any of the corpus spongiosum, prostate stroma and periurethral muscle
T3	Tumour invades any of the corpus cavernosum, beyond prostate capsule and bladder neck
T4	Tumour invades neighbouring organs

N – regional lymph nodes

NX	Regional lymph nodes cannot be assessed
N0	No regional lymph node metastasis
N1	Metastasis in a single lymph node: 2 cm or less in greatest dimension
N2	Metastasis in a single lymph node: >2 cm but <5 cm in greatest dimension or multiple nodes none >5 cm
N3	Metastasis in a single lymph node >5 cm in greatest dimension

M – distant metastasis

MX	Presence of distant metastasis cannot be assessed
M0	No distant metastasis
M1	Distant metastasis present

Histopathological grading

GX: Grade of differentiation cannot be assessed
G1: Well differentiated
G2: Moderately differentiated
G3: Poorly differentiated

Treatment

- *Male:* Surgical treatment should be optimised to achieve improved functional outcome and quality of life provided oncological safety and negative surgical margins.
- *Females:* Local radiotherapy is an alternative to urethral surgery for localised primary tumours.

In locally advanced urethral carcinoma, adjuvant cisplatinum-based chemotherapy prior to surgery may improve survival compared to surgery alone.

 KEYPOINTS

The urethra may be congenitally malformed requiring complex reconstruction in infancy; posterior urethral valve is a common initiator of renal transplant in children.

The urethra is prone to stricture formation due mainly to trauma and infection.

Dilatation and incision of strictures are rarely curative, and self-catheterisation usually worsens the stricture.

Urethroplasty has much better long-term results than urethrotomy but is associated with greater short-term morbidity.

Urethral cancer is rare but is diagnosed late and invades deeply. It should be suspected in patients with refractory urethral symptoms and negative investigations.

17

The penis

Surgical anatomy

The penis comprises two corpora cavernosa and the corpus spongiosum surrounding the urethra, which expands to form the glans penis (Figure 17.1). All three are surrounded by the tough deep fascia known as the Buck's fascia.

The spongy spaces of the corpora cavernosa are made of compartments lined with smooth muscle: those of the two corpora cavernosa intercommunicate freely, but not with the corpus spongiosum and the glans penis.

The penis is developed from the genital tubercle, while the urethra is derived from the urogenital sinus. At the 7th week of gestation, the urogenital sinus moves onto the penis as the urethral groove with the appearance of the urethral plate, which canalise to form the anterior urethra; by 15th week of gestation, the urethra closes with the ingrowth of ectoderm to form the tip of the penis and the terminal portion of the urethra.

A hood of skin then grows over the glans to form the prepuce, and in the later months of foetal life, this hood becomes adherent to the glans. This congenital adherence breaks down spontaneously during the first few years of childhood and infrequently causes trouble.

Blood supply

Arteries

The penis receives blood from three terminal branches of the internal pudendal artery (Figure 17.2) on each side: the deep arteries of the corpora supplying the corpus cavernosum, the dorsal arteries supplying the skin, fascia and glans and the bulbourethral arteries supplying the corpus spongiosum.

Veins

There are three groups of veins (Figure 17.3):

1. The deep dorsal veins drain the corpora cavernosa and lead under the symphysis pubis into the large veins, which surround the prostate and bladder.
2. The superficial veins, under the skin, mostly drain into the saphenous veins.
3. The intermediate veins, deep to Buck's fascia, drain blood from the glans penis into both deep and superficial systems.

Nerves

The penis is innervated via the sympathetic, the parasympathetic and the somatic nervous systems.

Urology Lecture Notes, Seventh Edition. Amir V. Kaisary, Andrew Ballaro and Katharine Pigott.
© 2016 John Wiley & Sons, Ltd. Published 2016 by John Wiley & Sons, Ltd.

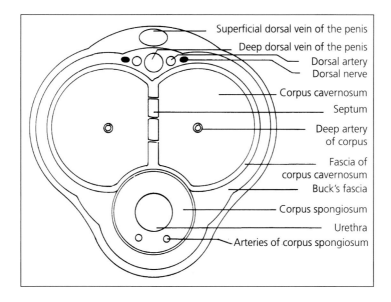

Figure 17.1 Transverse section through the penis.

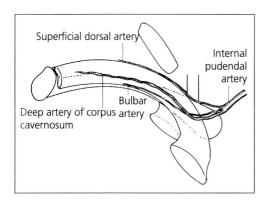

Figure 17.2 Arterial blood supply to the penis.

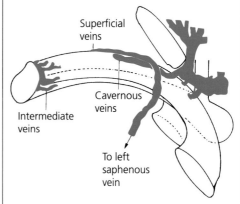

Figure 17.3 Venous drainage of the penis.

The sympathetic is mainly responsible for detumescence, the parasympathetic is mainly responsible for tumescence, and the somatic is responsible for sensory and motor function.

Anatomically, the parasympathetic fibres are joined by the nerves from the sympathetic system, which then enter the erectile tissue and are distributed alongside branches of internal pudendal arteries as the cavernous nerve. Care is taken to preserve them operatively during a radical nerve-sparing prostatectomy.

The somatic system of the penis is carried in the dorsal nerves, which are one of the terminal branches of the pudendal nerve (S2, S3). The pudendal nerve is composed of both afferent and efferent fibres: the afferent component from the dorsal nerve and the efferent component that innervates the ischiocavernosus and the bulbo-cavernosus muscles.

Physiology of erection

There are five phases of penile erection and detumescence:

1. Flaccid state: The flaccid penis has a relatively low blood flow through the corpus cavernosum.
2. Latent phase: Parasympathetic stimulation, mediated by neurotransmitter substances (whose action is imitated by papaverine, phentolamine and prostaglandin E), causes the small branches of the deep arteries within the corpora cavernosa to dilate and fill the spaces of the corpora cavernosa with blood while their smooth muscle walls are relaxed. This relaxation is affected by cyclic guanosine monophosphate (cGMP), which in turn is degraded by phosphodiesterase. The pressure inside the corpus cavernosum rises to about 40 mmHg (Figure 17.4)
3. Tumescence: With increasing pressure, the emissary veins are compressed and the venous outflow is reduced.
4. Full erection: An increase in pO_2 (to about 90 mmHg) and intracavernosal pressure (around 100 mmHg) raises the penis from the dependent position to the erect state.
5. Rigid erection: Occlusion of the veins leading out of the corpora cavernosa and spongiosum trapping blood inside these spaces. The pressure rises inside the corpora to over 150 mmHg, with contraction of the ischiocavernosus muscles.
6. Detumescence (initial, slow and fast phases)

Ejaculation

The physiology of ejaculation is divided into two phases: emission and expulsion (Figure 17.5).

Emission

This process commences with closure of the bladder neck, which prevents retrograde ejaculation, secretion of fluid from the prostate and seminal vesicle mixes with spermatozoa-rich fluid from the vas deferens in the prostatic urethra, with a minor component from both Cowper's glands and periurethral glands, making up the final ejaculate.

Expulsion

This follows the emission phase, resulting in the final product of emission/semen being expelled from the urethra, through the coordinated actions of bladder neck contraction and relaxation of the external urinary sphincter, followed by clonic contractions of the prostate, bulbospongiosus, ischiocavernosus, levator ani and transverse perineal muscles.

Circumcision

The arguments for and against neonatal circumcision have been raging for many centuries, with passion inversely proportional to evidence.

Phimosis is the inability to retract the prepuce. This may be physiological or pathological. Physiological phimosis is distinguished from pathological phimosis by an appearance of pouting of the inner prepuce on attempted retraction, which does not occur in pathological phimosis, but instead a scarred white ring appears.

Physiological phimosis is very common in young boys and will usually resolve without surgical intervention.

The absolute indication for circumcision is pathological phimosis, due to balanoposthitis xerotica obliterans (BXO) (Figure 17.6), also known as lichen sclerosus et atrophicus. This is very rare in children, affecting less than 1% of boys; it is more commonly seen in middle-aged man.

BXO. BXO is identical to lichen sclerosus atrophicus. It is common, and usually benign, but has been sporadically associated with squamous cell carcinoma (SCC). There is a whitish alteration in the skin of the prepuce causing it to become stiff, tight and difficult to retract. When the condition affects the glans penis, it produces a stenosis of the external urinary meatus, which

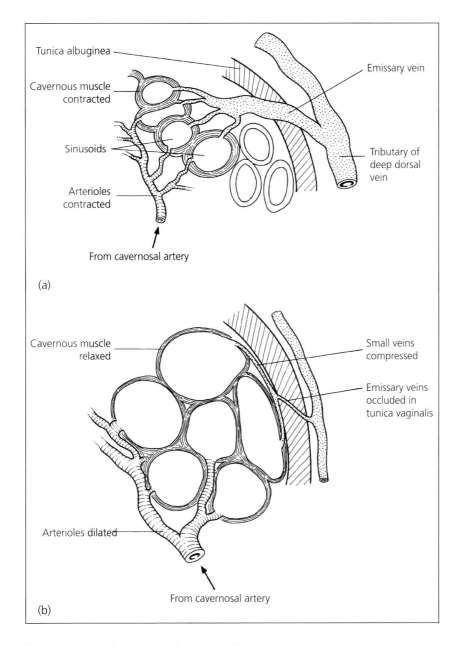

Figure 17.4 Mechanism of erection: (a) flaccid and (b) erect.

may require surgical correction. This is not a pre-malignant condition to SCC penis.

Other relative indications for circumcision in children are recurrent balanoposthitis and recurrent UTI. In boys with recurrent UTI, the number needed to treat is 11 and 4 in those with UTI and high-grade vesicoureteric reflux. The alternative to circumcision is preputioplasty where a small incision is made in the narrow band of the foreskin (Figure 17.7).

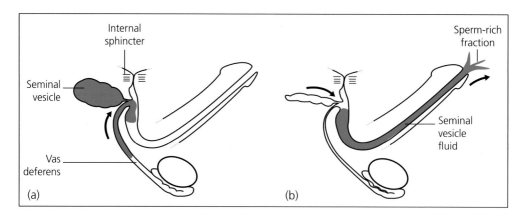

Figure 17.5 Mechanism of ejaculation: (a) resting normal phase and (b) ejaculation.

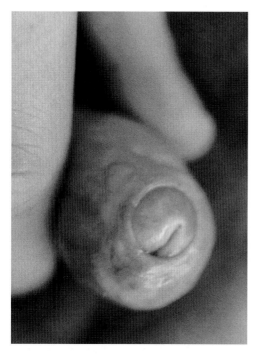

Figure 17.6 Balanoposthitis xerotica obliterans.

Acute balanoposthitis

Acute balanoposthitis is a condition characterised by redness and swelling of the foreskin and associated with purulent discharge from the preputial opening.

This occurs in children as well as men who cannot retract the foreskin to keep the preputial space and glans penis clean. It can be due to a specific infection, for example, *E. coli*; *Proteus vulgaris*; *Haemophilus ducreyi*, which causes chancroid; and *Candida albicans*, which occurs particularly commonly in diabetic men. However, culture may not grow any organism in up to 30% of the cases.

This condition is common and usually self-limiting; however if recurrent, circumcision may be warranted.

Ulceration on the glans penis may be due to primary infection with syphilis, in which case *Treponema pallidum* can be identified in the exudate. Diagnosis and treatment is usually in collaboration with a genito-urinary medicine (sexual health) team.

Peyronie's disease

Peyronie's disease is characterised by the development of plaques of fibrous tissue in Buck's fascia or the septum between the corpora cavernosa (Figure 17.8). The aetiology is unknown, but the pathological process may involve the result of acute inflammation, leading to the activation of fibroblasts and resulting in fibrotic plaque formation.

During an erection the part affected by fibrosis does not fill, so penile curvature results.

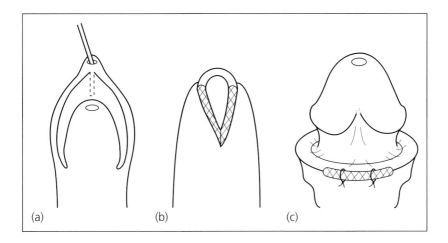

Figure 17.7 Preputioplasty (a, b and c are sequential surgery steps).

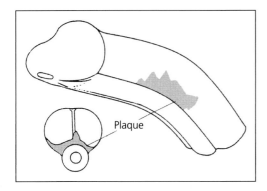

Figure 17.8 Peyronie's disease.

The association and risk factors with Peyronie's disease include Dupuytren's contracture, Ledderhose disease, tympanosclerosis, repetitive trauma, diabetes, smoking, erectile dysfunction (ED) that may pre-/post-date Peyronie's disease and hyperlipidaemia.

Patients usually present with either painful penis, both at rest and on erection (pain is present in 35% of patients, resolves in 90% of patients and usually lasts for 12 months), or painless, palpable plaque with a degree of penile curvature, which may impair intercourse. They may also complain of ED.

The disease is characterised by an acute inflammatory phase and a fibrotic phase, which results in disease stabilisation. The natural progression of the disease includes worsening curvature in 48%, stabilisation in 40% and improvement in 12%.

Non-surgical treatments of Peyronie's disease offer rich pickings – ranging from oral therapy including potassium para-amino benzoate (Potaba) which is possibly effective, acetyl-L-carnitine, vitamin E, tamoxifen, colchicine and pentoxifylline; intralesional injection of steroid, verapamil, collagenase and interferon; topical verapamil gel 15%; ESWL; traction device and vacuum device – none of which have offered a satisfactory result for the condition.

Surgical treatment is indicated in those where the disease is stable for 3 months, that is, without pain and without deteriorating deformities, usually around 12 months from the onset of symptoms, where sexual intercourse is compromised due to deformity.

In patients without ED or where ED is successfully treated, Nesbit or plication procedure (Figure 17.9) or tunical lengthening procedure, that is, plaque incision and grafting, should be considered. In those with ED or very complex deformities, penile prosthesis should be considered.

The choice of operation is usually made after thorough consultation with the patient. However a general rule is that in those with curvature <60°, adequate penile length and absence of complex deformities (hourglass or hinged deformities), a Nesbit or plication procedure is considered.

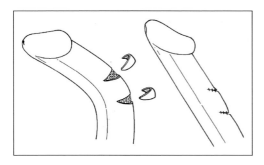

Figure 17.9 Correction of curvature in Peyronie's disease.

In those with curvature >60°, short penis and presence of complex deformities, tunical lengthening procedure should be considered.

The patient should be made aware of potential complications including ED, penile shortening, penile hypaesthesia and recurrent curvature.

Ejaculatory failure

- *Premature ejaculation*
  The causes of premature ejaculation are divided into two main categories: one being psychogenic, including anxiety, poor ejaculatory control techniques and early sexual experiences, and the other being organic, including penile hypersensitivities, hyper-excitable ejaculatory reflex, 5-HT receptor dysfunction and genetic predisposition.

  Treatments are divided into two forms: psychological/behavioural or pharmacological agents or a combination of both.

  Psychological/behavioural methods in the form of counselling and start–stop technique/stop–squeeze techniques.

  Pharmacological agents include topical local anaesthetic gel/spray and oral selective serotonin reuptake inhibitors (SSRIs), both long acting, for example, paroxetine, and newer shorter acting, for example, dapoxetine.

- *Anejaculation*
  Distinguish absence of antegrade ejaculation, characterised by the absence of fructose and sperm in the post-orgasmic urine

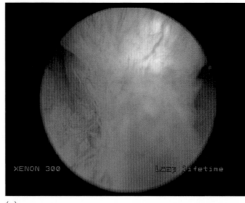

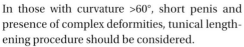

(a)

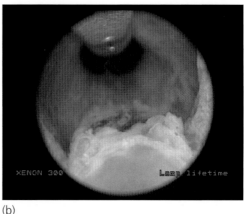

(b)

Figure 17.10 (a, b) Obstructed ejaculatory ducts openings at the verumontanum.

analysis from retrograde ejaculation, where sperm is found in post-orgasmic urine.

Anejaculation causes include spinal cord injury, retroperitoneal lymph node dissection or blocking of the seminal tract at the ejaculatory ducts. Ejaculation may be painful. Transrectal ultrasound may reveal distended seminal vesicles. It may be possible to unblock the ejaculatory ducts by incision or resection of their openings on the verumontanum (Figure 17.10).

- *Retrograde ejaculation*
  This is often the result of retroperitoneal lymph node dissection, diabetes mellitus, previous surgery at the bladder neck or destruction of the sympathetic innervation

Table 17.1 Erectile dysfunction pathophysiology

Anatomical	Micropenis, Peyronie's disease and hypo-/epispadias
Vasculogenic	Cardiovascular disease, diabetes mellitus, hyperlipidaemia, smoking and following major surgery/radiotherapy of the pelvis
Neurogenic	Degenerative disorders: MS, Parkinson's disease and stroke
	Spinal cord trauma and disease
	CNS tumours
Drug induced	Antihypertensive, antidepressants, antipsychotics, antiandrogens and recreational drugs
Hormonal	Hypogonadism, hypo-/hyperthyroidism, hyper-/hypocortisolism, hyperprolactinaemia and multiple endocrine disorders
Trauma	Fracture penis and pelvic fractures
Psychogenic	Variable elements include performance-related anxiety and lack of arousal

of the bladder neck by trauma or surgery in the pelvis, medication with an alpha-blocking action or a urethral stricture that may prevent the escape of semen.

Treatments include a sympathomimetic drug, for example, ephedrine or tricyclic antidepressants, for example, imipramine. Alternatively, if medical therapy fails, the sperm may be retrieved from alkalinised post-ejaculate urine.

Erectile dysfunction

ED has a high prevalence and incidence worldwide. Pathophysiology details are presented in Table 17.1. It should be emphasised that no single reason can be the sole factor to blame.

There is a high prevalence of cardiovascular diseases in patients who experience sexual dysfunction. The recognition of ED should be accepted as a warning sign of possible asymptomatic silent vascular disease, and investigating ED can result in identifying asymptomatic cardiovascular diseases. It is increasingly acknowledged that optimising sexual function and preserving cardiovascular health are a must. Cardiac risk stratification is a useful robust guide. The clinicians can estimate the risk of sexual activity in most patients with cardiovascular diseases from investigating their level of exercise tolerance falling in three cardiovascular risk groups (Table 17.2).

Clinical evaluation and history

It is important to take a comprehensive medical and sexual history of the patient and the partner, if in attendance, in a relaxed atmosphere.

The features of pathophysiological elements can be a useful guide. Previous consultations and treatments are valuable to obtain.

Sexual history should include details of sexual orientation and previous and current sexual relationships.

Frequency and details of nocturnal and morning tumescence.

Physical examination focusing on genitourinary, vascular, neurological and endocrinal features and secondary sexual characteristics is documented.

Table 17.2 Cardiac risk group stratification in erectile dysfunction

Low risk	Intermediate risk	High risk
Asymptomatic <3 risk factors	>3 risk factors	High-risk arrhythmias
Mild stable angina	Moderate stable angina	Unstable or refractory angina
Uncomplicated previous MI	Recent MI >2 weeks and <6 weeks	Recent MI <2 weeks
CHF/LVD: class I	CHF/LVD: class II	CHF/LVD: class III/IV
Successful coronary revascularisation	Non-cardiac atherosclerotic disease	Cardiomyopathies
Controlled hypertension		Uncontrolled hypertension
Valvular disease: mild		Valvular disease: moderate–severe

CHF, congestive heart failure; LVD, left ventricular dysfunction.
Adapted from cardiac risk stratification based on the second consensus conference (*Am J Cardiol* 2005 96(2): 175–181).

Laboratory testing: Investigation

The investigation of organic impotence should proceed in logical steps.

Haematological, biochemical and hormonal profiles addressing the related risk features are obtained. Lipid profile and fasting blood sugar or HbA1c need to be taken and diabetes excluded. Early morning total serum testosterone and calculated free testosterone may be needed to corroborate total testosterone measurements. Additional laboratory tests might be obtained should there be a relevant clinical finding, for example, serum prostate-specific antigen (PSA) in selected patients.

Introduction of oral selective inhibitors of phosphodiesterase type 5 (PDE-5) has made a major impact on the treatment of ED.

It is reasonable to commence one of these PDE-5 inhibitors before embarking on other investigations.

Penile vasculature can be assessed by Doppler studies or by a test injection into the corpus cavernosum of one of the substances that mimics parasympathetic stimulation, for example, papaverine or prostaglandin E. Nocturnal penile tumescence, which accompanies the rapid eye movement phase of sleep, can be assessed by simple stamp test (Figure 17.11), snap gauges,

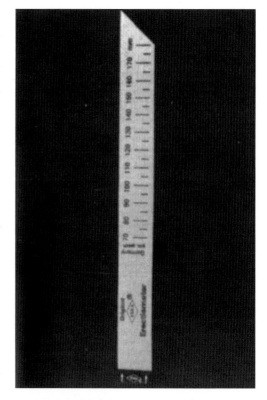

Figure 17.11 Paper strip to record the expansion of the penis during sleep.

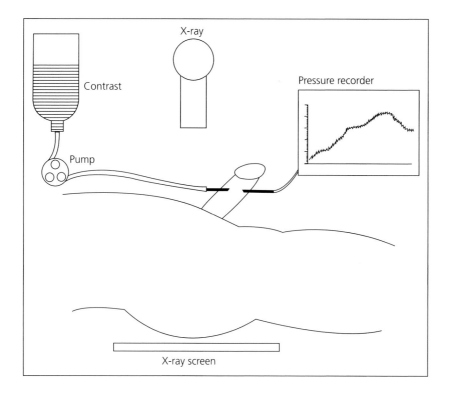

Figure 17.12 Corpus cavernosography.

formal sleep laboratory nocturnal penile tumescence and rigidity study.

Failure of the occlusion of the penile veins during rigid phase of erection – venous leakage –
can be diagnosed by injecting contrast into
the corpora cavernosa and monitoring the
pressure, while an artificial erection is produced by the injection of prostaglandin. This is
now being superseded by Doppler vascular
assessment.

The vast majority of patients with ED can be
managed adequately without additional specialised tests; however, some men might need additional investigations/evaluations:

1. RigiScan™ assessment of nocturnal tumescence and rigidity: should be done on at least
   two nights. Normal range of values includes
   between 3 and 6 erectile episodes per night,
   with each erectile episode from 10–15 min to
   longer than 30 min in duration in total, with
   penile tip rigidity of >80% and an increase in

circumference of >3 cm at the base and >2 cm
at the tip/coronal sulcus.

2. Intracavernosal injection test: A normal test is
   a rigid erectile response that appears within
   10 min and lasts for 30 min. It is not a diagnostic procedure for the assessment of vascular
   status.

3. Penile blood flow evaluation with dynamic
   duplex ultrasound:
   A normal study shows a peak systolic velocity
   of >35 cm/s; a peak systolic velocity of
   <25 cm/s indicates arterial insufficiency,
   within 10 min after a low-dose vasoactive
   agent (usually prostaglandin E). This provides
   valuable information about vascular status.
   Further vascular investigation is unnecessary
   after a normal result.

4. Arteriography and dynamic infusion cavernosography or cavernosometry (Figure 17.12) are
   performed only in patients who are being considered for vascular reconstructive surgery.

KEYPOINTS

Any asymptomatic man, who presents with erectile dysfunction (ED) and does not have an obvious cause, should be screened for vascular disease.

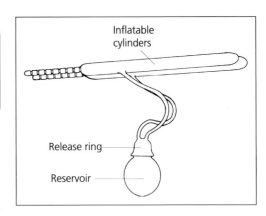

Figure 17.13 Inflatable penile prosthesis.

Treatment

- *Lifestyle modification*: Smoking, diabetes, hypercholesterolaemia, obesity and sedentary lifestyle are independent risk factors for both ED and cardiovascular disease. Counselling for lifestyle modification is encouraged.
- *Psychosexual counselling*.
- *Drugs*: Oral drug therapy is most widely used in view of its acceptability and effectiveness. PDE-5 inhibitors act by reducing the degradation of cGMP promoting blood flow into the penis and the restoration of erectile function. Oral drugs such as sildenafil, tadalafil, vardenafil and avanafil have differing half-lives that might prompt consideration of choice in patients. Recently topical alprostadil cream applied to the tip of the penis is claimed to give a firm erection within 5–30 min. Yohimbine is an alkaloid similar to reserpine and may in some cases restore erection if given a dose of 5 mg three times per day.
- *Vacuum devices*: These devices are available that creates a negative pressure environment and draws blood into the penis to produce a tumescence, which is then maintained with a rubber band placed around the base of the penis for no longer than 30 min.
- *Intracavernosal injection*: If a test injection of prostaglandin E produces a successful erection, the patient or partner can be taught to self-administer the injection. It is essential that patients are warned against the risks of developing priapism.
- *Medicated Urethral System for Erection (MUSE)*: Intra-urethral delivery of a pellet containing prostaglandin E1/alprostadil.
- *Implanted penile prostheses*: Devices are available that can be inserted into the corpora

 KEYPOINTS

ED stands for:
- **E**rectile dysfunction
- **E**ndothelial dysfunction
- **E**xercise and diet in prevention
- **E**arly detection of risk factors to prevent early death

  There is more to sex than an erect penis.

  Source: Princeton Consensus on Sexual Dysfunction

cavernosa to mimic erection. These are divided into malleable and inflatable devices. The malleable penile prosthesis can be manually manipulated to bent and straight position, while the inflatable penile prostheses are inflated from a concealed reservoir (Figure 17.13). Potential complications include infection, erosion and mechanical failure, in the case of inflatable penile prosthesis.
- *Vascular operations*: In selected group of patients, vascular operations may be considered. Arterial insufficiency: attempts to improve arterial blood flow have been tried, for example, the inferior epigastric artery is anastomosed to the dorsal artery of the penis. Venous insufficiency: the objective is to prevent blood leaking out of the penis with venous ligation surgery when a venous leak has been demonstrated.

Priapism

Priapism is prolonged unwanted penile erection in the absence of sexual stimulation and persists despite orgasm.

In priapism the corpora cavernosa are rigid, but the glans penis is soft.

Causes of priapism can be divided into several categories:

- Haematological – sickle cell disease, leukaemia, erythropoietin use, asplenism, in patients undergoing haemodialysis with heparin administration and stopping warfarin therapy.
- Neurological – spinal cord/brain injury, lumbar disc herniation, cauda equina. Anaesthetic agents.
- Non-haematological malignant neoplasm – penile, urethra, prostate, bladder, kidney and recto sigmoid malignancies.
- Trauma – blunt penile/perineal trauma and needle penetrating trauma.
- Pharmacological agents – intracavernosal agents for the treatment of ED, alpha adrenergic antagonist (prazosin) psychotropic and antidepressants, cocaine use.
- Idiopathic.

There are three types of priapism:

1. *Low-flow priapism* – ischaemic
   Corporal blood aspiration confirms low pO_2 and low pH.
2. *High-flow priapism* – *non-ischaemic*
   Corporal blood aspiration confirms arterial pO_2 and normal pH.
   Doppler study may show high blood flow and possible AV fistula.
3. *Stuttering priapism* – recurrent prolonged painful erections, usually self-limiting.

Treatment

Corporal cavernosal aspiration confirms diagnosis and is successful in the treatment of priapism in 24–36% of patients, depending on the duration of the priapism.

In ischaemic priapism, intracavernosal injection of phenylephrine or noradrenaline is given, with close blood pressure monitoring.

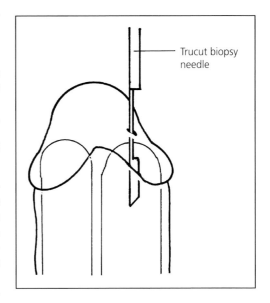

Figure 17.14 Hole made between glans penis and corpus cavernosum with biopsy needle.

If this fails, a shunt procedure is performed; this usually involves creating a communication between corpus cavernosum and corpus spongiosum, either with a biopsy needle (Figure 17.14) or by surgical anastomosis. However a variety of other surgical shunt techniques have also been described.

The treatment is urgent because delay may be followed by irreversible changes in corpora cavernosa smooth muscle, leading to penile fibrosis and ED.

In those with prolonged ischaemic priapism or where other treatments have failed, early insertion of penile prosthesis should be considered.

In sickle cell disease plasmapheresis can be used.

In high-flow priapism, corporal injection of sympathomimetic is not indicated; where AV fistula is demonstrated, selective angiography and embolisation may produce a cure.

In stuttering priapism, treatments options include cyproterone acetate, pseudoephedrine, etilefrine, PDE5I (in sickle cell disease), Aspirin 75 mg, LHRH analogue and self-injection of phenylephrine.

Cancer of the penis

Aetiology

Penile cancer is rare in most developed nations, where the rate is less than 1 per 100 000 men per year, with geographical variations, for instance, 3/100 000 in India and 8/100 000 in Brazil. Some studies demonstrated an association between human papillomavirus (HPV) infection and penile cancer, with observational studies demonstrating a lower prevalence of penile HPV in men who have been circumcised. Some, but not all, observational studies also suggest that male newborn circumcision is associated with a decreased risk of penile cancer. If the relationship is causal, the number needed to treat was about 909 circumcisions to prevent a single case of invasive penile cancer.

Childhood circumcision certainly does not prevent cancer of the penis; however, countries and cultures practising routine neonatal circumcision have a lower incidence of penile cancer (neonatal circumcision does not reduce the incidence of carcinoma in *situ* (CIS)) but have their own mortality and morbidity. It has been calculated that slightly more deaths would occur if all boys were to be circumcised than would occur from cancer of the penis, at least in the West.

Other known predisposing factors are smoking and previous recurrent balanoposthitis.

There are several well-recognised precancerous conditions:

- *Erythroplasia of Queyrat* (Bowen's disease): This is a form of CIS of the skin of the glans. It resembles balanoposthitis and is diagnosed by means of a biopsy. It can be cured with local coagulation with a $CO_{2 \text{ laser}}$ or 5-fluorouracil cream. If neglected, it progresses to overt cancer (Figure 17.15).
- *Condyloma acuminatum*: This is a benign wart caused by one of the family of papillomaviruses (Figure 17.16). It responds to local measures such as podophyllin, freezing and diathermy.
- *Giant condyloma acuminatum*: This is sometimes seen in a giant form, the *Buschke–*

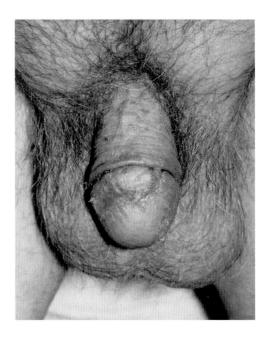

Figure 17.15 Erythroplasia of Queyrat.

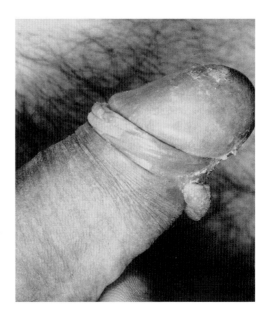

Figure 17.16 Condyloma acuminatum.

Löwenstein tumour. At first this contains papillomavirus and seems histologically to be benign, but if not treated radically always progresses to invasive cancer.

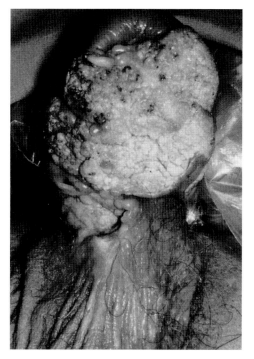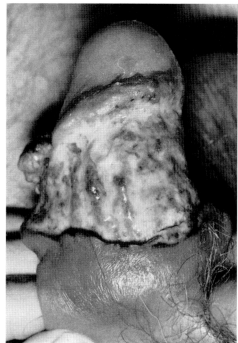

Figure 17.17 Papillary and ulcerated types of carcinoma of the penis.

- Intra-epithelial neoplasia grade 3.
- Paget's disease (intradermal).

Pathology

Cancer of the penis occurs in three macroscopic forms: an ulcer, a papilliferous cauliflower or a nodule (Figure 17.17). There is frequently secondary infection, and many of these cases present late in the course of the disease with a profuse, foul-smelling discharge from beneath an inflamed prepuce. The inguinal lymph nodes are often enlarged because of infection.

Grade

These are squamous cell carcinoma (Figure 17.18) and are graded into G1–G4 histological grades according to the frequency of mitoses that are present.

TNM classification

T – Primary tumour.

Tx – Primary tumour cannot be assessed.

Tis – Carcinoma *in situ*.

Ta – Non-invasive verrucous carcinoma not associated with destructive invasion.

T1 – Tumour invades subepithelial connective tissue.

T1a: Tumour invades subepithelial connective tissue without lymphovascular invasion and is not poorly differentiated or undifferentiated (T1 G1–G2).

T1b: Tumour invades subepithelial connective tissue with lymphovascular invasion or is poorly differentiated/undifferentiated (T1 G3–G4).

T2 – Tumour invades corpora cavernosa/spongiosum.

T3 – Tumour invades urethra.

T4 – Tumour invades other adjacent structures.

N – Regional lymph nodes

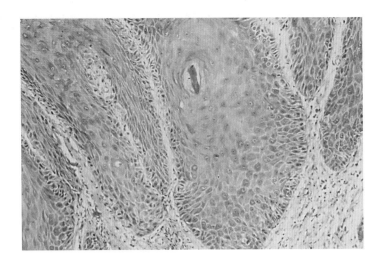

Figure 17.18 Squamous cell carcinoma of the penis.

Nx – Cannot be assessed.

N0 – No palpable or visibly enlarged inguinal lymph nodes.

N1 – Palpable mobile unilateral inguinal lymph node.

N2 – Palpable, mobile, multiple unilateral or bilateral inguinal lymph nodes.

N3 – Fixed inguinal nodal mass or pelvic lymphadenopathy, unilateral or bilateral.

M – Distant metastases

Mx – Cannot assess. Not assessed.

M0 – No distant metastasis.

M1 – Distant metastasis present.

Pathological classification

pT categories correspond to the clinical T categories.

pN categories are based upon biopsy or surgical excision.

pN – Regional lymph nodes

pNx – Regional lymph nodes cannot be assessed.

pN0 – No regional lymph node metastasis.

pN1 – Intranodal metastasis in a single inguinal lymph node.

pN2 – Metastasis in multiple or bilateral inguinal lymph nodes.

pN3 – Metastasis in pelvic lymph nodes, unilateral or bilateral or extranodal extension of regional lymph node metastasis.

pM – Distant metastasis

pM0 – No distant metastasis.

pM1 – Distant metastasis.

G – Histopathological grading

Gx – Grade of differentiation cannot be assessed.

G1 – Well differentiated.

G2 – Moderately differentiated.

G3–G4 – Poorly differentiated/undifferentiated.

Diagnosis

Punch biopsy may be sufficient for superficial lesions; an excisional biopsy is often preferred with a cuff of macroscopically normal surrounding tissue.

The treatment strategies in penile cancer are summarised in the Table 17.3.

Treatment of the primary tumour

The choice of treatment is partial amputation (Figure 17.19) or local radiotherapy. Both can produce 100% cure, but after radiotherapy there is a 20% chance of local recurrence that eventually requires partial amputation.

Table 17.3 Treatment strategies in penile cancer

Histology	Treatment options
Tis, Ta, T1a	• Wide local excision ± circumcision 　• CO_2/Nd : YAG Laser 　• Mohs micrographic surgery 　• 5-FU/5% imiquimod (high recurrence rate)
T1b (>1 mm depth)	• Excision and glans resurfacing 　• Glansectomy 　• Neoadjuvant chemotherapy (vinblastine, bleomycin, methotrexate) and CO_2 laser 　• In surgically treated patients, 3 mm surgical margins are required
T2 glans T2 cavernosum	• Glansectomy 　• Partial amputation 　• (In surgically treated patients, 5–10 mm surgical margins are required)
T3	• Penectomy ± perineal urethrostomy
T4	• Neoadjuvant chemotherapy and penectomy

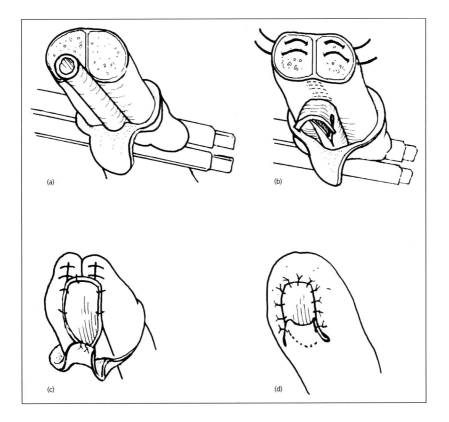

Figure 17.19 Partial amputation of the penis (a, b, c and d are sequential surgical steps).

Lymph node management

If on clinical examination, an inguinal lymph node is palpable, ultrasound guided fine needle aspiration biopsy should be carried out.

If inguinal lymph nodes are clinically impalpable and >G2T1 stage, then dynamic sentinel lymph node biopsy should be performed.

If the lymph node is negative for metastasis, clinical surveillance should be instigated.

If the lymph node is positive for metastasis, then inguinal lymphadenectomy should be performed.

Subsequent to the inguinal lymphadenectomy, if >pN2, or if the Cloquet lymph node is positive, or if extranodal metastasis is present, then one should proceed to pelvic lymph node dissection.

If unilateral lymph nodes are positive, then unilateral pelvic lymphadenectomy should be performed; or if they are bilateral (i.e., both sides are positive), pelvic lymphadenectomy, together with further staging investigations including CT-chest, abdomen and pelvis (±PET±bone scan), should be performed.

Prognosis

As with many types of cancer, the outcome of penile cancer depends on how advanced it is at presentation. For men with the very earliest stage – *penile CIS* – 5-year survival is over 9 out of 10 (90%). One of the most important factors that affect the outlook for people with penile cancer is whether lymph node metastasis is present. Recent studies have reported that 9 out of 10 men (90%) who do not have cancer in the lymph nodes will live for at least 5 years. For men who have cancer in their lymph nodes, but no spread to other parts of the body, it depends on which lymph nodes and how many lymph nodes have cancer cells in them. If there are cancer cells in only one lymph node in the groin, just over 8 out of 10 men (80%) will live for at least 5 years. If more than two lymph nodes in the groin have cancer cells in them or if the lymph nodes in the abdomen have cancer cells in them, around 4 out of 10 men (40%) will live for at least 5 years. If the cancer has spread further than the lymph nodes in the groin, the outlook is likely to be poorer.

Chemotherapy

Advanced bulky or metastatic penile cancer is highly lethal. Attempted treatment with cisplatin containing regimens has been considered, but no optimal chemotherapy regimen has been identified so far. Associated levels of toxicity encountered are discouraging for recommending therapy.

18

The testicle

Embryology

The germ cells arise in the yolk sac of the foetus, migrate along the umbilical cord, and bury themselves in the urogenital gonadal ridge on the back of the coelom (Figure 18.1). Later the future testis bulges forwards and then follows a lump of jelly called the gubernaculum downwards into the scrotum, carrying with it a bag of peritoneum in front and reaching the scrotum shortly before birth (Figure 18.2).

Surgical anatomy

The term testicle includes both testis and epididymis. The testis lies in front of the epididymis, slung from the external inguinal ring by the spermatic cord. In front of the testis and nearly surrounding it is the tunica vaginalis, remnant of the peritoneum. It contains only a trace of fluid.

Blood supply

The testicular artery arises from the aorta near the renal arteries and passes in front of the ureter and curls round lateral to the inferior epigastric vessels to enter the inguinal canal. The numerous large veins that drain the testicle form the pampiniform plexus, which joins together to enter the vena cava on the right and the renal vein on the left (Figure 18.3).

Structure

Testis

Each testis is made up of sets of tubules arranged in loops, which empty into a sac, the rete testis. This drains through a dozen *vasa efferentia* into the epididymis (Figure 18.4). The testicular tubule contains two types of cells – germinal cells and Sertoli cells. In between them is a packing of Leydig cells (Figure 18.5). The *germinal* cells divide into successive generations of spermatocytes, which ultimately developed by mitosis and meiosis into spermatozoa (Figure 18.6). The Sertoli cells secrete inhibin, which regulates the pituitary supply of luteinizing hormone (Figure 18.7). The Leydig cells secrete *testosterone*.

Epididymis

The epididymis is a long coiled tube lying behind the testis, which continues as the vas deferens. It is lined with microcilia (Figure 18.8).

Urology Lecture Notes, Seventh Edition. Amir V. Kaisary, Andrew Ballaro and Katharine Pigott.
© 2016 John Wiley & Sons, Ltd. Published 2016 by John Wiley & Sons, Ltd.

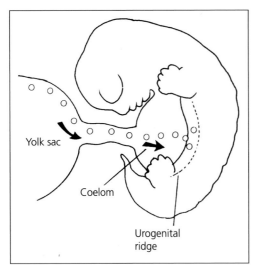

Figure 18.1 The incredible journey of the germinal cells from the yolk sac to the urogenital ridge.

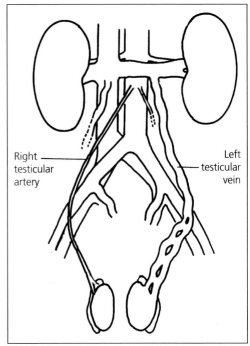

Figure 18.3 Blood supply of the testicle.

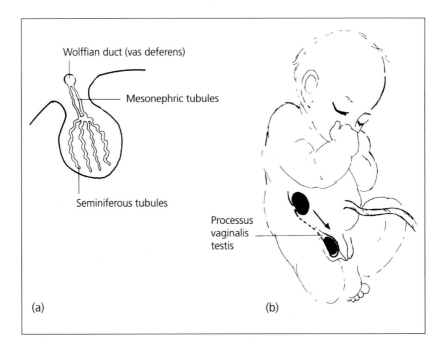

Figure 18.2 Normal descent of the testicle: (a) testicle embryology and (b) normal descent of the testicle.

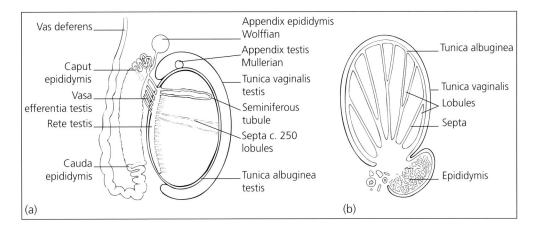

Figure 18.4 Structure of the testicle: (a) structure of the testicle and (b) structural arrangements.

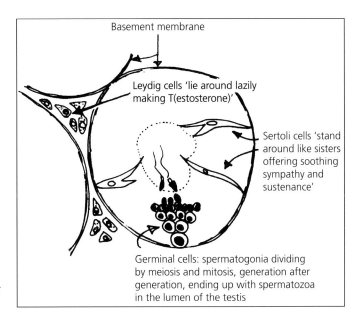

Figure 18.5 Diagram of testicular tubule.

Vas deferens

The vas deferens runs along the back of the spermatic cord, curls around the inferior epigastric vessels, crosses in front of the ureter and passes in the cleft between the inner and outer zones of the prostate to join the common ejaculatory duct and open into the prostatic urethra on the verumontanum. The vas deferens has a powerful muscular wall and is lined with columnar epithelium. It acts as a reservoir for sperms, emptying on ejaculation (Figure 18.9).

Seminal vesicle

The seminal vesicle lies superior to the prostate, just under the bladder. It is a long duct, coiled up so that on cross section it resembles a honeycomb (Figure 18.10). Its duct joins the vas deferens to form the *common ejaculatory duct.*

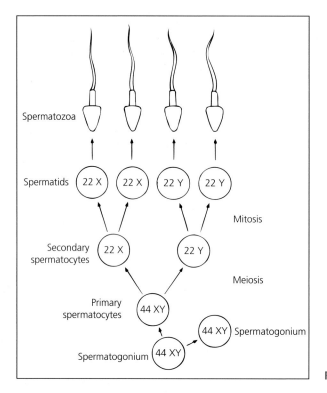

Figure 18.6 Spermatogenesis.

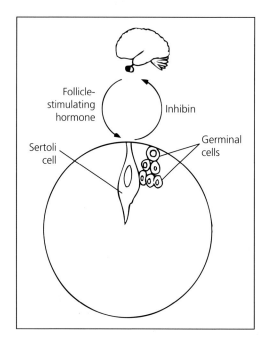

Figure 18.7 Sertoli cells and the pituitary.

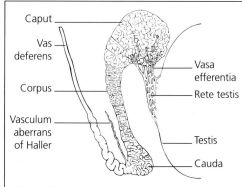

Figure 18.8 Anatomy of the epididymis.

Congenital anomalies

The gubernaculum opens the way for the testicle to follow the scrotum (Figure 18.11). There are two kinds of undescended testicles, those in which the gubernaculum has gone off course (ectopic) and those in which the descent to the bottom of the scrotum is incomplete (incomplete descent) (Figure 18.12).

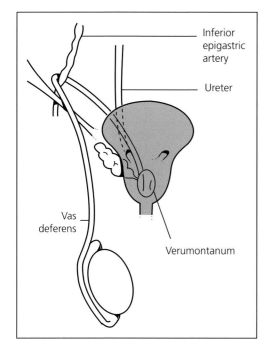

Figure 18.9 Surgical anatomy of the vas deferens.

- *Ectopic testicle*

  The errant gubernaculum may guide the ectopic testicle into one of four positions: *inguinal*, in the abdominal wall near the external inguinal ring; *perineal*; *penile*, near the base of the penis; and *crural*, in the thigh.
- *Incomplete descent*

  These testicles always move up and down and are defined according to their range of movement:
  - *Abdominal*, which may move in and out of the internal inguinal ring
  - *Inguinal*, which move along the inguinal canal
  - *Emergent*, when they appear at the external ring

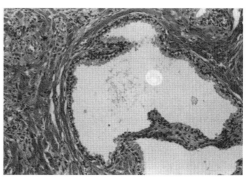

Figure 18.10 Histology of seminal vesicle.

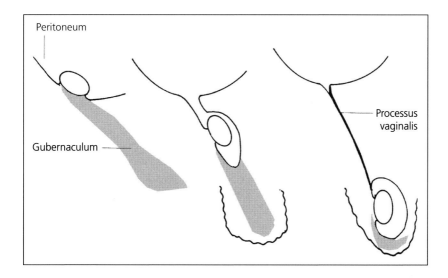

Figure 18.11 The gubernaculum opens the way for the testicle to follow into the scrotum.

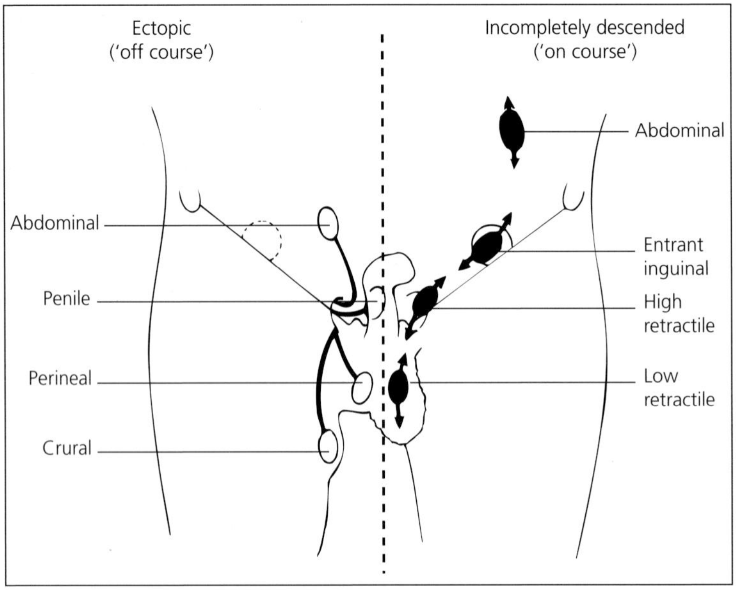

Ectopic ('off course')	Incompletely descended ('on course')
Abdominal	Abdominal
Penile	Entrant inguinal
Perineal	High retractile
Crural	Low retractile

Figure 18.12 Undescended testicles may be off course (ectopic) or on course (incomplete descent).

- *High retractile*, when they move up and down but cannot be made to go to the bottom of the scrotum
- *Low retractile*, when they descend to the bottom of the scrotum in a warm bath, under general anaesthesia or with gentle persuasion by a doctor's warm hand. Low retractile testes are essentially normal and will always end up in the scrotum with puberty.

Complications

1. *Torsion.* There is often a large loose sac of peritoneum in front of an emergent or retractile undescended testicle, which makes it prone to torsion (Figure 18.13).
2. *Infertility.* Infertility is common with bilateral undescended testicles, but not with unilateral undescent.
3. *Cancer.* About 1 in 10 testicular tumours is associated with maldescent.

Diagnosis

In most cases the diagnosis is made by inspection and palpation. Difficulty may arise with the low retractile testis: seldom is this difficult for an

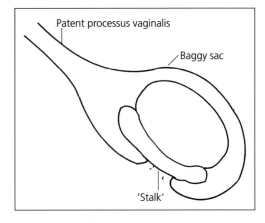

Figure 18.13 The baggy peritoneal sac associated with incomplete descent favours torsion.

experienced doctor with warm hands and a child who is not frightened. When in doubt, the child should be examined in a warm bath, and if there is still doubt, he may be given a general anaesthetic to see if the testicle descends to the bottom of the scrotum.

When no testicle can be felt on one side, it is often in the inguinal canal. The testicle is easily found with a computerised tomography (CT) scan, even in the abdomen.

Management

Ectopic testes

These never find their way into the scrotum and require orchidopexy.

Incomplete descent

1. *Abdominal.* These are now located by CT scan and, if necessary, are confirmed by laparoscopy. In prepubertal boys an effort should be made to preserve the testis. In the Fowler–Stephens procedure the testicular artery is divided as a first step, which may be performed through a laparoscope (Figure 18.14). Some 6 months later at a second operation, the testicle is mobilised and brought down into the scrotum, by which time it will have acquired a new blood supply from the artery to the vas (Figure 18.15) and it is safe to divide the testicular vessels.
2. *Inguinal.* Most of these are brought down by the routine operation of orchidopexy. Through a crease incision over the internal ring, the external oblique is opened and the testicle is mobilised, taking care not to injure its artery or the vas deferens. The testicular vessels are followed up behind the peritoneum and mobilised medially by dividing the fibrous bands. This allows the testicle to be placed in a sac between the dartos muscle and skin of the scrotum without tension (Figure 18.16).

Timing of orchidopexy

Although 90% of testicles are in the scrotum at birth, the next 9% do no descend until 12 months, after which no more do. Infertility, and possibly the late development of cancer, is thought to be prevented by orchidopexy performed before the age of 3, so there is a window of opportunity between 2 and 3, but at this age the technique is difficult. The best results are only obtained in specialised paediatric centres. After puberty the chance of improving fertility is minimal, and the risk of cancer increases rapidly, but most young men wish to keep both testes.

When an undescended testicle is found in a mature grown man, orchidectomy is the procedure that should be advised in view of the risks of malignancy. If the patient is concerned about his cosmetic appearance, he may be offered a silicone prosthesis.

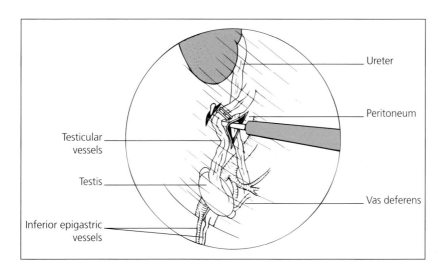

Figure 18.14 The first step in the Fowler–Stephens procedure: the testicular vessels are clipped laparoscopically.

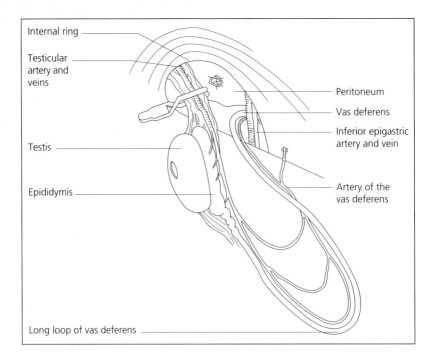

Figure 18.15 The second stage in the Fowler–Stephens procedure: the testicular vessels are divided and the testicle is brought down.

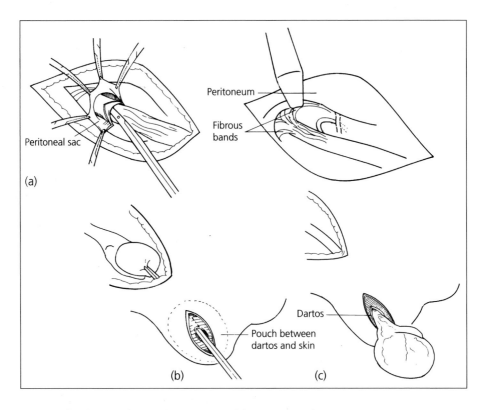

Figure 18.16 Orchidopexy (a, b and c are sequential surgery steps).

Hormone treatment

Puberty can be brought on early by giving pituitary gonadotrophins, which accelerate the descent of a low retractile testis but at the price of premature puberty and stunting of growth from early fusion of epiphyses. The method is no longer used.

Torsion

1. **Extravaginal**
   This is rarely seen in newborn boys. The testicle has rotated on the spermatic cord and it is almost never possible to save the testis by untwisting it (Figure 18.17).
2. **Intravaginal**
   The tunica vaginalis may be unusually roomy even with a normally descended testicle, and the testis and epididymis can twist on a stalk like a light bulb in its socket (Figure 18.18). Patients often recall attacks of pain that come on and are relieved equally suddenly, and a history of such warning attacks is sufficient reason to explore the testicle and fix it. Torsion may occur at any age, but is most common around puberty.

Clinical features

There is a sudden onset of pain and swelling in the testicle, which may wake the boy. On examination the scrotum is tender, red and swollen, and it is seldom possible to make out the testis from the epididymis (Figure 18.19).

The differential diagnosis is from:

1. *Mumps orchitis*, which never attacks boys before puberty
2. *Epididymitis*, which is always secondary to obvious urinary infection
3. *Fat necrosis*, which is occasionally seen in infants
4. *Cancer*, which in older boys and men can present with inflammation
5. *Torsion of an appendix testis*, which cannot be distinguished from torsion of the testis without exploration

Investigations

It is important to untwist the testicle before it dies from ischaemia, and no investigation should be allowed to delay surgical exploration. A Doppler or radioisotope scan may show absence of arterial circulation in the testicle but is justified only if it will not delay matters.

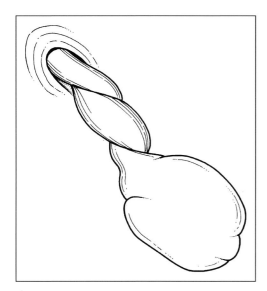

Figure 18.17 Neonatal extravaginal torsion.

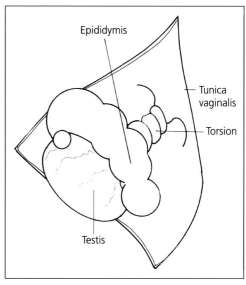

Figure 18.18 Intravaginal torsion of the testicle.

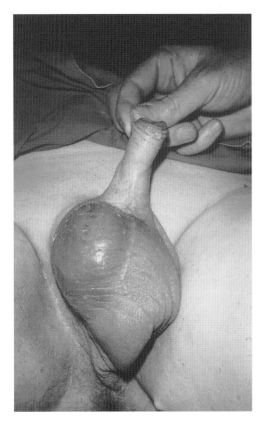

Figure 18.19 Appearance of torsion of the testicle.

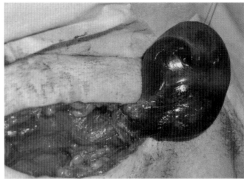

Figure 18.20 Nonviable necrotic testis.

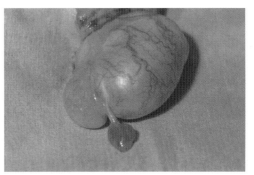

Figure 18.21 Torsion of appendix testicle.

Treatment

The testicle is explored through a transverse scrotal incision. The tunica vaginalis is opened, and the testicle is untwisted. If there is any doubt about the viability of the testis, it can be incised to see if it still bleeds. All too often it is necrotic and must be removed (Figure 18.20).

Because torsion occurs in about 10% of cases on the other side, the other testicle should be fixed then or at a later operation.

Torsion of the appendix testis

Tiny cysts are usually present at the upper pole, one on the epididymis (of Wolffian duct origin) and the other on the testis (of Müllerian duct origin). Apart from being of interest to embryologists, either can twist on its stalk, exactly mimicking torsion of the testicle and equally requiring urgent exploration (Figure 18.21).

> 🔑 **KEYPOINTS**
>
> - Time is important. Deal with the patient quickly.
> - If in doubt about diagnosis nature, seek urgent advice or proceed to surgical exploration.
> - Consent the patient for possible removal of the testis and plan to fix the other side.

Varicocele

The normal pampiniform plexus of veins draining the testicle has been thought to act as a heat exchanger to keep the testicle cool. A varicocele is a physiological dilatation of these veins (Figure 18.22). It is widely believed to depress spermatogenesis and lead to atrophy of the testis, and many operations are performed for this

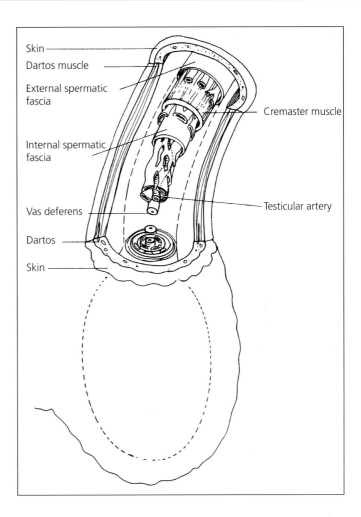

Skin
Dartos muscle
External spermatic fascia
Internal spermatic fascia
Vas deferens
Dartos
Skin
Cremaster muscle
Testicular artery

Figure 18.22 The veins of the spermatic cord.

reason although every controlled study so far has shown that the operations make no difference. The testicular vessels are approached through a short incision above and parallel to the inguinal ligament; the veins are separated from the testicular artery, ligated and divided. It has become fashionable to do the same thing via a laparoscope or even robotically.

 KEYPOINTS

- Nicknamed 'bag of worms'.
- Can be asymptomatic.
- Consider conservative management approach: tight underpants to lift the scrotum.
- Intervention is recommended if patient is symptomatic.
- Discuss all options available and help the patient to choose after full understanding is reached.

Hydrocele

Fluid accumulates in the cavity of the tunica vaginalis (Figure 18.23a and b). This may be primary or idiopathic (i.e. there is no obvious cause), or it may be secondary to obstruction to the lymphatic drainage of the testicle or may be part of widespread oedema caused by heart failure or as an inflammatory effusion from underlying disease in the testis or epididymis. The swelling is fluctuant and light shines easily through it.

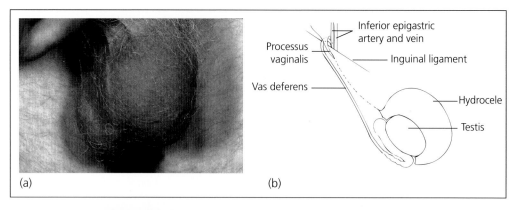

(a)

Inferior epigastric artery and vein

Processus vaginalis

Vas deferens

Inguinal ligament

Hydrocele

Testis

(b)

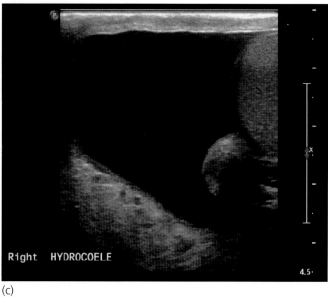

Right HYDROCOELE

4.5·

(c)

Figure 18.23 Hydrocele: (a) clinical presentation, (b) diagram and (c) ultrasound.

Neonatal

When a hydrocele in a neonate is associated with a hernia, it is operated on almost as an emergency in view of the risk of strangulation. The processus vaginalis is found at the external ring and ligated. There is no need to do anything about the tunica vaginalis testis (Figure 18.24).

Adult

In an adult there is always a suspicion that the hydrocele may be concealing some mischief in the testis. Ultrasound screening is performed to ensure that the underlying testis is healthy (Figure 18.23c), and if there is any doubt, tumour markers are measured to rule out cancer of the testis.

KEYPOINTS

- Testis is surrounded by fluid and thus cannot be felt separately.
- Light trans illumination possible.
- Swelling could be asymptomatic.
- Aspiration succeeds temporarily to relieve symptoms but re-filling quickly returns.
- Surgical correction is curative: eversion of the tunica vaginalis or eversion plication.

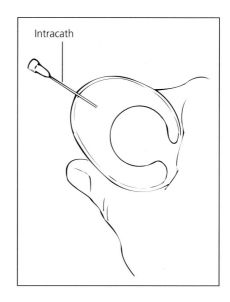

Figure 18.25 Tapping a hydrocele.

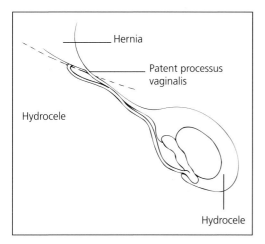

Figure 18.24 Infantile hydrocele.

Few hydroceles need any treatment: a good rule is to offer an operation if the patient's wife or his tailor complains. The options are to aspirate the fluid (Figure 18.25), warning the patient that it will fill up again, or evert the surplus tunica vaginalis (Figure 18.26).

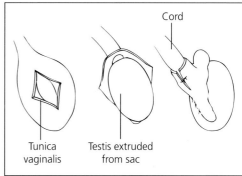

Figure 18.26 Jaboulay operation for hydrocele.

Cysts of the epididymis

A few tiny cysts are always present in the upper end of the epididymis, arising as diverticula of the vasa efferentia and epididymal tubules.

In middle age a few pea-sized cysts can usually be felt. Occasionally these cysts become large enough to be a nuisance. The swellings are always fluctuant and usually transmit light easily. If aspirated, the fluid may look opalescent, like limewater, because a few sperms are present. Occasionally there are so many to make the fluid look like cream. The diagnosis is easily confirmed by ultrasound (Figure 18.27). Treatment is seldom necessary. Aspiration is usually futile

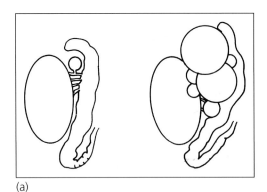

(a)

(b)

Figure 18.27 (a) Cysts of the epididymis (diagram) and (b) 18.27b (ultrasound).

KEYPOINTS

- Cyst is separate from testis.
- Tense on palpation and can be 'sore'.
- Could be multiple/bilateral.
- Could be asymptomatic; thus you can leave alone and follow up.
- Excise if asymptomatic.
- New cysts can form.

---

because the cysts fill up again and they are always multilocular. Excision of the cysts often results in a blockage of the vasa efferentia and should be postponed until the patient has completed his family (Figure 18.28).

Trauma to the testicle

The testis is easily injured in sport or at work. Blood collects in the tunica vaginalis cavity and the expansion of the clot may produce pressure atrophy of the rest of the testis. For this reason injured testes should all be explored, the clot evacuated, and the rent in the tunica albuginea sewn up (Figure 18.29).

Testicular tumours are notoriously apt to present after trauma and surgeons must always keep this possibility in mind because an orchidectomy may be needed.

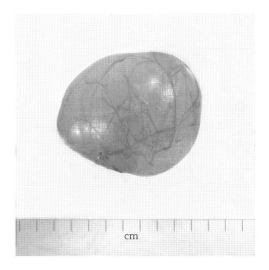

Figure 18.28 Cyst of the epididymis (a photograph).

Inflammation of the testicle

Acute

Acute orchitis

Most infections in the testis are caused by viruses, for example, Coxsackie or mumps. *Mumps orchitis* only occurs after puberty, when it may be bilateral and the oedema may lead to pressure necrosis and atrophy of the testis. When unilateral it may be impossible to distinguish it from torsion and therefore demands to be explored. There is some evidence that the *tunica albuginea* will decompress the testis and prevent atrophy.

Acute epididymitis

Bacterial infection finds its way down the vas deferens from the urinary tract to cause acute inflammation. This is seen after operations on the urinary tract especially if a catheter has been left in the urethra. The organisms are usually *Escherichia coli*. Acute epididymis arising out of the blue may be caused by *Chlamydia trachomatis*, which can be identified in fluid aspirated from the epididymis with special

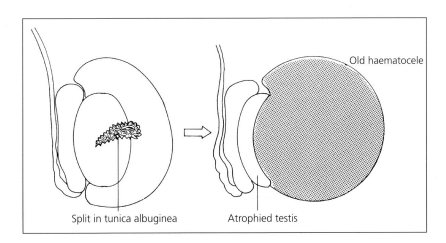

Figure 18.29 Closed injury of the testis: if not evacuated, the clot may cause atrophy of the testis.

culture techniques. Rarely, tuberculosis can cause surprisingly acute symptoms and should be excluded in every acute case where there is no obvious cause for infection such as a recent operation on the urinary tract.

Chronic

Chronic orchitis

Syphilitic gamma of the testis was for a generation only a pathological curiosity. Cancer is far more likely and in any event, orchidectomy is probably the right treatment. *Granulomatous orchitis* occurs with repeated urinary infections and does not always respond to antibiotics and usually requires orchidectomy.

Chronic epididymitis

Tuberculosis
Blood-borne infection with *Mycobacterium tuberculosis* occurs in the head of the epididymis, whereas urine-borne infection involves the tail along with the vas deferens (Figure 18.30). The epididymis is knobbly and hard, and there may be nodules along the vas. In late cases a sinus may form and discharge on the skin of the scrotum. Rectal ultrasound scanning may show tuberculosis elsewhere. After a full course of treatment, a residual mass in the epididymis may have to be removed.
Seminal granuloma
After vasectomy many men have induration in the epididymis caused by an inflammatory response to extravasated sperms. It may respond to prednisolone.

Orchialgia

There is a sad group of men who complain of persistent pain in the testicle. Often there has been some previous minor surgical operation, for example, vasectomy or hydrocelectomy, and pain persists. Careful clinical examination can find nothing wrong. An ultrasound scan is normal. Frequently the testicle is explored and nothing abnormal can be found. Before long the patient seeks a second opinion, and almost inevitably another surgeon will attempt to dener-

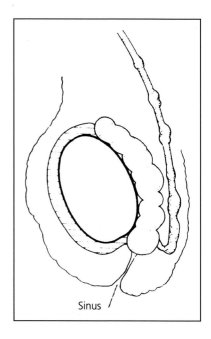

Figure 18.30 Tuberculosis of the epididymis and vas deferens.

vate the testicle. The result is instant relief of pain – for a while, but then it comes back.

Before long the patient has persuaded yet another surgeon to remove the testicle. This is done: once again the relief of pain is dramatic – for a while, and then it comes back on the other side. It is most important to recognise these unfortunate men because they need help, but from the psychiatrist, not the surgeon.

Cancer of the testis

Aetiology

There has been a dramatic increase in testicular cancer cases with 2286 new cases diagnosed in 2010. This has led to an intense search for causes but as of yet no preventative risk factor has been found. Both environmental and genetic factors are likely to be involved.

Known risk factors for testicular cancer are shown in Table 18.1.

Table 18.1 **Risk factors for testicular cancer**	
Demographic	**Age 24–49**
	Caucasian
Medical conditions	Carcinoma in situ
	Previous testicular cancer
	Cryptorchidism
	Inguinal hernia
	Subfertility
Genetic	Close family relative with testicular cancer

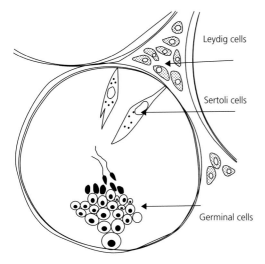

Figure 18.31 Cellular origin of testicular tumours.

Pathology

Cancer may arise from any of the cell types present in the testis; over 90% arise from germ cells (Figure 18.31).

Germ cell tumours

Gonadocytes and spermatocytes

These give rise to a spectrum of tumours, from highly anaplastic seminoma that shows nuclear polymorphism and may even stain for human chorionic gonadotrophin (hCG), to intermediate types with sheets of cells filled with glycogen that stain for placental alkaline phosphatase (PLAP),

to well-differentiated spermatocytic seminoma that seldom metastasises (Figures 18.32 and 18.33).

Embryonal carcinoma

Here the tissues attempt to form organs, with papillary and glandular elements. They stain for alpha-fetoprotein (AFP), which betrays the origin of germ cells from the foetal yolk sac. Pure yolk sac tumours are occasionally found in infants (Figure 18.34).

Teratocarcinoma

In this there is a spectrum, from the most benign-looking adult tissues, for example, cartilage and hair, to wildly malignant choriocarcinoma. Of all the possibilities, choriocarcinoma is the worst, spreading rapidly through the bloodstream (Figures 18.35 and 18.36).

Epidermoid cyst

A cyst containing mature tissue, mainly skin, is occasionally found. Some of them are possibly benign, but it can take very careful histological examination to distinguish it from teratocarcinoma.

Non-germ cell tumours

Leydig cell tumours

These arise from the Leydig cells that are packed in between the tubules of the testis and normally produce testosterone. They can give rise to precocious puberty.

Sertoli cell tumours

These are very rare, seldom metastasise and cause gynaecomastia.

Lymphomas

They may be confined to the testis and tend to occur in older men.

Small cell origin

These commonly metastasise.

Clinical features
Symptoms

- *Lump in the testicle*: this is in the body of the testis. It is not fluctuant or translucent. The

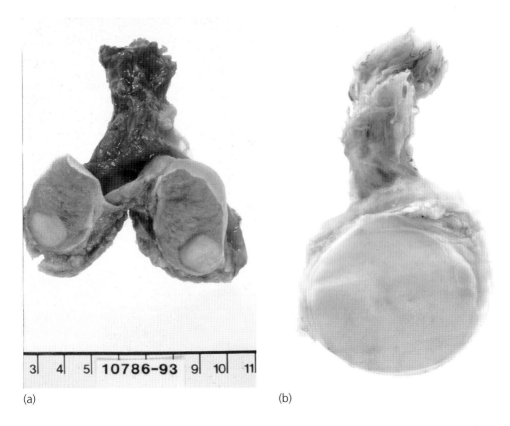

(a)   (b)

Figure 18.32 Seminoma: (a) a small tumour nodule within the testis and (b) a tumour replacing all normal testicular tissues.

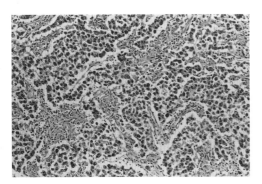

Figure 18.33 Seminoma. Microscopic appearance.

tragedy is that so many young men report this so late (see below).

- *Inflammation*: about 15% have signs of inflammation that are all too easily mistaken for epididymitis.

- *Trauma*: another 10–15% of men have a history of injury, which may lead to loss of valuable time in making proper diagnosis.
- *Gynaecomastia*: transient swelling of the breasts is common at puberty but can be due to trophoblastic elements secreting hCG, which should be measured in every case.
- *Back pain*: in a fit young man it should always make you think of metastases from a testicular tumour.

Physical signs

A hard lump is found in the body of the testis. Difficulty arises if the lump is near the epididymis, concealed in the body of the testis, or impossible to feel because of a tense hydrocele (Figure 18.37). Inflammation can be misleading. Always examine the breasts for gynaecomastia.

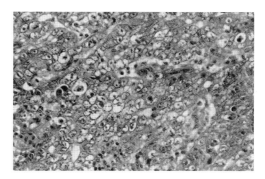

Figure 18.35 Teratocarcinoma. Macroscopic appearance.

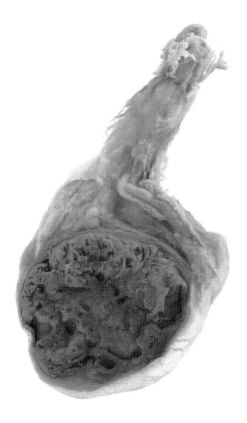

Figure 18.34 Embryonal carcinoma.

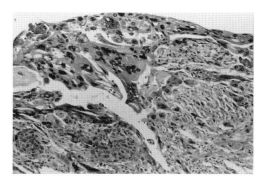

Figure 18.36 Teratocarcinoma. Microscopic appearance.

Investigations

1. *Ultrasound scan.* This investigation is so quick and painless that it should be performed on every suspicious testicle (Figure 18.38). Mistakes are rare. The ultrasound will show features suggestive of testicular cancer, such as increased vascularity accompanying a mass. There may be additional features of microlithiasis, suggesting that the tumour arose from carcinoma in situ. Carcinoma in situ is a bilateral condition associated with an increased risk of developing a secondary testicular cancer.

2. *Tumour markers.* Blood is sent for PLAP, which is secreted by gonadocytes; for hCG, which is secreted by trophoblastic cells; and AFP, which is secreted by yolk sac cells. (An ordinary 'pregnancy test' is a quick and cheap way of detecting abnormal amounts of hCG.)

Lactic acid dehydrogenase (LDH) has low specificity (high false-positive rate) and should be correlated with other clinical findings. High levels can be detected in smooth, cardiac and skeletal muscles, liver, kidney and brain. It is thought to have a direct relationship with tumour burden; thus it seems to be most useful as a marker for tumour bulk tissue.

3. *Exploration of the testicle.* The spermatic cord is clamped at the internal ring before the testicle is delivered: the diagnosis of cancer is usually obvious to the naked eye, but can be verified by frozen section if in doubt. The cord is transacted above the clamp (Figure 18.39).

4. *CT scan.* A CT scan of the chest and abdomen is performed to identify lymph node and pulmonary metastases (Figures 18.40).

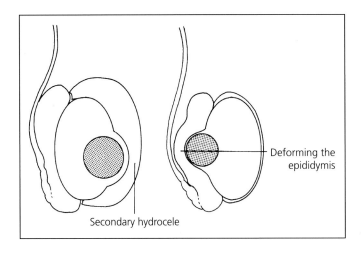

Secondary hydrocele

Deforming the epididymis

Figure 18.37 Some testicular tumours are difficult to feel.

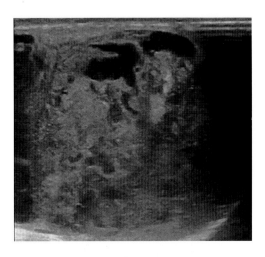

Figure 18.38 Ultrasound scan of a testicular teratoma.

 KEYPOINTS

Recommended tests for staging at diagnosis:
- Serum tumour markers: AFP
- hCG
- LDH
- CT abdomen, pelvis and chest
- Additional scans in case of symptoms.

TNM staging of testicular tumours

T stage (primary tumour)

The T stage is determined only after careful histological examination of the entire testicle.

TX	Tumour cannot be assessed
T0	No evidence of primary tumour
Tis	Testicular intra-epithelial neoplasia
T1	Tumour limited to the testis and epididymis. No vascular/lymphatic invasion
T2	Tumour limited to the testis and epididymis. Vascular/lymphatic invasion
T3	Tumour invades the spermatic cord. With or without vascular/lymphatic invasion
T4	Tumour invades the scrotum. With or without vascular/lymphatic invasion

N stage (regional lymph nodes, clinical)

The testis drains to the para-aortic lymph nodes at the level of the origin of the renal arteries and only later via the cisterna chyli into the thoracic

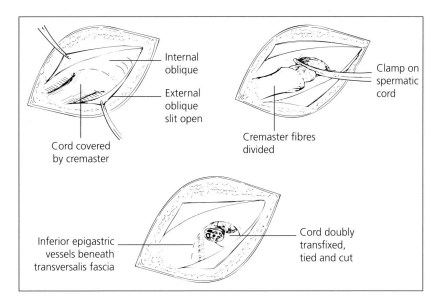

Figure 18.39 Left orchiectomy.

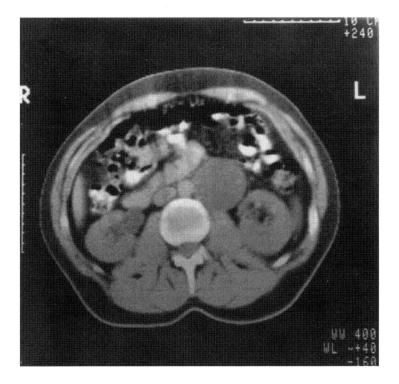

Figure 18.40 CT scan showing para-aortic mass on the left side of the aorta.

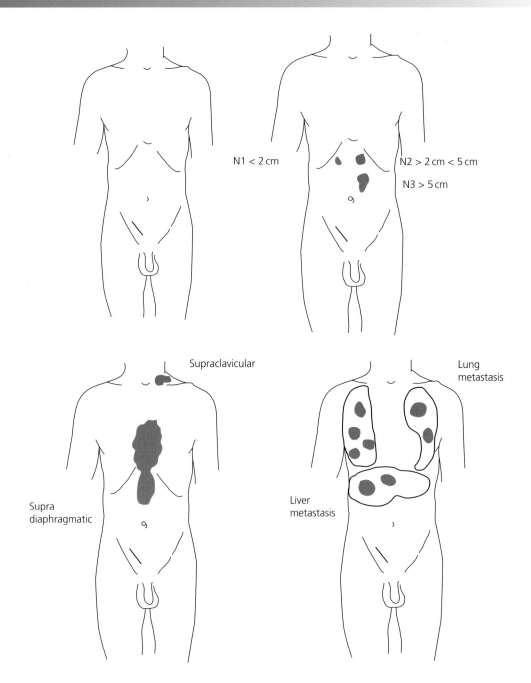

Figure 18.41 Lymph node (N) staging of testis tumours: (a) N0, (b) N1–N2–N3, (c) supra – clavicular and supra diaphragmatic and (d) liver and lung metastases.

duct and systemic circulation. The nodes are localised by CT scanning (Figure 18.41).

NX	Regional lymph nodes cannot be assessed
N0	No regional lymph node metastasis
N1	Lymph node metastases, single or multiple, none >2 cm in greatest dimension
N2	Lymph node metastases, single or multiple, >2 cm–<5 cm in greatest dimension
N3	Lymph node mass >5 cm in greatest dimension

M stage (distant metastasis)

Venous spread can occur early if trophoblastic elements are present.

MX	Distant metastasis cannot be assessed
M0	No distant metastasis
M1	Distant metastasis
M1a	Non-regional lymph nodes
M1b	Other sites

Serum tumour markers

	S1	S2	S3
LDH (U/l)	$<1.5 \times N$	$1.5–10 \times N$	$>10 \times N$
hCG (mIU/mL)	<5 000	5 000–50 000	>50 000
AFP (ng/mL)	<1 000	1 000–10 000	>10 000

Stage grouping

Stage		T	N	M	Serum markers
I		pT1–T4	N0	M0	SX
	IA	pT1			S0
	IB	pT2–T4			
	IS	Any patient/TX			S1–3
II			N1–3		SX
	IIA		N1/2/3		S0–1
	IIB				
	IIC				
III	IIIA		Any N	M1a	SX/0/1
	IIIB		N1–3	M0	S2
			Any N	M1a	
	IIIC		N1–3	M0	S3
			Any N	M1a	
				M1b	Any S

SX: Serum tumour marker studies not available.
S0: Serum tumour marker levels within normal limits.
S1/2/3: Elevated serum tumour marker levels.

Treatment

The treatment of testicular cancer represents one of the major triumphs of oncology, with a fall in death rates of 70% in the last 15 years and with 97.2% of patients now living more than 5 years. This is largely due to modern treatments such as the introduction of platinum-based chemotherapy.

Stage I

If the tumour is confined to the testis, then two options are available: surveillance and further therapy. If surveillance is followed in the absence of poor prognosis pathology features, then the likelihood of relapse is 13% in patients with a teratoma and 17% for those with a seminoma. Nearly all patients are salvaged with platinum-based chemotherapy.

Seminoma

Prophylactic radiation to the retroperitoneal lymph nodes can give 100% cure for stage I seminoma. However the use of radiotherapy has diminished due to well-documented long-term risks of secondary malignancies and cardiac disease. An identical rate of cure is obtained with a single course of single-agent carboplatin.

Other germ cell tumours

Stage I non-seminomas are highly curable (>99%). Orchiectomy will cure 70% with the remaining 30% relapsing and needing treatment. The relapses are highly curable with platinum-based chemotherapy. Surveillance is reasonable for non-seminomatous germ cell tumours without invasion of the veins or lymphatics of the testis, without yolk sac elements and without undifferentiated elements, but because of the higher rate of relapse, some centres have reverted to a policy of giving all these men prophylactic platinum-based combination chemotherapy.

Stage II

For some stage IIA seminoma, some clinicians still use radiotherapy although two cycles of platinum-based chemotherapy is as good. For all other patients, the standard of care to start with would be chemotherapy, which is followed carefully by serial tumour markers and CT scans.

Stage III

All patients are treated with chemotherapy. If a mass remains after the chemotherapy is completed, it is removed surgically. If the mass of lymph nodes is in the retroperitoneal tissue, this requires careful dissection of all the tumours off the aorta and inferior vena cava (Figure 18.42). Residual masses in the lungs or mediastinum are removed through the chest. Histological examination of the excised mass shows that in one third of cases, there is a residual necrotic tissue in another third differentiated teratoma and in the remaining third undifferentiated tumour. If necrotic tissue is found, no more treatment is needed. If undifferentiated tumour is found, further chemotherapy is given, with 30–40% of this group of patients being cured. It is important to remove all residual differentiated tumours, as over 5 years, 50% transform into an undifferentiated tumour.

Monitoring treatment

The effects of treatment are closely monitored by measuring serum levels of AFP, PLAP and hCG. These are hormones secreted by teratoma and seminoma. If the tumour is being treated effectively, levels of the hormones will decay over a known time period: 3–5 days for AFP and 12–36 h for hCG.

Prognosis

One of the most commonly used prognostic indices is that laid down by the International Germ Cell Cancer Collaborative Group. Non-seminoma germ cell tumours with good prognosis have a 5-year survival of 92–95%; those with intermediate prognosis, 72–80%; and those with poor prognosis, 48%. Seminoma tumours are classified as either good or intermediate in prognosis based on the presence or absence of non-nodal visceral metastasis and serum tumour marker levels.

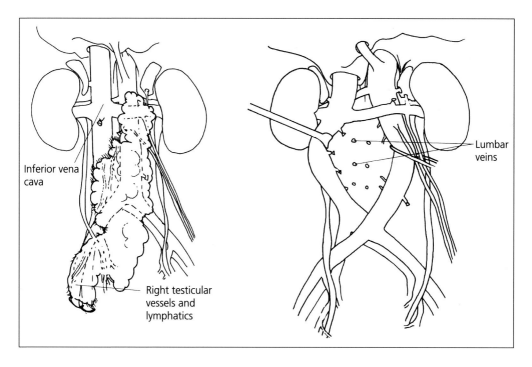

Figure 18.42 Removal of residual para-aortic nodes.

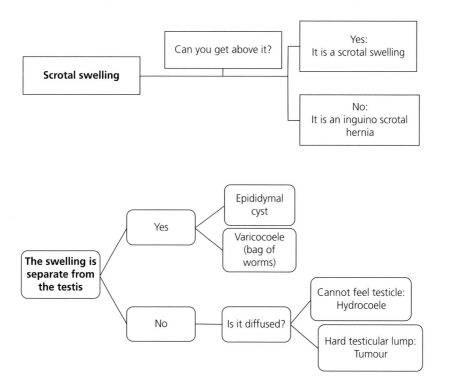

Scrotal swelling clinical examination guide.

19

Male infertility

History and general examination

Gross endocrine deficiencies are usually obvious: the young man who shaves and has a normal physique is unlikely to have a deficiency of androgens. Anabolic (androgenic) steroids taken by athletes and bodybuilders suppress the pituitary gonadotrophins luteinizing hormone (LH) and follicle-stimulating hormone (FSH) and result in testicular atrophy. A thorough drug history is important (e.g. sulfasalazine use, previous chemotherapy). Note any history of previous surgery to the bladder neck or pelvis that may have injured the autonomic nervous system, leading to probable retrograde ejaculation. Chronic illnesses such as diabetes, renal failure and liver failure can impair spermatogenesis. A past history of genitourinary infections may be relevant (e.g. mumps, gonorrhoea and non-specific urethritis). Endogenous toxins as a result of smoking and drinking alcohol could harm sperm production. Patients with recurrent sinusitis and chest infections may have epididymal destruction (cystic fibrosis) or Young's syndrome (immotile cilia syndrome).

It is important to establish if normal ejaculation occurs within the vagina. Sexual intercourse taking place around the point of maximal female fertility (i.e. ovulation) is optimal for fecundity, although some studies have shown that healthy sperms can remain in the genital tract for up to 96 h.

Investigations

Semen analysis

Semen is collected by masturbation after 72 h abstinence into a clean plastic container. The WHO reference range for seminal analysis is used in most laboratories (Table 19.1).

- *Volume*: the normal range is from 1 to 8 mL. (The most usual cause of a low semen volume is clumsy collection of the specimen!) Liquefaction time should be noted.
- *Sperm density and motility*: most traditional laboratory methods for measuring sperm density and motility are so inaccurate as to be useless. When the computerised Hamilton Thorne system is used, normal fertility is found with a sperm density as low as 1×10^6/mL provided motility is adequate.
- *Morphology*: there is very little correlation between morphological abnormalities and infertility. Many more are picked up by electron microscopy (Figure 19.1), but are of doubtful relevance.
- *Antibodies*: antibodies to the head and tail of the sperm may occur in blood, seminal plasma

Urology Lecture Notes, Seventh Edition. Amir V. Kaisary, Andrew Ballaro and Katharine Pigott.
© 2016 John Wiley & Sons, Ltd. Published 2016 by John Wiley & Sons, Ltd.

and cervical mucus. These may account for some of the immotile sperms sometimes found in the post-coital test.

Luteinizing hormone and follicle-stimulating hormone measurements

A grossly raised FSH level is a strong negative predictor of active spermatogenesis and is likely to be associated with azoospermia. However, modern microsurgical techniques such as micro-TESE can identify occasional foci of spermatogenesis

Table 19.1 Normal semen parameters

Colour	Grey-yellow
Volume	>2 mL
Sperm density	20–200 million/mL
Motility	>50% at 4 h
Abnormal forms	<96%
Fructose	Present
pH	>7.2

providing sperm for intracytoplasmic sperm injection (ICSI). Even very atrophic testes can harbour such foci. On the other hand, normal gonadotrophins associated with a normal testicular volume (15–25 cc) should raise suspicion of an obstructive cause for the azoospermia (a blockage somewhere between the testis and the ejaculatory ducts).

Testis biopsy

Although previously needle aspirations were taken from the testis or open biopsy methods were done to take tiny snippets of tubules (Figure 19.2), currently micro-TESE techniques may increase the probability of sperm retrieval. Biopsy tissue is put immediately into Bouin's preservative fluid to avoid distortion of the histology.

Infertility

Infertility is defined as the failure to conceive after regular unprotected intercourse for 18 months. The female partner should also be investigated,

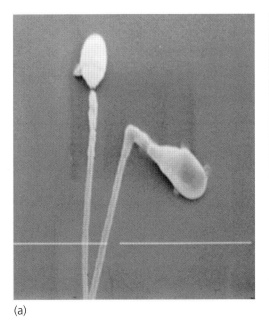

(a)

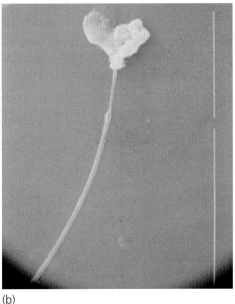

(b)

Figure 19.1 Scanning electron microscopy of 'abnormal' morphology of sperms (a and b shows different appearances).

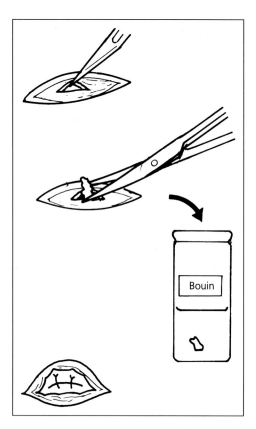

Figure 19.2 Biopsy of testis.

where appropriate, to ensure ovulation and tubal patency. Male infertility may be classified as:

(A) Non-obstructive
(B) Obstructive
(C) Coital

Non-obstructive

- Genetic disorders
- Hormonal
- Autoimmune
- Systemic diseases

Genetic disorders

Chromosomal abnormalities

Sex hormone abnormalities: Klinefelter's syndrome and variants
Very small testes should raise the suspicion of Klinefelter's syndrome (47, XXY, 46/XY) as seen

Table 19.2 **Klinefelter's syndrome**
• Tall and thin
• Gynaecomastia
• Small testes and penis
• Elevated gonadotrophins and hyalinised testicular tubules

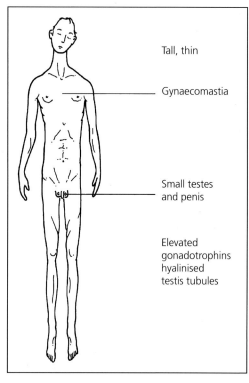

Tall, thin

Gynaecomastia

Small testes and penis

Elevated gonadotrophins hyalinised testis tubules

Figure 19.3 Klinefelter's syndrome.

in Table 19.2 (Figure 19.3). The presence of spermatogonia and sperm production is variable in men with Klinefelter's mosaicism. The diagnosis is easily confirmed by cytology of a scraping from the mucosa of the cheek, looking for the Barr body – the index of the extra X chromosome. Note the clinical features. Previous surgery for repair of a hernia, orchidopexy, may suggest damage to the vas deferens. Previous bilateral orchidopexy is often associated with testes that do not produce sperm. Follow-up of men with Klinefelter's syndrome is required and androgen replacement therapy should be started when testosterone levels are in the hypogonadal range).

Autosomal abnormalities

The most common autosomal karyotype abnormalities are translocations. These anomalies should be investigated as there is an increased associated risk of aneuploidy or unbalanced chromosomal complements in the foetus. Clearly when assisted fertility, in vitro fertilisation (IVF)/ICSI, is contemplated for men with translocations, amniocentesis should be performed. Embryos with known unbalanced translocation should not be implanted.

Sperm chromosomal abnormalities

Hybridisation analysis of spermatozoa remains currently as a research investigation. Techniques are needed to separate populations of genetically abnormal sperms from normal sperms for safety before assisted fertilisation, IVF and ICSI.

Genetic defects

Kallmann syndrome

Some 10 generic defects have been reported in patients with Kallmann syndrome (KS), the defining clinical features of which are hypogonadotrophic hypogonadism (HH; low gonadotrophins and testosterone levels) and anosmia. Other clinical features include facial asymmetry, cleft palate, deafness, maldescended testes and unilateral renal aplasia (X-linked KS). Euosmic forms account for over 50% of HH cases and a further 14 genetic lesions have been found to be present to contribute to the phenotype in these patients. The disorder may be oligogenic rather than monogenic.

Mild androgen insensitivity syndrome

The androgen receptor (AR) gene is located on the long arm of the X-chromosome. Mutations result in mild to complete androgen insensitivity. Patients with complete androgen insensitivity have female external genitalia and absence of pubic hair (Morris syndrome; testicular feminisation). In partial androgen insensitivity, several different phenotypes are encountered, ranging from predominantly female type with ambiguous genitalia to predominantly male phenotype with micropenis, perineal hypospadias and cryptorchidism (Reifenstein syndrome).

Y chromosome microdeletions

Y chromosome microdeletions (AZF a, b, c) are rare in men with a sperm concentration more than 5 million/mL. It is found in men with both azoospermia and severe oligospermia, more frequently with the former.

Cystic fibrosis mutations

Cystic fibrosis is an autosomal recessive disease. It occurs due to mutation in both alleles of the cystic fibrosis gene, which encloses the cystic fibrosis transmembrane conductance regulator (CFTR) protein. Men presenting with vas aplasia alone represent a mild form of cystic fibrosis that lacks the associated pulmonary and pancreatic symptoms and only presents with azoospermia.

Unilateral or bilateral absence/abnormality of the vas

Unilateral absence of the vas deferens is usually associated with an ipsilateral renal aplasia. Men with unilateral absence of the vas are usually fertile. An abdominal ultrasound examination is valuable in investigating these cases.

Sperm DNA fragmentation

Increased DNA damage in spermatozoa from men with oligozoospermia occurs. This is associated with reduced chances of natural conception and an increase in early pregnancy loss. Damage may improve after varicocele ligation.

Obstructive

Obstructive absence of spermatozoa and spermatogenic cells in semen and post-ejaculatory urine is due to bilateral obstruction of the seminal duct system.

Congenital

- Intratesticular: dysjunction between rete testis and efferent ductules
- Epididymis: idiopathic, detached
- Vas deferens: absence
- Ejaculatory duct: prostatic cyst, Müllerian cyst

Acquired

- Intratesticular: post-inflammatory or postsurgical obstruction
- Epididymis: post-infective, postsurgical
- Vas deferens: bilateral vasectomy, post-hernia/scrotal surgery
- Ejaculatory duct: post-infective, post-bladder neck surgery

Treatment

- Intratesticular obstruction: impossible. Assisted fertility is considered.
- Epididymal obstruction: reconstruction may be considered.

Microsurgical sperm aspiration for assisted conception could be considered.

- Vas deferens obstruction: corrective surgical techniques are considered, taking into account the aetiology of the obstruction and extent.

- Ejaculatory duct obstruction: the aetiology of obstruction will dictate the surgical approach chosen. A prostatic cyst obstructing the ejaculatory ducts (Figure 19.4) is amenable for resection of a part of the verumontanum, incision or deroofing.

> ### 🔑 KEYPOINTS
>
> - Obstruction should be suspected in azoospermia or severe oligospermia associated with a normal testicular volume with bulky epididymis.
> - Epididymal obstruction: scrotal exploration with standard reconstruction performed.
> - Microsurgical epididymal sperm aspiration and cryopreservation of spermatozoa considered.

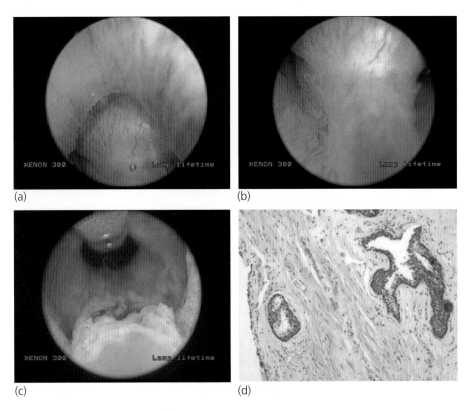

(a)　　(b)　　(c)　　(d)

Figure 19.4 (a–d) Prostate cyst obstructing ejaculatory ducts at the verumontanum.

Coital

1. ***Anorgasmia***: inability to reach orgasm. Usually psychological.
2. ***Premature ejaculation***: a male sexual dysfunction characterised by ejaculation that occurs prior to or within about a minute of vaginal penetration and inability to delay it. It could be related to prostatitis or could be psychogenic. It is a distressing feature and would only lead to infertility if extravaginal ejaculation occurs.
3. ***Anejaculation***: complete absence of ejaculation, both antegrade and retrograde. It is caused by failure of semen emission from the seminal vesicles, prostate and ejaculatory ducts. It is always associated with central or peripheral nervous system dysfunction. It can occur with alcohol, antihypertensive therapy, alpha-1 adrenoceptor antagonists, antipsychotics and antidepressants.
4. ***Retrograde ejaculation***: absence of antegrade ejaculation as a result of semen passing backwards into the bladder through the bladder neck region.

The aetiologies include:

- Bladder neck incompetence: following transurethral resection of prostate
- Urethra: hyperplastic verumontanum. Urethral valves and strictures
- Neurogenic: spinal cord injury, cauda equina lesions, multiple sclerosis and Parkinson's disease

Treatment

Azoospermia

If the FSH and LH are grossly elevated, testicular biopsy is unlikely to reveal live spermatozoa. If the biopsy shows maturation arrest (Figure 19.5), there is little evidence that any endocrine manipulation will be helpful. The presence of lymphocytes in the biopsies suggests an immunological problem as the aetiology or cause.

Blockage to the seminal tract may occur from a number of causes. There may have been exposure to mercury in childhood, once a common component of 'teething powders', which paralyse the microcilia in the bronchioles and in the epididymis. Congenital absence of vasa could occur. A blockage in the vas deferens can be demonstrated by vasography (Figure 19.6) and may be treated by epididymovasostomy (Figure 19.7). A transrectal ultrasound scan may show dilatation of the seminal vesicles, secondary to blockage of the ejaculatory ducts, which may be relieved by transurethral incision of the ejaculatory ducts.

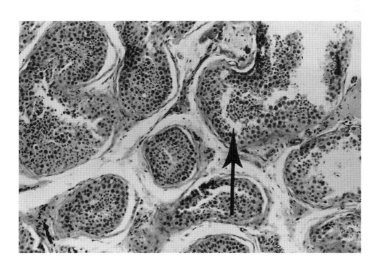

Figure 19.5 Maturation arrest: the arrow shows immature cells shed into the lumen of the tubule.

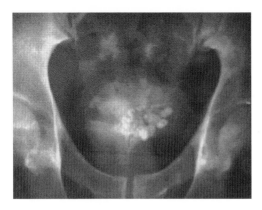

Figure 19.6 Vasogram showing filling of the vas deferens and seminal vesicle on the left side.

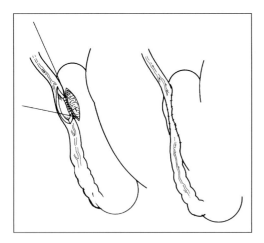

Figure 19.7 Epididymovasostomy.

Oligospermia

When a low sperm count has been reported, the first step must be to check it with a properly validated computerised technique. Because of the errors in the usual methods, claims that any form of treatment has been beneficial should be met with considerable scepticism. Loose underwear and trousers will reduce scrotal temperature and are usually advised, though the evidence basis for such recommendations is poor. Operations on varicoceles, whether they can be seen or have to be detected by Doppler studies in symptomless men, should be regarded with even more

scepticism. This is an area that cries out for 'evidence-based' decision-making.

Vasectomy

Consent

Both partners must understand that vasectomy is likely to be irreversible. It must also be explained that however carefully the vasa are divided, the ends may join each other again. Usually this is detected within the first few months after the vasectomy (early failure), but in something like 1:2000 cases, it occurs some years later (late failure) and takes place irrespective of what type of operation has been done. Until all the sperms have disappeared from the ejaculate, the couple must continue to use contraceptive precautions.

Because of the risk of medicolegal consequences, all these points should be fully discussed and spelled out on the consent form.

Procedure

Vasectomy can be performed under local or general anaesthesia. When there has been previous surgery in the inguinal region or scrotum, general anaesthesia may be preferable. The large number of different techniques described today shows that none of them are perfect. There is no objective evidence that any one method is superior to another in terms of preventing either early or late reunion (Figure 19.8). Usually a small length of vas is removed, and the ends are treated to seal them off in the hope of preventing spontaneous reunion. The ends may be ligated with absorbable or non-absorbable material or diathermised. Some surgeons seal one vas, others both. Some surgeons back one end, some both. Some stitch the sheath of the vas to interpose a layer of fascia between the two ends. Many do not. Both early and late recurrences have been reported after all of these methods, and it almost certainly takes place more frequently than is generally appreciated: in 10% of one series of men who came up to have their vasectomy reversed, it was found that spermatozoa were present in their pre-reversal specimens.

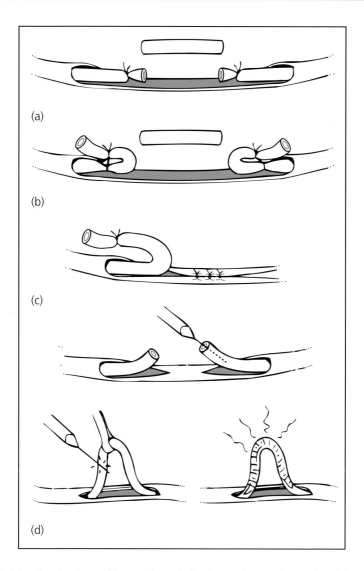

Figure 19.8 Variety of methods used in vasectomy in the hope of preventing early or late recanalisation. (a) Excise a segment and tie cut ends. (b) Excise a segment, fold away the cut ends and tie. Place the two ends in separate tissue planes. (c) Lumens of each cut end after excision of a segment needle cauterized. (d) Needle cautery of vas loop segment.

Complications

1. Haematoma is common from reactionary bleeding from small scrotal veins that go into spasm during the operation and escape notice. A large haematoma is dealt with by evacuation of the clot and haemostasis. Small collections usually resolve spontaneously.

2. Infection may take place, usually at the side of a skin suture but sometimes in a haematoma.

3. Pain in the scrotum: a small number of patients continued to complain of pain in the scrotum for which no cause can be found.

4. Sperm granuloma: sometimes a sperm granuloma is found at the side of the site of the

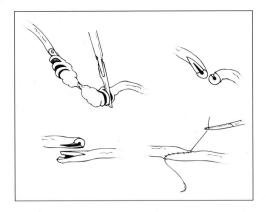

Figure 19.9 Reversal of vasectomy.

division of the vas or epididymis to give a typical tender nodular swelling.

Reversal of vasectomy: Re-anastomosis of the vas

The ends of the vas are found, trimmed back to the lumen and sewn together (Figure 19.9). Most surgeons use magnification when performing this operation. Success in terms of sperms finding their way through the anastomosis can be expected in over 80%, but only about 50% will father children. There are many possible reasons for this, including the possible development of autoantibodies during the time that sperms have been abstract in the epididymis.

Part 6

Additional therapeutic modalities

20

Radiotherapy

Radiotherapy involves the use of high-energy ionising radiation to cause DNA damage and ultimately cell death. Ionising radiation acts by ejecting an electron from an atom to yield an ion pair. This may result in direct damage to DNA via molecular excitation or indirect damage via the hydrolysis of water into free radicals. Radiation can have an effect anywhere in the cell cycle but it is only at the time of mitosis that cell death occurs. There can therefore be a time lag between treatment and its full effect. Typical radical doses are given as multiple fractions 5 days a week over several weeks at a dose per fraction of 2 Gy. This is to allow normal cells to recover from sublethal damage and to cycle into the more radiosensitive part of the cell cycle, G2 and M phases.

The dose of radiation is defined as the amount of energy deposited in tissues and is measured in grays (Gy).

Radiotherapy is delivered in three ways: external beam radiation, brachytherapy and radioisotope therapy. External beam radiation involves the use of linear accelerators or isotope sources to deliver radiation from a distance. Brachytherapy involves the implantation of radioactive sources into the patient such as the case of iodine-125 low-dose brachytherapy in early stage prostate cancer. The radioactive sources release gamma rays locally. Finally radioactive isotopes are administered orally or intravenously and are preferentially taken up by target organs. An example is strontium-89 in the palliative treatment of prostate cancer patients with bone metastases.

Delivery

Radical radiotherapy can be offered as sole treatment or with surgery being given before treatment, neo-adjuvant or after surgical resection in the adjuvant setting.

Side effects of radiotherapy

Radiation side effects are divided into acute and late effects.

- Acute: These occur within hours or weeks and include both systemic effects, such as lethargy and fatigue, and localised effects depending on the site treated. They occur in tissues that are rapidly dividing. In the case of irradiating the bladder, patients may experience diarrhoea, cystitis and proctitis. Acute radiation side effects resolve within 3 months of treatment but could become chronic.
- Late: These occur 3 months or later after treatment and can progress with time they are permanent. They depend on the area treated and occur when slowly dividing tissues attempt

Urology Lecture Notes, Seventh Edition. Amir V. Kaisary, Andrew Ballaro and Katharine Pigott.
© 2016 John Wiley & Sons, Ltd. Published 2016 by John Wiley & Sons, Ltd.

to divide. In some cases the effects are believed to be mediated by fibrosis of the vascular endothelium. An example is erectile dysfunction seen in about 30% of patients treated with brachytherapy.

Carcinogenic: Radiation can cause secondary malignancies. This is of particular relevance when treating men and younger patients with testicular tumour. Subsequent cancer risk can occur in relation to treatment volume and dose.

Pelvic radiotherapy

Variable dose fractionation according to the site treated. For example:

Prostate cancer 74 Gy in 37 fractions over 7½ weeks

Bladder cancer 64 Gy in 32 fractions over 6½ weeks

Pre-existing morbidities

When considering pelvis radiotherapy, there are several conditions where radiotherapy would be advised against. These include ulcerative colitis and previous radiotherapy in this area.

Steps in delivering radiotherapy

- Consent: All patients receive written and verbal information regarding radiotherapy and its side effects. Informed consent must be obtained prior to commencing radiotherapy planning.
- Planning CT scan: Three-dimensional CT imaging is obtained through the area to be treated with the patient in the treatment position. Following this, patients are given small permanent marks the size of a pinhead to act as reference marks for treatment.
- Physics planning: The volume to be treated is outlined on the planning CT scan along with organs at risk (bladder and rectum if treating

prostate) by the clinician. Other imaging modalities such as PET scans and MRI may be fused to the planning CT scan to aid definition of the target volume and organs at risk. The planning radiographers or physicists will then come up with the best radiotherapy plan, which will be transferred to the treatment machine.

- Treatment machines: Most treatments are delivered by linear accelerators that can produce megavoltage photons. These machines are capable of delivering conventional, conformal and intensity-modulated radiotherapy (IMRT) with on-board image guidance and verification. Treatment times are approximately 10 min; most of this time is spent on setting the patient up in the treatment position.

External beam radiotherapy

Conventional radiotherapy

- Uses a small number of beams
- Uniform intensity across the field

Conformal radiotherapy

The introduction of multileaf collimators composed of small metal leaves (5 mm thick or less) allows the radiation field to be shaped as each leaf moves independently. This accurate shaping of the radiation field to encompass the tumour minimises the dose to the surrounding normal tissue, resulting in a reduction in long-term toxicity and allowing for dose escalation and improved tumour control.

Intensity-modulated radiotherapy

IMRT is a further refinement. By moving the leaves during the delivery of the dose, this allows the intensity of radiation to vary across the target.

- Creates concave treatment shapes and steep dose gradient.

- Aims at sparing normal surrounding tissue and structures.
- The beam is divided into multiple beamlets. Doses can be varied in intensity. Can be delivered to different parts of the field.
- Disadvantages: Despite normal tissue being spared from higher doses, a greater volume of tissue receives a lower dose.

Image-guided radiotherapy (IGRT)

This links continuous imaging of the target to the delivery of the radiation, allowing compensation for any movement of the target (Figure 20.1). For example, the prostate can move by up to 1 cm depending on the bladder and rectal fill. The insertion of fiducial markers into the prostate can act as a surrogate for any movement during radiation treatment. Patients can be imaged on the treatment bed using KV or MV portal imaging or cone beam prior to treatment and any correction in positioning adjusted before the delivery of the radiation.

The introduction of IMRT and IGRT has resulted in not only improvements in local tumour control but also a significant reduction in both acute and late radiation toxicity. These are now used routinely in the treatment of prostate cancer with a reduction in the incidence of radiation proctitis and cystitis.

CyberKnife

CyberKnife is a frameless robotic system consisting of a linear accelerator mounted on a robotic arm. It can deliver treatment with a higher accuracy and uses real-time image guidance to track the tumour. This modality requires implantation of markers/transducers in the tumour. Accurate delineation of the tumour is essential.

It is being used to treat low-risk prostate cancer, with patients typically being treated with 35 Gy in five fractions over 1 week. Referral pathways and protocols are established. We do not at present have long-term survival and local tumour control data.

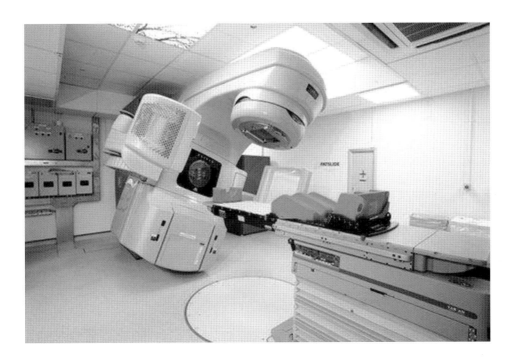

Figure 20.1 Linear accelerator with on-board imaging used to deliver image-guided external beam radiotherapy.

Proton beam therapy

This modality uses protons, rather than photons, to deliver the radiation dose. It enables the dose to be deposited up to, but not beyond, a specific depth within the tissue, thus allowing improved target coverage and reduced dose to the surrounding normal tissue. There is no proton facility within the United Kingdom although plans are going ahead to site 2 units in the country. There is at present no evidence to show it has a role in adult urological tumours.

Brachytherapy

Brachytherapy employs sealed radionuclide sources that are implanted directly into a tumour or body cavity to deliver localised radiotherapy. Iodine-125 seed brachytherapy is increasingly being used to treat low-risk prostate cancer. In this procedure small radioactive seeds the size of a grain of rice are implanted permanently transperineally into the prostate gland. Iodine-125 has a half-life of 60 days and delivers a mean x-ray energy of 0.03 MeV. The main disadvantage of this procedure is the risk to staff of handling radioactive sources and caring for the patient. Another method used to reduce exposure to radiation is remote afterloading. An example is high-dose rate (HDR) brachytherapy in prostate cancer. Here under anaesthetic inactive source holders are implanted into the prostate gland. Once the patient has recovered, live radioactive sources are remotely loaded into the source holders in a shielded room.

Radioisotope therapy

Radioisotopes can be given orally or by injection and are taken up by a particular tissue where they remain. Once there, they release radiation locally. However, a disadvantage is that once given, the source cannot be recovered, limiting the degree of total exposure. Strontium-89 is a beta particle emitter with a half-life of 50 days; it is used to treat prostate cancer with bone metastases. It is preferentially taken up in the bone and is used to relieve bone pain. However, patients must have sufficient bone marrow reserve as this receives part of the dose and can result in anaemia and thrombocytopenia.

Palliative radiotherapy

Radiotherapy is often used to palliate symptoms.

21

Minimally invasive urology

Surgery is a therapeutic approach adopted by surgeons to enter the body's cavities to perform remedial management of various pathological ailments. Incisions are needed to allow surgeons access into these cavities and utilise direct vision and their hands to carry out therapeutic manoeuvres. Advances in surgical technique and medical engineering have enabled surgeons to change the way in which they access the body and reduce these incisions and offer significant improvements in surgical treatments performed under magnification. Wherever possible, minimally invasive surgery is the preferred approach for most surgery today.

Laparoscopy

Laparoscopy is a surgical procedure in which a fibre-optic instrument is inserted through the abdominal wall to view the organs in the abdomen or permit small-scale surgery. In general, the surgeon has a two-dimensional view rather than the three-dimensional view of open surgery. The introduction of instruments through fixed trocars or ports in the abdominal wall means that the movement is limited and counter-intuitive due to the 'fulcrum effect'.

Patient selection

Adequate history and physical examination are the cornerstones for patient selection for laparoscopy.

Contraindications

- Relative:
- Prior abdominal and pelvic surgery, pelvic fibrosis, obesity, hiatus hernia, non-reducible herniation of the abdomen/inguinal hernia, umbilical abnormalities and abdominal aortic/iliac aneurysm
- Absolute:

    Abdominal wall infections, generalised peritonitis, bowel obstruction and uncorrected coagulopathy

Anaesthetics

The ideal anaesthetic technique should aim to optimise patient safety. The technique should provide adequate muscle relaxation and analgesia and allow for rapid post-operative recovery. Laparoscopic procedures often employ the Trendelenburg position and frequent alteration in the position of the operating table. Thus precautions to safeguard against the risk of peripheral neuropathy and protect bony prominences by adequate padding and secure strapping are required. Over 4 h of Trendelenburg position puts the patient at risk of lower limb compartment syndrome. This risk can be minimised by keeping the blood pressure high enough to perfuse the lower limbs, using self-adjusting leg supports that eliminate pressure on the calf as the patient goes head down and beanbags that mould to the patient when a vacuum is applied and so

Urology Lecture Notes, Seventh Edition. Amir V. Kaisary, Andrew Ballaro and Katharine Pigott.
© 2016 John Wiley & Sons, Ltd. Published 2016 by John Wiley & Sons, Ltd.

preventing patient movement. Laparoscopic surgery has been performed under local, regional and general anaesthesia. The technique chosen should be based on the medical condition of the patient, the indication for the procedure, the preference or choice of the patient and the surgeon's needs.

Pneumoperitoneum

Insufflation of CO_2 aims at instilling approximately 3–6 L of CO_2 into the abdomen:

1. **Insufflator**
   This is a piece of equipment that has a CO_2 gas cylinder attached to it and has an insufflation tube line to be attached to the patient. Readouts indicate clearly the total CO_2 delivered, actual and set CO_2 flow rate, pressure set point and intra-abdominal pressure. A spare tank of CO_2 should always be available in the operating room.
2. **Trocars/ports**
   A laparoscopic trocar is a means through which access into the abdomen is secured. All trocars have two common components: a sharp or dilating obturator to facilitate access into the abdominal cavity and a sheath through which the obturator passes. The sheath may have a side port for CO_2 insufflation. The sheath has a valve or a membrane through which instruments may be introduced without loss of CO_2 from the abdomen. Trocars are reusable or disposable. A primary trocar is the first trocar to be placed after a pneumoperitoneum is obtained. Secondary trocars follow. Sites for trocar placements are chosen to facilitate access to the organ to be operated upon (Figure 21.1).
3. **Laparoscopic instruments**
   A wide assortment facilitates all laparoscopic procedures. They are available in both reusable and disposable types. Laparoscopic lenses come in 0° and 30° versions, the latter to allow looking round corners. Most standard laparoscopic instruments are available in diameters ranging from 3 to 12 mm and 35 cm in length. These diameters allow their passage through a given trocar and are of a sufficient length to reach the operative site. They include graspers, incising instruments, retractors, needle holders, knot pushers, specimen entrapment sacks and aspiration/irrigation devices. Surgical clips and staplers have been adapted for use through the laparoscopy ports to secure/ligate vessels, close luminal structures and re-approximate tissue edges.

Improvements in design and material are an ongoing hallmark of laparoscopy equipment and instruments. Instruments for cutting and sealing simultaneously have been developed making surgery safer. These include instruments that cut and seal through vibration at a lower temperature than traditional electrical diathermy (Harmonic) or by pressure and energy transmission (LigaSure).

Accessing the site for surgery

Trans-peritoneal surgery requires access to the intra-peritoneal space either blind through a Veress needle insufflation approach or under direct vision using the Hasson approach. Using a Veress needle, a suitable site is found for inserting a spring-loaded needle to insufflate the abdomen and then insert the primary port, which will be used to pass the camera. This should allow the needle to approach without injuring neighbouring structures. Where there are adhesions, a Veress needle risks injury to bowel and blood vessels (e.g. common iliac vein or aorta). The advantage is that the port site is tight and gas leakage is unusual. Under direct vision using an open approach, a 1–1.5 cm incision is made in the skin, allowing the peritoneum to be opened and bowel avoided if it is close. In general, the direct vision approach is preferable.

For extra-peritoneal surgery, a direct vision approach is usually the main way access is achieved, as there is no natural space to fill with gas.

After the primary port with the camera is inserted, additional ports are placed while inspecting the port pass into the abdomen.

Exiting the site of surgery

Before exiting, it is important to check for bleeding. The insufflation pressure should be reduced to 4–6 mmHg and the site of surgery carefully

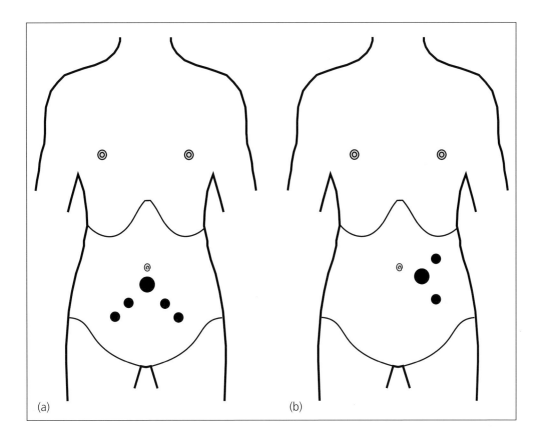

Figure 21.1 Trocar placement: (a) prostate surgery and (b) renal surgery.

expected for bleeding. All bleeding should be stopped before exiting. The scrub nurse should confirm that the needle and swab counts are correct. Port site hernias do not develop if port diameters are less than 5 mm in diameter. All port sites 10 mm or greater should be closed with a suture.

Complications of laparoscopy

These mainly fall into two main categories: intra-operative and post-operative groups. These risks are shared also with robotic-assisted laparoscopy:

1. Intra-operative: These are either associated with anaesthesia or related to laparoscopic technique.
   (a) Cardiovascular:
   - Gas embolus can cause cardiovascular collapse. It is usually due to inadvert-

ent placement of the insufflation needle into a blood vessel or vascular organ. When a large volume of gas reaches the right ventricle, an airlock impedes the pulmonary circulation. Consequent cascade of events could lead to a catastrophic right ventricular failure, drop in venous pulmonary flow and left ventricular drop of output.
- Hypotension: Intra-peritoneal abdominal insufflation up to pressure of 20 mmHg is tolerated but should be kept as low as possible to perform the surgery safely. This is typically about 10–12 mmHg. Intra-abdominal pressure more than 30 mmHg could decrease the cardiac output and arterial blood pressure. Higher pressures

may be needed for extra-peritoneal laparoscopy but are tolerated better.

- Hypertension: Hypercapnia due to absorption of CO_2 may stimulate the sympathetic nervous system leading to tachycardia and hypertension. Patients with essential hypertension are vulnerable.
- Arrhythmias: Bradycardia, tachycardia and premature ventricular contractions could occur.

(b) Pulmonary:
- Hypoxemia: Ventilation–perfusion imbalance can be caused by a contribution of Trendelenburg position and the abdominal contents resting on the diaphragm. This could in turn lead to decreased lung volume, atelectasis and blood pooling in the dependent parts of the lungs.
- Acidosis: Absorption of insufflated CO_2 and ventilation–perfusion imbalance could lead to autonomous stimulation of the central nervous system. This could lead to acidosis, myocardial depression, vasodilatation and hypotension.
- Aspiration: Trendelenburg position and increased intra-abdominal pressure could put the anaesthetised patient at risk of regurgitation and aspiration of gastric contents.
- Pneumothorax, pneumomediastinum and pneumopericardium: These could occur if a trocar is placed above the 12th rib or there is presence of diaphragmatic defects or positive pressure trauma to the lungs.

(c) Miscellaneous:
- Shoulder pain from CO_2 irritation of the diaphragm.
- Subcutaneous emphysema.
- Vascular injuries range from haematoma formation in the abdominal wall to laceration of the abdominal aorta and common iliac vessels.
- Perforation of a solid organ or a hollow viscus.

- Diathermy injury through breaks of the insulation covering instruments allowing metal to touch or arc across bowel or other organs. Capacitance injury is also possible.
- Compartment syndrome after prolonged Trendelenburg position necessary for trans-peritoneal laparoscopic pelvic surgery. This is more common after Trendelenburg more than 4 h, in older men with peripheral vascular disease and in men with dense muscles.
- Raised intraocular pressure is more common after prolonged Trendelenburg position, and so all glaucoma medications need to be taken before surgery.
- Peripheral nerve damage.

2. Post-operative:
(a) Fever/peritonitis: May represent the first sign of a missed intra-operative bowel perforation or urinary leakage. Often there will be pain localised to the nearest port site.
(b) Delayed haemorrhage: Could be one of the causes of post-operative haemodynamic instability.
(c) Incisional hernia: Risk of abdominal content herniation via a small-diameter trocar (≤5 mm) is low but could occur via a trocar ≥10 mm site.
(d) Impaired renal function: Could be secondary to intra-operative unrecognised bladder perforation or clipping or other injury to the ureter.
(e) Loin pain may indicate an obstructed ureter from a clip, diathermy or other energy sources used to stop bleeding.

Establishing a consistent laparoscopy team with an experienced surgical assistant and a scrub nurse is a must. The role played by an attentive anaesthetic team cannot be underplayed. Meticulous attention to details plays the most important role in successful laparoscopy procedures.

Trans-peritoneal compared to extra-peritoneal approaches for laparoscopy

Most general surgical procedures are performed through the peritoneum, where there is a natural space. However, extra-peritoneal structures (e.g. adrenal, kidney and prostate) can be reached more directly by extra-peritoneal approach. For trans-peritoneal access to the right kidney or adrenal, the ascending colon, duodenum and liver need to be mobilised. On the left side, the descending colon and tail of pancreas need to be mobilised. None of these steps are necessary when performing extra-peritoneal laparoscopy. As there is no natural space in the retroperitoneum, a balloon is inflated behind and lateral to the kidney in the extra-peritoneal fat to create a working space. Then the target is accessible very easily. Similarly, for the prostate, a space needs to be created in front of the prostate by inflating a balloon in the retropubic space. For trans-peritoneal approaches to pelvic organs, for example, the prostate, a steep Trendelenburg position is required, which is not true for the extra-peritoneal approach. As such, there is a greater risk of ileus, bowel injury and compartment syndrome, although the underlying risk is itself very small.

Although access is more direct and quicker by the extra-peritoneal approach, the working space is smaller than the intra-peritoneal space, and the landmarks used for orientation are often unfamiliar with surgeons. This can make extra-peritoneal laparoscopy more difficult for the inexperienced.

Robotics

Robotics is a branch of technology concerned with the design, construction, operation and application of robots. A robot is a mechanical device that can perform preprogrammed repetitive tasks creating a 'master–slave' system. In industry, robots are used for mass production and improved efficiency. Advances in the field led to the creation of robotic integrated surgical systems, which can assist surgeons in performing surgical procedures in real time with improved vision and surgical precision. It allows computer control of laparoscopic instruments with enhanced degree of manoeuvrability and stereoscopic vision.

The following procedures are performed regularly by robotic surgery:

- Radical prostatectomy, partial nephrectomy, pyeloplasty and radical cystectomy
- Hysterectomy, myomectomy and sacrocolpopexy
- Nissen fundoplication, Heller myotomy, gastric bypass and bowel resection
- Mitral valve prolapse and endoscopic atrial septal defect closure
- Trans-oral resection of the tonsil, tongue and larynx and trans-axillary thyroidectomy
- Coronary artery bypass graft

In urology, radical prostatectomy for early prostate cancer was probably the first attractive urological procedure to attract application of robotic-assisted surgery.

Only one company creates a robot that is commonly used (Intuitive Surgical) known as the da Vinci robot (Figure 21.2), which is now in its third generation. In this system, the surgeon sits at a console, while the robot is positioned over the patient controlling specific instruments. There is usually a patient-side assistant who sees a two-dimensional screen and may operate additional instruments to those controlled by the robot. Twin consoles have been developed in which the assistant handles instruments in a second console in a similar way to the primary surgeon action in the main console. This also facilitates training.

The robotic system provides much clearer vision than standard laparoscopy. The view can be magnified 10-fold and is seen with high definition in three dimensions, unlike most laparoscopic operations, in which the view is visible in two dimensions. Furthermore, it is possible to incorporate other imaging into the

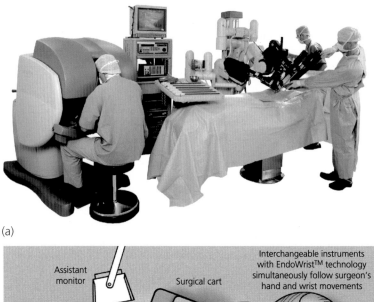

(a)

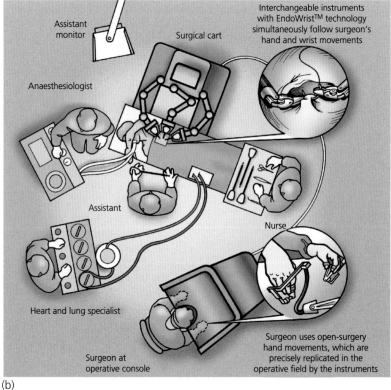

(b)

Figure 21.2 da Vinci robot: (a) system, (b) theatre layout, (c) EndoWrist, (d) hand control and (e) operator view. Photos courtesy of Intuitive Surgical Inc.

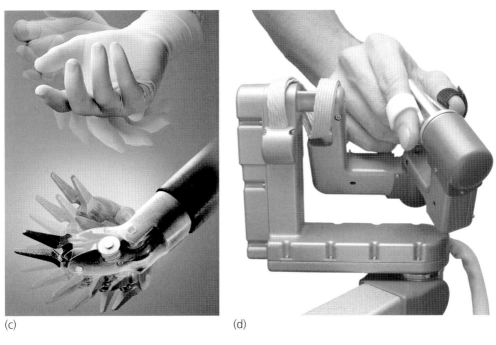

(c)

(d)

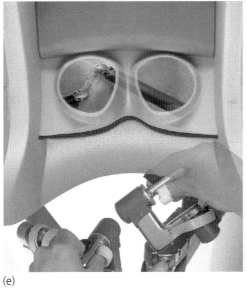

(e)

Figure 21.2 (*Continued*)

surgeons view, for example, MRI or other images onto the organ of interest. This would be useful for the removal of tumours while sparing normal tissues, for example, in partial nephrectomy. Robotic instruments can be moved with greater dexterity than standard laparoscopic instruments. This is because the robotic instruments have wrists that allow articulation like the human hand, which traditional laparoscopic instruments do not have. Furthermore, there are tremor filters and there is the ability to scale motion. These properties mean that operating deep inside the body, such as in the pelvis, can be much more precise, intuitive and easier to perform than by standard laparoscopy. However, there is no tactile feedback unlike open surgery and visual cues are necessary to replace 'feel', which most robotic surgeons develop and find an accurate substitute.

As with all laparoscopic surgery, there are less pain, less blood loss and a faster return to normal activities after robotic-assisted laparoscopic surgery compared to open surgery. Advantages in long-term outcomes have been more difficult to demonstrate. In part, this is because the successful performance of surgical techniques or steps is the key to long-term outcomes irrespective of whether the surgery is performed by open, laparoscopic or robotic means. Long-term outcomes depend more on the individual surgeon's ability to perform the techniques necessary for good outcomes than on the use of the robot. Furthermore, there are learning curves for complex surgery, which seem to be shortest for open surgery and longest for pure laparoscopy. The robot shortens the learning curve for laparoscopic surgery, which is why it has become so popular among surgeons and less so by those who pay the bills! The relevant question is whether the robot with all its technological advances facilitates the delivery of new or existing surgical steps to a level that allows better outcomes than traditional open or laparoscopic surgery. There is some evidence that this might be true, but irrespective of this, robotic procedures have increased every year.

Single-port laparoscopy versus multi-port laparoscopy

This is a minimally invasive procedure performed through a single port rather than multiple ports. As such, there is less scarring and pain than by typical multi-port laparoscopy or open surgery. Typically, the single port is placed through or near the umbilicus, but it can be performed elsewhere. There are many designs for the port, and these usually allow multiple instruments to pass through. Technically, it is much more difficult to operate with all the instruments through one than multiple ports. In traditional laparoscopy, triangulation of instruments is the key to accurate surgery. In single-port surgery, surgery is performed by moving the instruments in the same axis as the port making it very difficult, but robotic-assisted single-port surgery is much easier than pure laparoscopy (Figure 21.3).

Complications of robotic surgery

Robotic surgery shares the same risks of pure laparoscopic surgery described previously. Additional risks include those of equipment failure and human error when using the robot. Training is required to use the robot and then practice to become fluent with the motions required to use the robotic instruments. This risk was underestimated in the past but has

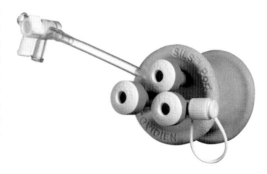

Figure 21.3 The SILS™ Port multiple access port. An advanced surgical product designed to perform laparoscopic surgery through a single incision, as well as through the anus to provide access for rectal procedures. This product is designed to give surgeons the ability to use multiple instruments with maximal manoeuvrability through adjustable cannulae all within a low-profile malleable blue port.

become recognised now. Patient positioning is as important in laparoscopy with the same risk. The time it takes to convert from robotic to laparoscopy or open surgery is rarely a problem except in extreme emergencies. If there is an urgent need to open, the robotic instruments are removed, the robotic arms released from the ports, the robot undocked and the patient turned supine. This can sometimes take several minutes, which may be important in extreme emergencies.

As there is no direct tactile feedback with the robot, it is possible to apply excessive force unless visual and other cues are used to substitute for touch. Also, all instruments inside the patient need to be kept in the view of the surgeon at all times, as unintentional movements by instruments off screen might result in injury as they could penetrate organs unknowingly or release energy (e.g. diathermy) onto bowel or other structures.

Training in laparoscopy and robotics

'See one, do one, teach one' was the aphorism for surgical training years ago, but is no longer acceptable and training has improved dramatically in recent years. As there are reduced learning opportunities in theatre nowadays, simulation has emerged as an important way to supplement clinical exposure and can be used to assess operative proficiency. Simulation occurs in a risk-free environment such that the consequence of errors can be seen and theoretically unlimited repetition is possible to develop mastery. Subsequent rehearsal of learned skills is important for retention, but sometimes the opportunity to use simulators can be limited for reasons such as access.

A simple way to develop laparoscopic skills at home uses just a webcam, a black box with holes to pass laparoscopic instruments and sutures and other materials to manipulate. More complex virtual reality systems provide haptic (sense of touch) and kinaesthetic (sense of position in space) feedback. Commercially available systems include the minimally invasive surgery trainer (MIST) to perform procedures such as a laparoscopic cholecystectomy and a more high-fidelity version called LapSim. The latter comprises a virtual abdomen allowing virtual surgery. The da Vinci robotic system can be attached to a simulator, such that the operator performs training exercises and operates in exactly the same way as she would in a patient. Similarly, separate from the traditional da Vinci robotic platform itself exists the SimSurgery Education Platform (SEP).

There are many advantages to incorporating simulation in training and everyday surgery. Training and assessment modes are available providing feedback on time to completion, accuracy, collisions, efficiency of movement and other parameters. Skills learned in a skills lab are transferable to live surgery. Furthermore, simulators can be used by trained surgeons to 'warm up' and rehearse steps before starting on the patient. This can reduce error and operative time, even in a trained surgeon. Simulation tools can be used also in pre-operative planning and intra-operative localisation.

Appendix A: ECOG performance status

Grade	ECOG
0	Fully active, able to carry on all pre-disease performance without restriction
1	Restricted in physically strenuous activity but ambulatory and able to carry out work of a light or sedentary nature (e.g. light house work, office work)
2	Ambulatory and capable of all self-care but unable to carry out any work activities. Up and about more than 50% of waking hours
3	Capable of only limited self-care, confined to bed or chair more than 50% of waking hours
4	Completely disabled. Cannot carry on any self-care. Totally confined to bed or chair
5	Dead

Source: Oken MM et al. *Am J Clin Oncol* 1982; 5: 649–655. Reproduced with permission from Wolters Kluwer Health.

Urology Lecture Notes, Seventh Edition. Amir V. Kaisary, Andrew Ballaro and Katharine Pigott.
© 2016 John Wiley & Sons, Ltd. Published 2016 by John Wiley & Sons, Ltd.

Appendix B: TNM classification of malignant tumours

Classification of cancer cases by the extent of disease provides a method of conveying clinical experience of the disease applicable to all sites regardless of treatment. It can be supplemented later by the information that becomes available from surgery, histopathology or both.

The TNM system for describing the anatomical extent of the disease based on the assessment of three components:

1. **T** – Extent of the primary tumour
2. **N** – Absence or presence and extent of regional lymph nodes metastases
3. **M** – Absence or presence of distant metastases

Clinical classification is based on pretreatment evidence acquired: **TNM**.

The addition of numbers to these three components indicates the extent of the malignant disease:

TX – Primary tumour cannot be assessed
T0 – No evidence of primary tumour
Tis – Carcinoma *in situ*
T1, T2, T3, T4 – Increasing size and/or local extent of the primary tumour

NX – Regional lymph nodes cannot be assessed
N0 – No regional lymph node metastasis
N1, N2, N3 – Increasing involvement of regional lymph nodes

MX – Distant metastasis cannot be assessed
M0 – No distant metastasis
M1 – Distant metastasis

Pathological classification is based on evidence acquired from pathological examination of tissue obtained **pTNM**.

Sentinel lymph node

This is the first lymph node to receive lymphatic drainage from a primary tumour. If it contains a metastatic tumour, other lymph nodes may contain a tumour. If it does not contain a metastatic tumour, other lymph nodes are not likely to contain a tumour. Occasionally there is more than one sentinel lymph node.

Histopathological grading: G

GX – Grade of differentiation cannot be assessed
G1 – Well differentiated
G2 – Moderately differentiated
G3 – Poorly differentiated
G4 – Undifferentiated

Stage grouping

A tumour with four degrees of **T**, three degrees of **N** and two degrees of **M** will yield 24 TNM

Urology Lecture Notes, Seventh Edition. Amir V. Kaisary, Andrew Ballaro and Katharine Pigott.
© 2016 John Wiley & Sons, Ltd. Published 2016 by John Wiley & Sons, Ltd.

categories. It will be necessary to condense these categories into a convenient number of TNM stage groups:

Stage 0	Tis/Ta	N0	M0
Stage I	T1	N0	M0
Stage II	T1	N1	M0
	T2	N0, N1	M0
Stage III	T1, T2	N2	M0
	T3	N0, N, N2	M0
Stage IV	T4	Any N	M0
	Any T	N3	M0
	Any T	Any N	M1

Appendix C: Response evaluation criteria in solid tumours

Response Evaluation Criteria in Solid Tumours (RECIST) is a set of published rules that define when cancer patients improve 'respond', stay the same 'stabilise' or worsen 'progress' during treatments. The criteria were published in February 2000 by an international collaboration including the European Organisation for Research and Treatment of Cancer (EORTC), National Cancer Institute of the United States and the National Cancer Institute of Canada Clinical Trials Group. Today, the majority of clinical trials evaluating cancer treatments for objective response in solid tumours are using RECIST.

Eligibility

Only patients with measurable disease at baseline should be included in protocols where objective tumour response is the primary end point:

- Measurable disease – the presence of at least one measurable lesion. If the measurable disease is restricted to a solitary lesion, its neoplastic nature should be confirmed by cytology/histology.
- Measurable lesions – lesions that can be accurately measured in at least one dimension with longest diameter (LD) ≥20 mm using conventional techniques or ≥10 mm with spiral CT scan.

Non-measurable lesions – all other lesions, including small lesions (LD <20 mm with conventional techniques or <10 mm with spiral CT scan), that is, bone lesions, leptomeningeal disease, ascites, pleural/pericardial effusion, inflammatory breast disease, lymphangitis, cystic lesions and also abdominal masses that are not confirmed and followed by imaging techniques.

All measurements should be taken and recorded in metric notation, using a ruler or callipers. All baseline evaluations should be performed as closely as possible to the beginning of treatment and never more than 4 weeks before the beginning of the treatment.

The same method of assessment and the same technique should be used to characterise each identified and reported lesion at baseline and during follow-up.

Clinical lesions will only be considered measurable when they are superficial (e.g. skin nodules and palpable lymph nodes). For the case of skin lesions, documentation by colour photography, including a ruler to estimate the size of the lesion, is recommended.

Methods of measurement

CT and MRI are the best currently available and reproducible methods to measure target lesions selected for response assessment. Conventional CT and MRI should be performed with cuts of 10 mm or less in slice thickness contiguously. Spiral CT should be performed using a 5 mm

Urology Lecture Notes, Seventh Edition. Amir V. Kaisary, Andrew Ballaro and Katharine Pigott.
© 2016 John Wiley & Sons, Ltd. Published 2016 by John Wiley & Sons, Ltd.

contiguous reconstruction algorithm. This applies to tumours of the chest, abdomen and pelvis. Head and neck tumours and those of extremities usually require specific protocols.

Lesions on chest X-ray are acceptable as measurable lesions when they are clearly defined and surrounded by an aerated lung. However, CT is preferable.

When the primary end point of the study is objective response evaluation, ultrasound (US) should not be used to measure tumour lesions. It is, however, a possible alternative to clinical measurements of superficial palpable lymph nodes, subcutaneous lesions and thyroid nodules. US might also be useful to confirm the complete disappearance of superficial lesions usually assessed by clinical examination.

The utilisation of endoscopy and laparoscopy for objective tumour evaluation has not yet been fully and widely validated. Their uses in this specific context require sophisticated equipment and a high level of expertise that may only be available in some centres. Therefore, the utilisation of such techniques for objective tumour response should be restricted to validation purposes in specialised centres. However, such techniques can be useful in confirming complete pathological response when biopsies are obtained.

Tumour markers alone cannot be used to assess response. If markers are initially above the upper normal limit, they must normalise for a patient to be considered in complete clinical response when all lesions have disappeared.

Cytology and histology can be used to differentiate between PR and CR in rare cases (e.g. after treatment to differentiate between residual benign lesions and residual malignant lesions in tumour types such as germ cell tumours).

Baseline documentation of 'target' and 'non-target' lesions

All measurable lesions up to a maximum of five lesions per organ and 10 lesions in total, representative of all involved organs, should be identified as target lesions and recorded and measured at baseline.

Target lesions should be selected on the basis of their size (lesions with the LD) and their suitability for accurate repeated measurements (either by imaging techniques or clinically).

A sum of the LD for all target lesions will be calculated and reported as the baseline sum LD. The baseline sum LD will be used as reference by which to characterise the objective tumour response.

All other lesions (or sites of disease) should be identified as non-target lesions and should also be recorded at baseline. Measurements of these lesions are not required, but the presence or absence of each should be noted throughout follow-up.

Response criteria

Evaluation of target lesions

Complete response (CR): Disappearance of all target lesions

Partial response (PR): At least a 30% decrease in the sum of the LD of target lesions, taking as reference the baseline sum LD

Stable disease (SD): Neither sufficient shrinkage to qualify for PR nor sufficient increase to qualify for PD, taking as reference the smallest sum LD since the treatment started

Progressive disease (PD): At least a 20% increase in the sum of the LD of target lesions, taking as reference the smallest sum LD recorded since the treatment started or the appearance of one or more new lesions

Evaluation of non-target lesions

CR: Disappearance of all non-target lesions and normalisation of tumour marker level

Incomplete response/SD: Persistence of one or more non-target lesion(s) or/and maintenance of tumour marker level above the normal limits

PD: Appearance of one or more new lesions and/or unequivocal progression of existing non-target lesions

Evaluation of best overall response

The best overall response is the best response recorded from the start of the treatment until disease progression/recurrence (taking as reference for PD the smallest measurements recorded since the treatment started). In general, the patient's best response assignment will depend on the achievement of both measurement and confirmation criteria

Patients with a global deterioration of health status requiring discontinuation of treatment without objective evidence of disease progression at that time should be classified as having 'symptomatic deterioration'. Every effort should be made to document the objective progression even after discontinuation of treatment.

In some circumstances it may be difficult to distinguish residual disease from normal tissue. When the evaluation of CR depends on this determination, it is recommended that the residual lesion be investigated (fine needle aspirate/biopsy) to confirm the CR status.

Confirmation

The main goal of confirmation of objective response is to avoid overestimating the response rate observed. In cases where confirmation of response is not feasible, it should be made clear when reporting the outcome of such clinical studies that the responses are not confirmed.

To be assigned a status of PR or CR, changes in tumour measurements must be confirmed by repeat assessments that should be performed no less than 4 weeks after the criteria for response are first met. Longer intervals as determined by the study protocol may also be appropriate.

In the case of SD, follow-up measurements must have met the SD criteria at least once after study entry at a minimum interval (in general, not less than 6–8 weeks) that is defined in the study protocol.

Duration of overall response

The duration of overall response is measured from the time that measurement criteria are met for CR or PR (whichever status is recorded first) until the first date that recurrence or PD is objectively documented, taking as reference for PD the smallest measurements recorded since the treatment started.

Duration of SD

SD is measured from the start of the treatment until the criteria for disease progression are met, taking as reference the smallest measurements recorded since the treatment started.

The clinical relevance of the duration of SD varies for different tumour types and grades. Therefore, it is highly recommended that the protocol specify the minimal time interval required between two measurements for determination of SD. This time interval should take into account the expected clinical benefit that such a status may bring to the population under study.

Response review

For clinical trials where the response rate is the primary end point, it is strongly recommended that all responses be reviewed by an expert(s) independent of the study at the study's completion. Simultaneous review of the patients' files and radiological images is the best approach.

Reporting of results

All patients assessed for response to treatment should be assigned one of the following categories: (i) CR, (ii) PR, (iii) SD, (iv) PD, (v) early death from malignant disease, (vi) early death from toxicity, (vii) early death because of other cause or (viii) unknown (not assessable, insufficient data).

Appendix D: The Clavien–Dindo classification of surgical complications

Assessment of quality of outcome in medicine is of paramount value to patients and healthcare providers. Evaluation of surgical performance and outcome based on a methodology for reporting is crucial to gather credible data collection for benchmarking. Since 1992 several approaches to rank complications by severity based on therapy used to treat the complications were attempted. To avoid subjective interpretation of adverse events and possible tendency to downgrade complications, several researchers attempted to reach a tool for quality assessment. A valuable tool should be simple to utilise in audits and everyday practice.

The Clavien–Dindo Classification of Surgical Complications was the outcome of efforts undertaken by several researchers and endorsed by several societies and investigators. It is feasible to be used for retrospective and prospective studies.

Grades	Definition
Grade I	Any deviation from post-operative course without the need for pharmacological treatment or surgical, endoscopic and radiological interventions: • Therapeutic regimens accepted: drugs: anti-emetics, antipyretics, analgesics, diuretics and electrolytes • Physiotherapy • Wound infections opened at the bedside
Grade II	Pharmacological treatment with drugs required other than those allowed in grade I: • Blood transfusion • Parenteral nutrition
Grade III	Surgical, endoscopic or radiological intervention required
Grade III-a	Intervention not under general anaesthesia
Grade III-b	Intervention under general anaesthesia

(Continued)

Urology Lecture Notes, Seventh Edition. Amir V. Kaisary, Andrew Ballaro and Katharine Pigott.
© 2016 John Wiley & Sons, Ltd. Published 2016 by John Wiley & Sons, Ltd.

(Continued)

Grades	Definition
Grade IV	Life-threatening complication requiring intermediate care (IC)/intensive care unit (ICU) management: • Includes CNS complications: brain haemorrhage and subarachnoid bleeding • Excludes transient ischaemic attacks (TIA)
Grade IV-a	Single organ dysfunction – including dialysis
Grade IV-b	Multiple organ dysfunctions
Grade V	Death of patient

Source: Clavien PA et al. *Ann Surg* 2009; 250: 187–196. Reproduced with permission from Wolters Kluwer Health.

Appendix E: Adverse effects of cancer treatment

The National Cancer Institute Common Toxicity Criteria grading system for the adverse effects of cancer treatment was first created in 1983 aiming at the recognition and grading of adverse effects of chemotherapy in cancer patients. Continuous efforts at improving and upgrading the system are ongoing international efforts.

Grade	Definition of effects
Grade 1	• Minimal • Usually asymptomatic effects that do not interfere with functional end points (interventions or medications are generally not indicated for these minor effects)
Grade 2	• Moderate • Usually symptomatic. Interventions such as local treatment or medications may be indicated (they may interfere with specific functions but not enough to impair activities of daily living)
Grade 3	• Severe and very undesirable • There are usually multiple, disruptive symptoms (more serious interventions, including surgery or hospitalisation may be indicated)
Grade 4	• Potentially life threatening, catastrophic, disabling or result in loss of organ, organ function or limb

Source: Trotti et al. *Semin Rad Oncol* 2003: 13(3); 176–181. Reproduced with permission from Elsevier.

Urology Lecture Notes, Seventh Edition. Amir V. Kaisary, Andrew Ballaro and Katharine Pigott.
© 2016 John Wiley & Sons, Ltd. Published 2016 by John Wiley & Sons, Ltd.

Appendix F: Urinary catheters

Endoscopy of the lower urinary tract and the establishment of urinary tract drainage are basic skills required by all urologists and uniquely define the specialty of urology. There are three main types of catheters:

1. Condom catheter
2. Indwelling catheter
3. Intermittent (short-term) catheter

Condom catheters

Condom catheters are most often used in elderly men with dementia. There is no tube placed inside the penis. Instead, a condom-like device is placed over the penis. A tube leads from this device to a drainage bag. The condom catheter must be changed every day (Figures F.1, F.2 and F.3).

Indwelling catheters

An indwelling urinary catheter is one that is left in the bladder. You may use an indwelling catheter for a short time or a long time.

An indwelling catheter collects urine by attaching to a drainage bag. A newer type of catheter has a valve that can be opened to allow urine to flow out.

An indwelling catheter may be inserted into the bladder in two ways:

1. Most often, the catheter is inserted through the urethra. This is the tube that carries urine from the bladder to the outside of the body.

2. Sometimes, the healthcare provider will insert a catheter into the bladder through a small hole in the lower belly (suprapubic). This is done at a hospital or healthcare provider's office.

An indwelling catheter has a small balloon inflated on the end of it. This prevents the catheter from sliding out of your body. When the catheter needs to be removed, the balloon is deflated.

Indications

The most common indications for the use of a bladder catheter can be broadly divided into two main categories: to obtain drainage or to allow the instillation of diagnostic or therapeutic agents:

- To monitor urinary output and the collection of microbiologic clean urine.
- The relief of acute or chronic urinary retention due to either bladder outlet obstruction or neurogenic bladder dysfunction.
- After lower urinary tract surgery/trauma: continuous drainage or simultaneous irrigation (post transurethral resection and clot evacuation).
- To provide access to the bladder for urinary tract imaging studies such as cystography; this requires the instillation of radiographic contrast material.
- Catheterisation is used during urodynamic testing for assessment of voiding function. It is also used to allow instillation of pharmacologic agents for local therapy of some bladder pathologies such as chemo/immunotherapy.

Urology Lecture Notes, Seventh Edition. Amir V. Kaisary, Andrew Ballaro and Katharine Pigott.
© 2016 John Wiley & Sons, Ltd. Published 2016 by John Wiley & Sons, Ltd.

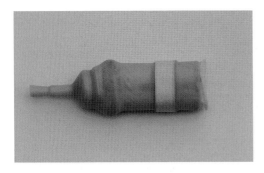

Figure F.1 Conveen sheath.

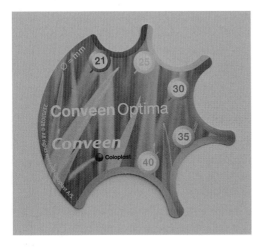

Figure F.2 Conveen size measuring tool.

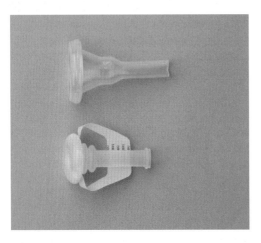

Figure F.3 A clear silastic Conveen sheath.

Catheter selection

The size and type of urinary catheter used depend on the indication for catheter insertion, age of the patient and type of fluid expected to be drained. Currently there is a wide variety of catheter types. Catheters can be classified on the basis of size, material, coating, number of channels and tip form.

Size

Catheter size is measured in the Charrière or French scale, whereby one French or Ch is equal to 0.33 mm. This measurement indicates the total diameter of the catheter and not the lumen size.

Joseph Charrière was born on 19 March 1803 in Switzerland and moved to Paris as an apprentice to a cutler. He was a great craftsman and innovator, who devised the scale and improved many medical instruments (Table F.1).

As a general rule, catheter size should be the smallest size that can accomplish the desired drainage (i.e. 12–14 Fr for clear urine and 20–24 for thick pus- or blood-filled urine).

Material

Modern urinary catheters are most frequently made of latex, rubber, silicone and polyvinyl chloride (PVC). Rubber and latex catheters are often chosen for short-term drainage. Silicone catheters are indicated when there is rubber/latex sensitivity or allergy and are particularly suited for patients requiring a longer period of indwelling time. Silicone is relatively inert, causing less tissue reaction, and is associated with less bacterial adherence than other catheter materials. The use of silicone catheters seem to be associated with a lower incidence of urinary tract infections compared with those made of latex.

Coating

Various coatings on urethral catheters have been applied in an attempt to reduce urethral trauma and infection risks. The use of hydrophilic coatings has been advocated among patients on chronic self-intermittent catheterisation.

Table F.1 Charrière catheter sizes and diameters										
Charriere (Ch)	30	27	24	21	18	15	12	9	6	3
Diameter (mm)	10	9	8	7	6	5	4	3	2	1

Number of channels

The most basic catheters are constructed with a single lumen to permit urinary drainage. Additional lumens are added to permit addition of a retention balloon (two-way catheter) and for simultaneous drainage and irrigation (three-way catheter). The insertion of a three-way catheter for continuous bladder irrigation is most often performed after transurethral resection procedures of the bladder or prostate, which additionally can be combined with a large-volume retention balloon (30–50 mL), which under slight traction can often achieve complete haemostasis of the resected prostatic fossa. It should be borne in mind, however, that the addition of a multi-channel catheter is accomplished by decreasing the overall internal diameter or lumen of the main drainage channel; a 24 Fr three-way catheter has a smaller internal drainage diameter than a 24 Fr two-way catheter, which has a narrower lumen than a 24 Fr one-way catheter (Figure F.4).

Tip shape

Most catheters are designed with a blunt straight tip that is blind ending. Catheters with curved tips or with an end hole have specific utility in certain clinical scenarios (e.g. a coudé tip for patients with a high bladder neck or prominent median prostate lobe). Introducing a catheter over a guide wire is to be practiced by doctors trained to do so and requires supervision (Figure F.5).

Technique of catheter insertion

Once the need for urethral catheterisation has been established, the procedure should be described to the patient and potential complications discussed. Clinical history including allergies, urologic pathology, previous urologic

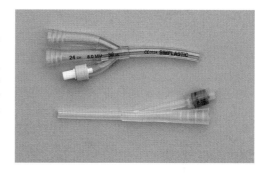

Figure F.4 A three-way irrigation catheter and a Foley drainage catheter.

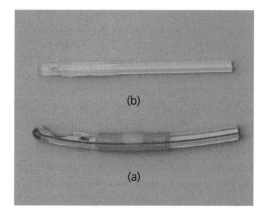

Figure F.5 A haematuria catheter has a wide opening near the tip to allow improve drainage of blood clots and debris.

interventions and catheterisation attempts are valuable in preparation. Catheterisation should be carried out in a sterile fashion with antiseptic preparation and draping of the patient's meatal and genital area. The use of topical anaesthetic gels before urethral catheterisation is widely practiced (e.g. 2% lidocaine gel).

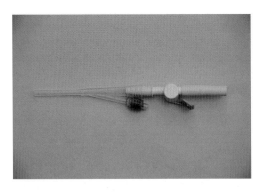

Figure F.6 A catheter valve allows the patient to dispense with a urinary bag and empties the bladder at will. A simple lever has an 'open' and 'close' positions that can be used by the patient.

Male patients

Anatomic considerations are important. The adult male urethra is approximately 18–20 cm in length, and its diameter is variable.

After sterile skin preparation and draping, grasp the shaft of the penis with the left hand in a right-handed operator. The male urethra course mimics a horizontal clockwise letter J. Hold the penis at a 90 degree angle or perpendicular to the patient. Remember the letter J path. Insert the lubricated tip of the catheter into the urethral meatus and gently but firmly continue to advance the catheter for 7–10 cm while simultaneously bringing the shaft of the penis to the horizontal plane or parallel to the patient. Continue to advance the catheter while expecting to feel a slight increase in resistance as the membranous urethra is being passed through. Once the entire length of the catheter has been introduced (up to the juncture of the two-way catheter bifurcation), wait for spontaneous urine passage, confirming proper placement of the catheter. Only when the position of the catheter has been verified should the retaining balloon be inflated, with the amount of fluid indicated on the catheter. The catheter should be attached to a sterile closed bag system as soon as urine is draining. The drainage bag should be placed below the level of the bladder to encourage one-way gravity flow with the tubing as straight as possible and avoiding kinks that might impair drainage.

In patients with acute urinary retention with significant bladder distension, rapid bladder drainage might precipitate decompression-induced haematuria. In these patients the catheter should be intermittently clamped and released to permit gradual bladder decompression over 30–60 min. If the patient is uncircumcised, insure returning the foreskin to its normal reduced position to avoid paraphimosis. Secure the catheter to the patient, allowing for a normal range of motion and without tension, using adhesive tape or a commercial securing device.

Female patients

The female urethra is approximately 3.5–4 cm long. After antiseptic preparation and sterile draping, use the left hand in a right-handed operator to spread the patient's labia to reveal the urethral meatus. After lubrication, insert the tip of the catheter and gently advance using a slightly downward direction, until about half the length of the catheter has been inserted. Check for urine return and the retaining balloon can then be inflated with the amount of fluid indicated on the catheter (Figure F.6).

Complications of catheter use include:

- Allergy or sensitivity to latex
- Bladder stones
- Blood infections (septicaemia)
- Blood in the urine (haematuria)
- Kidney damage (usually only with long-term, indwelling catheter use)
- Urethral injury
- Urinary tract or kidney infections

Drainage bags

A catheter is usually attached to a drainage bag. There are two types of bags:

1. A leg bag is a small device that attaches by elastic bands to the leg. It holds about 300–500 mL

of urine. The bag is utilised during the day time because it can be hidden under pants or a skirt. The patient can easily empty it into the toilet.

2. A larger drainage device can be used during the night. It holds 1–2 L of urine. The bag can be hung on the bed or placed on the floor.

Catheter valve

How to care for a catheter

To care for an indwelling catheter, the area where the catheter exits the body and the catheter itself are washed with soap and water every day. Also clean the area after every bowel movement to prevent infection.

In case of a suprapubic catheter, clean the opening in the abdomen and the tube with soap and water every day. Then cover it with dry gauze.

Plenty of fluids to drink will help prevent infections.

Wash your hands before and after handling the drainage device. Do not allow the outlet valve to touch anything. If the outlet gets dirty, clean it with soap and water.

Intermittent (short-term) catheter

Patients, who have impaired voiding due to neurological causes that may not be amenable for surgical intervention corrections or possible response to pharmacological medical therapy, are candidates to learn intermittent self-catheterisation. They are counselled in full with regards to the technique and have available soft lubricated catheters, short and long lengths, so they can be used by men and women who are trained for introducing the catheter through the urethra into the bladder for urinary drainage. These catheters are disposable single use individually packaged. The clinician introducing the technique to the patient concerned can help to identify the appropriate most suitable catheter from an extensive available range to choose from. The patient is taught to perform the procedure ensuring cleanliness and steps to achieve catheterisation without mishaps.

Appendix G: Evidence-based medicine

Clinicians are increasingly looking up available materials to aid decision-making related to the medical care of each patient. With the enormous increase in articles and publications in paper and electronic formats, clinicians at all levels and medical specialties should exercise serious and explicit cautious approach to utilise the best available evidence-based medical information. References used ought to be assessed according to their Levels of Evidence. Grading recommendations aims at providing transparency between the underlying evidence and the recommendation given.

Levels of evidence

1a	Evidence obtained from meta-analysis of randomised trials
1b	Evidence obtained from at least one randomised trial
2a	Evidence obtained from one well-designed controlled study without randomisation
2b	Evidence obtained from at least one other type of well-designed quasi-experimental study
3	Evidence obtained from well-designed non-experimental studies, such as comparative studies, correlation studies and case reports
4	Evidence obtained from expert committee reports or opinions or clinical experience or respected authorities

Grades of recommendation

A	Based on clinical studies of good quality and consistency addressing the specific recommendations and including at least one randomised trial
B	Based on well-conducted clinical studies but without randomised clinical trials
C	Made despite the absence of directly applicable clinical studies of good quality

Source: Oxford Centre for Evidence-Based Medicine – Levels of Evidence (March 2009). http://www.cebm.net/index.aspx?o=1025 (Accessed on 26 August 2015).

Urology Lecture Notes, Seventh Edition. Amir V. Kaisary, Andrew Ballaro and Katharine Pigott.
© 2016 John Wiley & Sons, Ltd. Published 2016 by John Wiley & Sons, Ltd.

Multiple choice questions

1 The genito-femoral nerve supplies all of the following EXCEPT:

A Sensory to genitalia

B Motor to dartos muscle

C Motor to cremaster muscle

D Sensor to lower thigh

2 Calcium reabsorption is stimulated by all of the following EXCEPT:

A Hypocalcaemia

B Metabolic alkalosis

C Hypermagnesemia

D Phosphate loading

E Vitamin D

3 The hormonal regulation of spermatogenesis is carried out primarily by:

A FSH

B LH

C Testosterone

D GnRH

E Seminiferous growth factor

4 The symptom that is least specific for bladder outlet obstruction is:

A Hesitancy

B Intermittent stream

C Nocturia

D Post-void dribbling

5 Which of the following statements is true?

A Haemospermia usually results from malignancy of the prostate.

B Pneumaturia is most frequently due to gas-forming infections in diabetic patients.

C Diabetic patients have high concentrations of urinary sugar.

D A thick, purulent, profuse urethral discharge is usually seen in non-gonococcal urethritis.

E Cloudy urine most commonly results from phosphate crystal precipitation in alkaline urine.

6 Which of the following is typically seen microscopically in a normal expressed prostatic secretion?

A Macrophages

B Clumps of leukocytes

C Oval fat macrophages

D Secretory granules

7 In long-term hospitalised patients with incontinence, which method is preferable?

A Indwelling urethral catheter

B Incontinence pants or pads

C Intermittent catheterisation

D Urinary diversion

8 All of the following statements are true regarding retrograde pyelography EXCEPT:

A An abdominal X-ray film should be routinely performed.

B Urethral catheterisation should be performed gently without force.

Urology Lecture Notes, Seventh Edition. Amir V. Kaisary, Andrew Ballaro and Katharine Pigott.
© 2016 John Wiley & Sons, Ltd. Published 2016 by John Wiley & Sons, Ltd.

C Flushing of air bubbles is important to the quality of the study.

D Urine cytology may be obtained from ureters at any point of the study.

9 All of the following statements are true regarding prostate cancer EXCEPT:

A Tumour volume correlates strongly with pathological stage.

B The higher the grade, the more likely the cancer is to be detected by ultrasound.

C The prevailing pattern of hypoechoic appearance is thought to be due to the decrease in sonographically detectable interfaces in the tissue.

D Haematomas from prior biopsies are rarely confused with possible cancer.

10 Involuntary bladder contractions are most commonly seen in association with:

A Inflammation of the bladder

B Bladder outlet obstruction

C Neurologic disease or injury

D Indwelling catheters

E Urethral hypermobility

11 The penile cavernosal artery is a branch of:

A Hypogastric artery

B Obturator artery

C External iliac artery

D Internal pudendal artery

E Inferior gluteal artery

12 All of the following are indicated in a 65-year-old man with epididymitis and bacteriuria EXCEPT:

A Scrotal elevation

B Quinolone antibiotics

C CT IVU

D Cystoscopy

E Prednisone

13 The most common cystoscopy finding in interstitial cystitis is:

A Reduced bladder capacity

B Hunner's ulcers

C Pinpoint petechial haemorrhages of mucosa after hydrodistension

D Bladder trabeculation

14 Which of the following statements regarding the natural history of BPH is true?

A Most men with significant amounts of residual urine after voiding develop urinary tract infections.

B The symptom most strongly predictive of a subsequent prostatectomy is nocturia.

C Recovery of upper urinary tract function in patients with uraemia is usually good following catheter drainage.

D Bladder instability rarely resolves with prostatectomy.

E Once obstructive symptoms develop, spontaneous improvement is rare.

15 Which of the following statements regarding the symptoms associated with BPH is true?

A It is not possible to use symptom scores, IPSS, preoperatively to predict response to therapy.

B Haematuria is more common in carcinoma of the prostate than in BPH.

C Detrusor instability is uncommon in men with clinical prostatism.

D The symptom of nocturia correlates well with urodynamic findings of obstruction.

E The symptom of hesitancy does not correlate with the urodynamic findings of obstruction.

16 Which of the following regarding the evaluation of patients with BPH is false?

A Maximum flow is the most useful measurement with uroflowmetry.

B CT–intravenous urography is indicated only in patients who have associated haematuria.

C Urinary tract infection should be ruled out in all patients at the time of initial evaluation.

D The size of the prostate on rectal examination cannot be used to predict the degree of bladder outlet obstruction.

E Cystoscopy should be performed on most patients suspected of having bladder neck obstruction.

17 Metastatic disease involving the kidney is most commonly discovered by:

A Ultrasound

B CT scan

C MRI

D   Autopsy

E   Intravenous urogram

18 Which of the following is the most accurate means of staging bladder cancer patients for regional lymph node involvement?

A   CT scan

B   MRI

C   Ultrasound

D   Lymphangiogram

E   Pelvic lymphadenectomy

19 A 74-year-old white male with a 40 pack per year smoking history complained of gross haematuria. IVP revealed urinary tracts without filling defects but left-sided hydronephrosis and a large filling defect on the left wall of the bladder. Transurethral resection of bladder tumour revealed deep muscle invasion of grade 3 transitional cell bladder cancer. Metastatic workup was without evidence of extra vesicle disease. After radical cystectomy and urinary diversion, the final pathology report reveals a deeply muscle-invasive transitional cell carcinoma without metastasis to regional lymph nodes. The stage of the patient's tumour is:

A   T2N0M0

B   T3aN0M0

C   T3bN0Mx

D   T1

E   T4

20 Which of the following statements regarding prostate-specific antigen (PSA) is true?

A   It is the glycoprotein that causes coagulation of the ejaculate.

B   The PSA level is proportional to the volume of prostate cancer.

C   PSA is not organ-specific.

D   The preoperative PSA level is very helpful as a predictor of pathologic stage.

E   The PSA level rises at an average rate of 0.35 ng/mL/g of intracapsular cancer.

21 The most common pure histologic type of testicular cancer is:

A   Embryonic cell

B   Teratoma

C   Yolk sac tumour

D   Choriocarcinoma

E   Seminoma

22 The primary lymphatic drainage of the left testis is via:

A   Pre-aortic nodes above the left renal vein

B   Inter-aorto-caval nodes at the level of the left renal vein

C   Precaval nodes at the level of the left renal vein

D   Left common iliac nodes

E   Para-aortic nodes below the left renal vein

23 A 27-year-old white male undergoes right radical orchiectomy for a solid intra-testicular mass. Pathology reveals teratocarcinoma invading the epididymis. The patient's T stage is:

A   T1

B   T2

C   T3

D   T4a

E   T4b

24 Which of the following precludes the diagnosis of pure seminoma?

A   Elevated beta-hCG

B   Elevated alpha-fetoprotein level (AFP)

C   Elevated lactate dehydrogenase (LDH)

D   Elevated gamma-glutamyl transpeptidase (GGT)

E   Elevated placental alkaline phosphatase (PLAP)

25 Bartholin's glands in the female are homologues of the male:

A   Prostate

B   Cowper's glands

C   Utricle

D   Seminal vesicles

E   Seminal colliculus

26 All of the following types of urinary calculi are radiolucent EXCEPT:

A   Uric acid

B   Matrix

C   2,8-Hydroxyadenine

D   Cysteine

E   Xanthine

27 The most important etiological factor for bladder calculi in the developed world is:
A Hypercalciuria
B Urinary tract infection
C A foreign object in the urine
D Urine pH
E Bladder outlet obstruction

28 Indications for diagnostic ureteroscopy include the following EXCEPT:
A A radiographic filling defect of the ureter or renal pelvis
B A tumour found near or at the ureteral orifice
C Unilateral upper tract haematuria
D Upper tract cytology findings suggestive of malignancy
E Multiple bladder tumours suggestive of upper tract seeding

29 Risk factors for deep vein thrombosis (DVT) include all of the following EXCEPT:
A Anaesthesia duration greater than 1 h
B Age greater than 60 years
C Presence of malignant disease
D Use of oestrogens
E Race

30 The most common cause of anaemia is:
A Vitamin B_{12} deficiency
B Iron deficiency
C Folic acid deficiency
D Haemolytic anaemia
E Chronic renal insufficiency

31 The right adrenal vein drains into the:
A Right renal vein
B Inferior phrenic vein
C Inferior vena cava
D Right gonadal vein
E Lumbar vein

32 The only source of aldosterone production is the:
A Zona glomerulosa
B Zona fasciculata
C Zona reticularis
D Adrenal medulla
E Macula densa

33 The hallmark of Cushing's syndrome secondary to adrenal carcinoma is:
A Purple striae
B Virilisation
C Temporal hair loss
D Hypertension
E Thin skin

34 In addition to nephrotoxicity, side effects of cyclosporine include the following EXCEPT:
A Hirsutism
B Gingival hypertrophy
C Pruritus
D Hypertension
E Breast fibroadenomas

35 The most immediate postoperative complication after TURP is:
A Bleeding requiring transfusion
B Infection
C Failure to void
D Clot retention
E Myocardial infarction

36 The greatest risk of ureteral injury in the laser treatment of ureteral calculi is associated with:
A Ureteroscopy itself
B Use of power greater than 20 mJ
C Thermal injury
D Discharge frequencies greater than 5 Hz
E Inadvertent firing of the probe while it is in contact with the ureteral mucosa

37 On semen analysis, all of the following indicate the absence of the seminal vesicles EXCEPT:
A Lack of fructose
B Liquefaction of semen
C Low sperm count
D Low semen volume
E Lack of carbohydrate

38 In urethral carcinoma, palpable inguinal adenopathy is most commonly due to:
A Inflammation
B Infection
C Nodal metastasis

D Lymphatic obstruction from radiation therapy

E Lymphatic obstruction from chemotherapy

39 The most common complication of a hydrocele surgical correction is:

A Infection

B Recurrence

C Testicular artery injury

D Haematoma formation

E Epididymal injury

40 The most common form of bladder cancer is:

A Squamous cell carcinoma

B Transitional cell carcinoma

C Glandular adenocarcinoma

D Small cell carcinoma

E Neuroendocrine carcinoma

41 A 55-year-old woman has irritative, voiding and urge incontinence symptoms. Video urodynamic investigation demonstrates normal bladder capacity, maximal flow rate of 7 mL/s, detrusor peak flow pressure of 45 cm H_2O and minimal bladder neck opening during voiding. Postmicturition residue is 180 mL. Clinical examination showed no bladder base decent and no stress incontinence, with normal cystoscopy. The next step recommended is:

A Urethral dilation

B Anticholinergic therapy

C Transurethral bladder neck incision

D Biofeedback

E Alpha-blocker therapy

42 A 52-year-old man reports a recent onset of passing gas in his urine. He has diabetes and receives hypoglycaemic therapy with good control. The next step in investigating his case is:

A Cystoscopy

B Barium enema

C Pelvic CT scan

D Cystogram

E Urine culture

43 A 22-year-old man presents with a 2-week history of pain in the right hemiscrotum. On examination he has a tender 2 cm mass that is in either the tail of the epididymis or lower pole of the right testis. The most appropriate procedure to consider is:

A Surgical exploration

B Testicular radionuclear scan

C AFP and hCG serum levels

D MRI

E Scrotal ultrasound scan

44 A healthy fit 25-year-old female reports 10 afebrile urinary tract infection episodes over the past year. The factor most likely to increase her risk of UTI is:

A Parity

B Daily bicycle riding

C Tampon use

D Vaginal spermicide usage

E Oral contraceptive pill

45 Patients who have von Hippel–Lindau disease most frequently have:

A Glioblastomas

B Café au lait skin spots

C Retinal angiomas

D Renal angiomyolipoma

E Thyroid carcinoma

46 Renal calculi could contain all of the following EXCEPT:

A Cholesterol

B Oxalate

C Cysteine

D Phosphate

E Urate

47 In renal cell carcinoma, stage III indicates:

A Tumour limited to the renal capsule

B Lung metastases

C No involvement of regional lymph nodes

D None of the above

E All of the above

48 A fall astride injury could be associated with:

A Rupture of the bulbar urethra

B Rupture of the posterior urethra

C A risk of subsequent stricture

D   None of the above
E   All of the above

49 **A 6-week-old boy has a large palpable left-sided abdominal mass. An ultrasound examination revealed a large fluid-filled left mass harbouring multiple cysts. A nuclear renal isotope study showed no uptake in the left kidney and normal right kidney. He has respiratory distress and an elevated left hemidiaphragm. The most appropriate treatment is:**
A   Observation and systemic antibiotic therapy
B   Cystoscopy and left retrograde pyelography
C   Percutaneous aspiration of the mass
D   Left pyeloplasty
E   Left nephrectomy

50 **A 72-year-old man underwent TUR prostatectomy 5 months ago. Histology confirms benign features. Although he voids well with minimal IPSS, he continues to have haematuria with clot retention in need of cystoscopy and clot evacuation. He does not wish to have any further surgical treatment. The next step in management would be:**
A   Bicalutamide
B   Tamsulosin
C   Antibiotic therapy for 6 weeks
D   Vitamin K supplements
E   Finasteride

51 **The most relevant advice to give to a patient who has gout as prophylaxis against urinary stone formation is:**
A   Dietary calcium restriction
B   Increased oral fluid intake
C   Alkalinising agents
D   Allopurinol
E   Thiazides

52 **Endocrinal evaluation in an infertile male patient is warranted in all of the following features EXCEPT:**
A   Erectile dysfunction
B   Decreased libido
C   Gynaecomastia
D   Premature ejaculation
E   Oligospermia with a total count less than 10 million/mL

53 **A hyperdense renal cyst may be:**
A   Probable angiomyolipoma
B   Probable malignancy
C   Bosniak II cyst
D   Bosniak III cyst
E   Bosniak IV cyst

54 **Which food is associated with a low risk of urethral cancer?**
A   Citrus
B   Apples
C   Tomatoes
D   Carrots
E   All of the above

55 **Serum prostate-specific antigen (PSA) levels are specific for the presence of:**
A   Prostate cancer
B   Prostate disease
C   Prostate enlargement
D   Prostate inflammation
E   None of the above

Answers

1-D The genito-femoral nerve arises from the first to the third lumbar nerves and is primarily a sensory nerve to the genitalia. The genital branch of the genito-femoral nerve also supplies the cremaster and dartos muscles in the scrotum.

2-C Reabsorption of calcium is inhibited by hypermagnesemia.

3-C The primary hormonal regulation of spermatogenesis is by testosterone, which probably acts via an effect on the Sertoli cells.

4-C Obstructive symptoms include hesitancy, decreased force of stream, intermittent stream and post-void dribbling. Those are usually secondary to benign prostatic hyperplasia, urethral stricture or neurogenic bladder and less commonly due to malignant prostatic obstruction, urethral carcinoma or a foreign object. Nocturia is an irritative symptom secondary to increased urine output or decreased capacity.

5-D The most common cause of cloudy urine is alkaline pH, which causes the precipitation of phosphate crystals, although it may occur in the presence of infection. Although haemospermia can occur with malignancies, it is usually due to nonspecific inflammation of the prostate or seminal vesicles. Pneumaturia is almost always due to a fistula between the intestine and bladder. In rare instances it is due to infection with gas-forming organisms in diabetic patients. Urethral discharge is the most common symptom of venereal infection. A purulent, thick, profuse discharge is commonly seen with gonococcal urethritis, whereas a scant and watery discharge is generally associated with nonspecific urethritis.

6-D In normal prostatic fluid, there should be few, if any, leukocytes but numerous secretory granules of various sizes. Macrophages and clumps of leukocytes are indicators of inflammation. Oval fat macrophages characterise postinfection prostatic fluid.

7-C Clean intermittent catheterization or condom catheter drainage is preferable to manage patients with urinary incontinence in the long-term hospitalised setting due to risk of infection with long-term indwelling urethral catheters.

8-D Ureteral urine specimen for cytology should be obtained prior to injection of hyperosmolar contrast to avoid poorly preserved cytology specimens. All of the other statements are correct.

9-D All of the statements are true except D. Perhaps the most frequently encountered artefact simulating prostate cancer is haematoma from recent biopsy. It appears hypoechoic, is in the peripheral zone, and may even cause bulging of the boundary echo, reminiscent of a cancer penetrating the capsule.

10-C Involuntary contractions are almost commonly seen in association with neurologic disease or injury.

11-D The penile cavernosal artery is a branch of the internal pudendal artery.

12-E Epididymitis is usually caused by the spread of infection from the urethra or bladder and as such usually responds to the same antibiotics commonly used to treat UTIs. Bed rest with scrotal elevation improves lymphatic drainage. Oral nonsteroidal anti-inflammatory drugs may be

Urology Lecture Notes, Seventh Edition. Amir V. Kaisary, Andrew Ballaro and Katharine Pigott.
© 2016 John Wiley & Sons, Ltd. Published 2016 by John Wiley & Sons, Ltd.

of symptomatic benefit. Prednisone has been found to be of no value as an adjunct to antibiotic therapy. Structural urologic abnormalities often exist and radiographic investigations and cystoscopy evaluation ought to be considered.

13-C The characteristic cystoscopy finding in patients with interstitial cystitis is the development of pinpoint petechial haemorrhages of mucosa after hydrodistension. The two cystoscopic findings often classically associated with interstitial cystitis – reduced bladder capacity and Hunner's ulcers – are frequently not found.

14-C The absolute indications for the treatment of BPH include uraemia, hydronephrosis and bladder decompensation with overflow incontinence. Fortunately, recovery of upper urinary tract function in this group of patients is usually quite good following initial catheter drainage. The recovery of lower urinary tract function is largely dependent upon the severity and duration of bladder decompensation. Bladder instability will resolve in most patients following treatment. In most men with significant amounts of residual urine after voiding, urinary tract infections do not develop. Once the urine becomes infected, however, it is difficult to clear the infection without the relief of outlet obstruction.

15-A Symptom scores are valuable for the following progression of BPH and quantitating response to therapy. However, it is not possible to use these scores preoperatively to predict response to therapy in individual patients because some patients with low scores do as well after transurethral resection of the prostate as patients with higher scores. Only the symptoms of hesitancy and slow stream have been consistently correlated with urodynamic findings of obstruction. Nocturia is a difficult symptom to evaluate because many elderly men experience increased diuresis at night associated with an alteration in their diurnal secretion of antidiuretic hormone. It is estimated that 50–80% of men with clinical prostatism have some degree of detrusor instability. Haematuria is more common in BPH than in carcinoma of the prostate.

16-E To properly evaluate bladder neck obstruction, there is no adequate substitution for cystourethroscopy. Therefore, when the diagnosis is uncertain or a urethral stricture is likely, cystoscopy may be performed initially. In the patient who is markedly symptomatic, however, this examination is best performed immediately prior to prostatectomy to guide the surgeon in choosing an operative approach. The examination should include a complete evaluation of the interior of the bladder, with special reference to trabeculation, and diverticula. The bladder neck is examined for the presence of a contracture or intravesical intrusion of the prostate. The length of the posterior urethra is measured from the bladder neck to the verumontanum to aid in estimating the size of the prostate.

17-D Due to its profuse vascularity and high blood flow, the kidney is a frequent site of metastatic deposits from a variety of solid tumours and haematologic malignancies. Metastases to the kidney are seldom clinically identified and are most often discovered at autopsy. The most common solid tumour metastasizing to the kidney is lung carcinoma. Virtually every other solid neoplasm may metastasize to the kidney. The principal method of detection of symptomatic metastatic lesions within the kidney is CT scan. With pyelography or ultrasonography identification, it is difficult to distinguish metastatic tumours from primary renal neoplasms.

18-E CT scanning, ultrasonography and MRI have been used but are inaccurate in determining the presence or absence of microscopic muscle invasion or minimal extravesical tumour spread. Pelvic lymphadenectomy is the most accurate means of staging bladder cancer patients for regional lymph node involvement and is usually performed in conjunction with cystectomy rather than as an independent procedure. In patients with limited pelvic lymph node metastases, the performance of cystectomy and pelvic lymph node dissection may be associated with cure rates of 10–35%.

19-B The TNM staging system is the tumour, node, metastasis system. This staging system is seen below.

T – extent of the primary tumour

N – absence or presence and extent of regional lymph nodes metastases

M – absence or presence of distant metastases

TX – primary tumour cannot be assessed

T0 – no evidence of primary tumour

Tis – carcinoma *in situ*

T1, T2, T3, T4 – increasing size and/or local extent of the primary tumour

NX – regional lymph nodes cannot be assessed

N0 – no regional lymph node involvement

N1, N2, N3 – increasing involvement of regional lymph nodes

MX – distant metastasis cannot be assessed

M0 – no distant metastasis

M1 – distant metastasis

20-B PSA is a serine protease, produced only by prostatic epithelial cells, which hydrolyzes the coagulum of the ejaculate. PSA is an important marker for monitoring patients with prostatic cancer. PSA level rises at an overall rate of 3.5 ng/mL/g of intracapsular cancer, whereas in prostates without cancer, BPH causes serum levels of PSA to rise by only 0.3 ng/mL/g of BPH.

Although PSA level is proportional to the volume of prostate cancer present, preoperative serum PSA levels are not found to be very helpful as a predictor of pathologic stage.

21-E The highest incidence of testicular cancers is noted in young adults (20–40 years). Seminoma is the most common histologic type overall, with a peak incidence between the ages of 35 and 39 years. Embryonic carcinoma and teratocarcinoma occur predominately between the ages of 25 and 35 years. Choriocarcinoma occurs more often in the 20–30-year age group. Yolk sac tumours are the predominant lesions of infancy and childhood, rarely occurring in pure form in the adult. Malignant testicular lymphomas are predominantly tumours of men over the age of 50.

22-E The primary drainage of the left testis is to the left para-aortic nodes just below the level of the left renal vein and, subsequently, to the pre-aortic nodes.

23-C TNM staging system is Tx unknown status

T0 – no tumour

T1 – tumour confined to the testis

T2 – tumour beyond the tunica

T3 – tumour invasion of the rete testis or epididymis

T4a – tumour invasion of the cord

T4b – tumour invasion of the scrotum

24-B The detection of an elevated AFP level strongly suggests the presence of a non-seminomatous element. LDH is a non-specific tumour marker in patients with germ cell testicular neoplasms and may be helpful as a marker substance in the surveillance of patients with advanced seminoma. GGT and PLAP are also non-specific tumour markers that may be elevated in patients with seminoma and those with non-seminomatous testis tumour.

25-B In the female, the phallic portion of the urogenital sinus remains a vestibule because the ureteral plate does not extend as far to the genital tubercle as in the male. The urethra and vagina open into the vestibule. The labial swellings grow posterior to the vestibule and meet to form posterior commissure. The swellings also grow lateral to the vestibule to form the labia majora. Urethral folds that flank the urogenital sinus develop into the labia minora. After the 9th week of development, Bartholin's glands begin as an invagination of the vestibule endoderm and then grow into the labia majora. These glands are the homologues of Cowper's glands in the male.

26-D Cysteine stones, contrary to the relatively common misconception, are not radiolucent, but have a radiodensity that often results in a ground glass appearance. Cysteine stones are approximately 0.45 times as radiopaque as calcium oxalate calculi. With the exception of uric acid, all of the other radiolucent stones are very rare.

27-E Obstruction due to prostate enlargement, bladder neck contracture or urethral stricture is the most important factor in the formation of bladder stones. Bladder stones are much less common in women than men.

28-E The presence of multiple bladder tumours is not an indication for ureteroscopy without other evidence for upper urinary tract tumours such as suspicious cytology results from ureteral samples.

29-E All of the statements are true except E.

30-B Iron deficiency anaemia is the most common cause of anaemia. Both the mean corpuscular volume and mean corpuscular haemoglobin content are decreased resulting in microcytic, hypochromic peripheral smear. The reticulocyte percentage index is less than 1%.

31-C The adrenal glands are paired retroperitoneal organs that lie within perinephric fat at the antero-superior and medial aspects of the kidneys. The adrenals have a delicate and rich blood supply without a dominant single artery. The venous drainage is usually a common vein. On the right the vein exits the apex of the gland and enters the posterior surface of the IVC. The left adrenal vein empties directly into the left renal vein often opposite to the gonadal vein.

32-A The zona glomerulosa is the only source of the major mineralocorticoid, aldosterone, which regulates sodium resorption in the kidney, the gut and salivary and sweat glands. The other zones produce and secrete cortisol and the principal androgens dehydroepiandrosterone (DHEA), dehydroepiandrosterone sulfate (DHEAS) and androstenedione.

33-B Adrenal carcinoma is a rare disease with an incidence of approximately two cases per million and a poor prognosis. Adrenal malignancies are usually larger than 6 cm in size at diagnosis, and approximately 80% of these tumours are functional. Adrenal carcinoma is one of the causes of corticosteroid excess. Virilisation is the hallmark of Cushing's syndrome secondary to adrenal carcinomas. Also, virilisation without evidence of cortisol excess is indicative of carcinoma except in children.

34-C The primary disadvantage of cyclosporine is its nephrotoxicity. This is a dose-related effect and is potentially reversible. The side effects of cyclosporine include hepatotoxicity, hypertension, hirsutism, breast fibroadenomas, gingival hypertrophy and immunosuppression. Pruritus is not reported to be a significant side effect of cyclosporine.

35-C The most common problem in the postoperative period is failure to void occurring in 6.5% of patients. In patients with severely hypotonic bladders, catheter drainage may be required for 1–2 weeks, during which time bladder tone seems to return.

A The term pulsed-dye laser generally refers to lasers that utilise coumarin green dye. When excited, this dye generates a wavelength of 504 nm that is well absorbed by the yellow colour of most calculi but poorly absorbed by body tissues. The laser fibre may be employed with a rigid or flexible ureteroscope. When the calculus is visualised, the laser fibre is placed in direct contact with the stone. The laser beam is fired at a discharge rate of 5 Hz. Higher frequencies may impair the surgeon's visual field because of the light flash. The laser energy is absorbed by the stone, which results in the formation of a 'plasma' bubble on the surface of the stone.

This expansion bubble of a column of electrons mechanically disrupts the stone along stress lines. The pulsed-dye laser has proved to be effective in the treatment of the ureteral calculi. Even if the probe is inadvertently fired on the ureteral mucosa, no discernible damage is done. The greatest risk of ureteral injury comes from the ureteroscopy itself. The most easily fragmented calculi are those of struvite and calcium oxalate dihydrate. Cystine and pure calcium oxalate monohydrate stones are more resistant to fragmentation.

36-C The seminal vesicle is responsible for the majority of the volume of ejaculate, and therefore a low semen volume would be an indication of absence of the seminal vesicles. The seminal vesicles do produce secretions rich in carbohydrate, primarily fructose, and lack of fructose or carbohydrate in ejaculate would again indicate absence of the seminal vesicles. Finally, the seminal vesicle secretion also contains coagulation factor responsible for the initial coagulation of semen. Liquefaction of semen would indicate absence of the coagulation factor and imply absence of the seminal vesicles. The sperm count would not necessarily be related to the seminal vesicle secretion.

37-C The incidence of metastatic inguinal adenopathy from distal male cancers is about 50–60%. In contradistinction to penile primary lesions, there is little inflammation associated with these seven lesions. Clinical adenopathy in this setting is a highly reliable sign of metastasis.

38-D The most common complication of hydrocele surgical correction is haematoma formation. Meticulous haemostasis can help decrease the incidence. All other choices are well-known complications of hydrocele surgical correction, although less common.

39-B

40-E Video urodynamic investigations indicate bladder neck obstruction. She underwent no previous pelvic surgery. The bladder peak flow pressure and increased post-micturition volume are most consistent with bladder outlet obstruction. Biofeedback is useful in patients with pelvic floor spasticity. Urethral dilation has no effect on the bladder neck. Anticholinergic therapy is contraindicated in patients with increased post-micturition bladder residue. A medical trial of medical therapy (alpha-blocker) is indicated.

41-E Pneumaturia is the passage of gas in the urine. It could be due to gas-forming urinary tract infection or a fistula between the bladder and intestine. Urine analysis and culture showing multiple organisms is suggestive of a colovesical fistula. Patients with diabetes mellitus may have gas-forming infections due to fermentation of high concentrations of sugar in urine. The most common organism is *E. coli*. Additional investigations can be performed subsequently based on the urine analysis and culture results.

42-E Scrotal ultrasound has more than 99% accuracy to differentiate testicular from extra-testicular abnormality (epididymis) and is simple and quick to do.

43-D Spermicide usage increases urinary tract infections' risk by decreasing normal vaginal flora and decreasing vaginal pH.

44-C Patients with von Hippel–Lindau disease may have haemangioblastomas of the cerebellum, renal cell carcinomas and cystadenomas of the epididymis. Diagnosis can be easily made with inspection of the retina where angiomas can be identified.

45-A

46-D

Stage I	T1 N0 M0
Stage II	T2 N0 M0
Stage III	T1, T2, T3 N1 M0
	T3 N0 M0
Stage IV	T4 N0, N1 M0
	Any T N2 M0
	Any T Any N M1

47-E

48-E The diagnostic findings are sufficient to confirm that the left kidney is multicystic, dysplastic and nonfunctioning. Nephrectomy is preferred.

49-E Finasteride has been shown to be effective in treating post-prostatectomy haematuria. Prolonged antibiotic therapy is only advocated if urinary tract infection of prostatic origin is suspected.

50-C Raising urine pH to be maintained between 6.0 and 6.5 above the dissociation constant of uric acid is the key to prevent recurrent uric acid stone formation.

51-D Endocrinal evaluation of an infertile male patient is performed in all of the afore-mentioned cases except premature ejaculation.

52-C

53-E All contain several active compounds that are important in detoxification.

54-E PSA is organ-specific and not disease-specific.

Index

Note: Page references in *italics* refer to Figures; those in **bold** refer to Tables

Urology Lecture Notes, Seventh Edition. Amir V. Kaisary, Andrew Ballaro and Katharine Pigott.
© 2016 John Wiley & Sons, Ltd. Published 2016 by John Wiley & Sons, Ltd.